School Nurse Resource Manual

A GUIDE TO PRACTICE

NINTH EDITION

I. CLINICAL GUIDELINES

II. CLINICAL PROCEDURES

III. SCHOOL NURSE MANAGEMENT

IV. MANAGEMENT of VULNERABLE POPULATIONS

EDITORS
VICKI TALIAFERRO
CHERYL RESHA

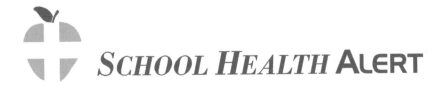

SCHOOL HEALTH ALERT

SCHOOL HEALTH ALERT
P.O. Box 150127
Nashville, TN 37215

SCHOOL NURSE RESOURCE MANUAL 2016-17
Copyright © 2016-17 School Health Alert.

NOTICES

Nursing, including school nursing, is a dynamic, constantly changing field. The publisher, editors and contributors have made a diligent effort to ensure any procedures or recommendations outlined in this manual are accurate, based on latest evidence, and in accordance with accepted school nursing practices at the time of publication. It is, of course, necessary for readers to apply their professional judgment, experience, knowledge of the patient, and any new research to determine the best treatment for a specific case. Additionally, it is the responsibility of the school nurse to adhere to their individual state nurse practice act when administering any treatment or medication.

Several websites are included in this manual to provide additional information, resources and references on a particular topic. However, listing these websites does not imply endorsement. Note that with any internet site, addresses and content may change and information therein updated.

Mentions of any specific products within this book are for informational purposes and also do not constitute endorsements.

Phone: 866-370-7899
Fax: 615-370-9993

ABOUT THIS MANUAL

"School nursing is a specialized practice of professional nursing that advances the well-being, academic success, and life-long achievement and health of students. To that end, school nurses facilitate positive student responses to normal development; promote health and safety including a healthy environment; intervene with actual and potential health problems; provide case management services; and actively collaborate with others to build student and family capacity for adaptation, self-management, self- advocacy, and learning" (NASN, 2010)[1]. School nursing services uniquely address health and safety needs of students individually, as a population, and as a subspecialty of community/public health nursing.

School nurses' work focuses directly on three areas: health services, health education, and the school environment. Their services require diverse knowledge including, but not limited to, pediatric and adolescent health, infectious diseases, mental health, chronic diseases, and emergency care. They can influence health and safety aspects of schools and can provide leadership to a district's or campus' coordinated school health program that in addition to health services, health education, and the school environment addresses mental health and social services, nutrition services, physical activity, family and community involvement, and staff health promotion.

This resource serves as a quick reference for school nurses and can assist them, their administrators, and consulting physicians to develop policies and procedures for safe student care. This manual offers brief summaries of conditions that most school nurses encounter but is not intended to be a substitute for any comprehensive pediatric or emergency care textbook.

The *school nurse guidelines* were developed through cooperative efforts of school nurses and physicians. We strongly recommend a similar process at the district or system level with adaptations that account for state laws and regulations as well as the unique needs of students in a school district. The registered nurse plans student health services; however, vocational/practical nurses, or unlicensed staff such as office personnel or clinic assistants may perform certain tasks within state nursing practice guidelines. The registered nurse is responsible for training persons assigned to perform a delegated nursing task, monitoring their performance, and ensuring their compliance with the procedures. State school nurse consultants are an invaluable resource regarding laws, regulations and nurse practice acts in each state.

---

[1] National Association of School Nurses. (2010). *Definition of school nursing.* Retrieved from http://www.nasn.org/RoleCareer

PHYSICIAN CONSULTATION

The availability of a physician's services to schools varies across communities. Some large districts have full-time medical directors or consultants, while others have part-time physician services. Small districts may engage a physician to consult for a set number of hours or on-call. Some physicians volunteer as a community service.

Regardless of the arrangement, it is sound medical-legal practice for the school nurse to have written guidelines to standardize assessment and management decisions. Such guidelines with input from the school physician complement professional school nursing practice standards and the nursing process and should incorporate accepted pediatric care recommendations.

We suggest that students who have conditions that are likely to require treatment or emergency care during school hours or activities, have individual written orders from their own healthcare provider. These orders should be reviewed and updated at least each school year or as necessary and incorporated into the student's individualized healthcare plan. The most common individual orders are for students with asthma, life threatening allergies, or diabetes. Some students with seizure disorders, migraine headaches, or other chronic conditions also need individual orders each school year.

DESCRIPTION OF SCHOOL NURSE GUIDELINES

We offer an outline format so that important features of each condition and guidelines for action can be seen at a glance. Each guideline includes a definition or etiology of the disease or condition, presenting signs and symptoms, management strategies and follow-up. This format provides the registered nurse a quick reference for student care and offers information to educate and train staff who may assist the school nurse.

Registered nurses apply their professional skills and judgment in the management of each individual case, but each school and district or system should provide care for all students in a consistent manner guided by local policies and procedures, e.g., criteria for referral or exclusion and return to class.

Usual procedures, such as Standard (Universal) Precautions, parent notification, record keeping, confidentiality, etc. may not be repeated in all guidelines but is understood to be a standard practice in all aspects of care.

STANDING ORDERS

Although standing orders are not addressed in this edition, the distinction between the two types of orders should be understood.

General orders are written by a physician, often the school medical consultant, which apply to all students for whom the order may be applicable. They should be reviewed annually and updated when necessary. It is not necessary for the school physician to have previously examined the student. Dosage is based on weight or age. Common examples of general orders are acetaminophen for fever, ibuprofen for minor headache, etc. These orders are issued with the understanding that a registered nurse will administer these medications after an assessment of the child.

Some state boards of nursing do not allow general standing orders in school settings. Other boards may allow a "physician directed nursing protocol" which requires signatures of both a physician and a nurse (usually a nursing administrator or manager). If the administration of nonprescription products is permitted, the school's policy (for discretionary medications) should be in writing and parents must be informed. Parents should sign a written request for each school year indicating that their child may receive any of the named medications in the discretionary medication policy from school personnel according to the district's policy.

Specific orders are written and signed by a physician *for an individual child.* The parents should also sign a medication authorization form for school personnel to administer any medicine at school. These specific orders contain the drug or treatment, dose, route, time and duration of administration. For example for a child with diagnosed with ADHD: "Methylphenidate 20 mg (one tablet) by mouth daily between 11 A.M. and noon after lunch or with food through December 20, 2016". Most districts require that individualized orders be renewed annually.

Each school/district should have a medication policy that guides medication administration and documentation of both specific, individual orders for medication and for any discretionary medications orders by the school physician that are allowed.

We welcome your suggestions for future editions and wish you success in caring for our nation's children. You may contact us on the Internet at *www.schoolnurse.com.*

Robert Andrews, Publisher
School Health Alert
P.O. Box 150127, Nashville, TN 37215
(866) 370-7899
www.schoolnurse.com

ACKNOWLEDGMENTS

This 9th Edition was edited by Vicki Taliaferro, BSN, RN, NCSN with Cheryl Resha, Ed.D. M.S.N., R.N., FNASN.

Contributors and reviewers include:

Patricia K. Bednarz, RN, MN, FNASN

Patricia Bednarz is a health and education consultant. Ms. Bednarz has a successful 25 plus year career of diversified, progressive experience as a school nurse, project manager and nursing educator in Lansing School District and Michigan State University. She has expertise in managing state and federal grants that includes writing and contributing to proposals, implementation, fiscal management and evaluation. In 2010, Patricia was named a Fellow in the National Academy of School Nurses. Ms. Bednarz was a member of the Michigan State School Nurse Task Force and continues to serve as the co-chair of the Public Awareness Advisory Committee. She has published articles in peer-reviewed journals and presented at state and national school nurse conferences.

Jane Borr, BSN, RN, NCSN

Jane Borr is the manager for a hospital funded school nurse program that partners with area school districts for nursing services in the schools. She served on the Michigan Association of School Nurses board as treasurer from 2010 – 2014 and was a member of the Michigan School Nurse Task Force from 2011 – 2014 where she co-chaired the data and staffing committee. She is a nationally certified school nurse.

Hendrina Cuprey, RN, MSN, NCSN

Hendrina Cuprey works as school nurse for Holland Hospital/Holland School System in Michigan. She has worked in nursing for the past 22 years, eleven of which have been in school nursing. She serves as the Membership Chair of the Michigan Association of School Nurses. She is a nationally certified school nurse.

Rosemary Dolatowski, MSN, RN

Rosemary Dolatowski is in her 29th year as the Director of School Health Services for the Burlington Area School District. Rosemary has worked in a variety of clinical settings and has co-authored a chapter in the book Cardiac Rehabilitation & Clinical Exercise Programs: Theory & Practice; she has also authored articles on Cardiac and School Nursing and has presented at local, state and national conferences. She has served as an adjunct Nursing Professor at both Gateway Technical College and Cardinal Stritch University. As the Director of School Health Services in Burlington, Wisconsin, she is responsible for Policy & Procedure development, training and education of health services staff, and developing and monitoring students' Individual Healthcare Plans. She was instrumental in developing the statewide data collection tool for all Wisconsin School Nurses. She was named the Wisconsin School Nurse of the Year in 2006 and currently serves as the Wisconsin Director to the National Association of School Nurses.

Mary Patricia Kohl Lamberti, DNP, APRN, ANP - BC

Dr. Lamberti is currently an Assistant Professor of Nursing at Southern Connecticut State University (SCSU). She holds a Doctorate in Nursing Practice and is ANA certified as an Adult Nurse Practitioner. In addition to teaching at the university, Dr. Lamberti works as an APRN in the Student Health Center at the university, serving students for acute and chronic healthcare needs.

Julia Lechtenberg, MSN, RN, NCSN

Julia Lechtenberg serves as a District Nurse and has over 16 years of experience as a school nurse. She is a member of the National Association of School Nurses, Michigan Education Association and Sigma Theta Tau International. She is a nationally certified school nurse and a Johnson and Johnson School Health Leadership Fellow. Ms. Lechtenberg's school nursing experience includes district level consultative services in an urban school district, preschool through 12th grade. Ms. Lechtenberg has published articles in school nursing publications and presented at state and national school nurse conferences. She currently serves as the Michigan Director to the National Association of School Nurses.

Suzanne Levasseur, MSN, APRN

Suzanne Levasseur is the Supervisor of Health Services for the Westport Public Schools District in Connecticut. She is an Advanced Practice registered nurse and a Certified Pediatric Nurse Practitioner and is on staff at Danbury Hospital in Danbury, Connecticut. She is currently the President for the Association of School Nurses of Connecticut and is the editor of the texts, *Pediatric Nursing Secrets* and *Perinatal Nursing Services*.

Julianna Putman, MS, CCC-SLP, TSLI

Julianna Putman is an ASHA certified speech and language pathologist. She received her Bachelor of Arts in Communicative Sciences and Disorders at Michigan State University. She then received her Master of Science in Speech and Language Pathology from The University of Tulsa. She is in her fourth year of school-based speech language pathologist. Her focus is currently on students with moderate-severe cognitive and physical impairments.

Suzanne Putman, BSN, MEd, RN

Suzanne Putman is a Nurse Consultant-Special Education and earned her Bachelor of Science degree in nursing from Oakland University and her master of education specializing in school nursing from Cambridge College. She has over 30 years of maternal-child nursing experience including 20 years of experience as a school nurse consultant for students with cognitive and physical impairments.

Cheryl Resha, EdD, MSN, RN, FNASN

Dr. Resha is currently an Associate Professor of Nursing at Southern Connecticut State University (SCSU). She holds a Doctorate in Educational Leadership. Prior to joining SCSU, Dr. Resha worked for the Connecticut State Department of Education as a manager and state school nurse consultant; and for a large suburban school district as the school nurse supervisor. With over 18 years' experience in the field of school nursing, Dr. Resha has provided leadership and advocacy for school nurses, safe school nurse practice and quality school health programs. Professionally, Dr. Resha has also been a member of ASNC and NASN since 1998. As an active member of NASN for several years, Dr. Resha was inducted as a Fellow in the National Academy of School Nursing in June 2012. Dr. Resha has authored and contributed to articles and publications regarding school nursing, such as the *Scope and Standards of Professional School Nurse Practice and Delegation: Is It a Safe Practice in Schools?* Dr. Resha is the co-editor of the monthly *School Health Alert*.

Dona R. Roberts, BSN, RN

Dona R. Roberts is adjunct faculty serving as an instructor in the Simulation and Fundamentals Skills Lab of the Practical Nursing program at Brown Mackie College, Indianapolis, Indiana. She has authored and contributed to articles in nursing journals and resource publications for school nurses. Professionally, Ms. Roberts served as school nurse in a school system for several years and during that time was selected "School Nurse of the Year" for the State of Indiana. She spent more than a decade at the Indiana State Department of Education, first as Health Services/School Nurse Consultant and later as the Physical Activity, Nutrition, and Tobacco director for the Coordinated School Health CDC grant. Her regular participation as a member of the Indiana University School of Nursing Alumni Association, Board of Directors bespeaks to her advocacy for nursing.

Vicki L. Taliaferro, BSN, RN, NCSN

Ms. Taliaferro is an independent School Health Consultant. She has authored and contributed to articles, texts and publications regarding school nursing, position papers and state and local guidelines on school health topics and initiatives. She is a speaker and a consultant to various state education, hospital and community agencies and professional organizations. Ms. Taliaferro has been the editor for *School Health Alert's School Nurse Resource Manual* for the last three editions. She is a consultant to the National Association of School Nurses and editor of the *School Nurse Digest* and the *Administrator's Risk Alert* electronic newsletters. Previously, she served as the State School Nurse Consultant with the Maryland State Department of Education for 10 years. She has served as president of the National Association of State School Nurse Consultants and received their Outstanding State School Nurse Consultant award in 2004.

Antoinette Towle MSN, PNP BC, SNP BC

Dr. Towle is presently an Assistant Professor of Nursing at Southern Connecticut State University (SCSU) teaching across the curriculum nursing to undergraduate, RN to BSN, Accelerated and graduate nursing students. She has over 34 years' experience as a registered nurse, and over 15 years' experience as an Advanced Practice registered nurse. She holds a Doctorate in Nursing Education, is ANCC board certified as a Pediatric and School Health Nurse Practitioner. Dr. Towle has extensive experience working in school health, in a variety of roles, school nurse, school nurse practitioner, and the Director of Health Services.

Susan Zacharski, MEd, BSN, RN

Susan Zacharski is currently a School Nurse Consultant with over 40 years of experience as a registered nurse and over 27 years' experience as a school nurse. Her school nursing experience includes Department Head of Health Services in an urban school district, preschool – 8th grade general education with a focus on special needs students including the medically fragile, participation in state level committees and leadership positions at both the state and national level. She was a member of the Michigan School Nurse Task Force from 2011 – 2014 where she co-chaired the school nurse practice committee.

TABLE OF CONTENTS

This page intentionally left blank.

SECTION I

CLINICAL GUIDELINES

This page intentionally left blank.

CLINICAL GUIDELINES INDEX

CLINICAL GUIDELINES INDEX

ABDOMEN: Blunt Injury

DEFINITION/ETIOLOGY:
Following a hard blow to abdomen (by rock, fist, bicycle handlebar, etc.) an internal organ may be ruptured and bleed into the abdominal cavity slowly but continuously. Injured abdominal organs may include the spleen, liver, retroperitoneum, small intestines, colorectal, bladder, kidney, diaphragm and/or pancreas.

SIGNS AND SYMPTOMS:
- History of blow to abdomen
- Possible bruise visible
- Pain and tenderness to mild pressure
- Abdominal distention
- Vomiting
- Rapid, weak pulse with low blood pressure
- If kidney is bruised or torn, there may be blood in urine shortly after trauma or next day (more likely, if injury is to the lumbar area of the back)
- Shoulder pain (Kehr's sign). Kehr's sign is pain at the tip of the shoulder due to internal bleeding in the abdominal cavity. A positive Kehr's sign is a medical emergency. **Call 911 immediately!**
  - If spleen is ruptured there may be complaints of left shoulder pain
  - If liver is injured there may be complaints of right shoulder pain
- Gradual onset of shock and coma
- Symptoms may appear a day or two following the blow

MANAGEMENT/TREATMENT:
1. Identification of trauma may not be obvious with initial evaluation.
2. Notify parent. Tell what to watch for in the next 48 hours.
3. Keep in clinic for 15 minutes after blow to abdomen.
4. Allow to rest in position of comfort.
5. Monitor pulse and blood pressure.
6. If student has none of the above symptoms, may return to class. Send a note to the teacher to have the student return to clinic before close of school and sooner, if symptoms appear.
7. Reassess the student.
8. If any symptoms ensue, refer to emergency room or physician.
9. Record on injury report, including what parent/guardian was told.

ABDOMEN: Blunt Injury *(continued from previous page)*

FOLLOW-UP:
Check student again on following day.

POTENTIAL COMPLICATIONS:
- Ruptured spleen: can be life-threatening without immediate treatment.
- Hypovolemic shock: symptoms include rapid pulse, cold-moist-clammy skin, alteration of consciousness, low blood pressure.

NOTES:
Bicycle handlebar injury:
Abdominal injury may occur when handlebars are turned so they punch the abdomen with force. Bicycle handlebar injuries are often considered trivial; alarming symptoms may not develop for 24 hours. Symptoms of serious injury are severe pain, vomiting or collapse.

References

ACEP News. (2011). *ACEP clinical policy: Blunt abdominal trauma.* Retrieved from
http://www.acep.org/News-/Publications/ACEP-News/ACEP-Clinical-Policy--Blunt-Abdominal-Trauma

Bodhit, A.N., Bhagra, A., & Ganti Stead, L. (2011). *Abdominal trauma: Never underestimate it.*
Retrieved from http://www.hindawi.com/crim/em/2011/850625/

Emergency Medical Paramedic. (2013). *What is kehr's sign?* Retrieved from
http://www.emergencymedicalparamedic.com/what-is-kehrs-sign/

Legome, E.L., Geibel, J. (2015). Blunt abdominal trauma. *Medscape.* Retrieved from
http://emedicine.medscape.com/article/1980980-overview#a2

ABDOMINAL PAIN/APPENDICITIS

DEFINITION/ETIOLOGY:
Pain or discomfort located between the bottom of the diaphragm and the top of the pelvic region. Acute abdominal pain: less than 2 weeks' duration. Chronic recurrent abdominal pain: three or more episodes, severe enough to affect normal activities, occurring more than 12 weeks.

Abdominal pain may be due to a variety of conditions, including but not limited to:

Intra-abdominal causes:

Gastrointestinal tract
- Dietary (excessive or inappropriate intake, food-borne pathogens)
- Constipation
- Appendicitis
- Lactose intolerance (recurrent)
- Irritable bowel syndrome (discomfort for at least 12 weeks within past 12 months plus at least two of the following: altered frequency and/or appearance of bowel movements, pain relief with bowel movement)
- Peptic ulcer (recurrent)
- Incarcerated inguinal hernia
- Celiac disease (recurrent)

Liver/Gall Bladder/Spleen
- Hepatitis
- Pancreatitis
- Cholecystitis (inflammation of the gall bladder) and cholelithiasis (gall stones)
- Contusion/rupture spleen (trauma)
- Sickle cell anemia (recurrent)

Urinary tract
- Cystitis (inflammation or infection of the bladder)
- Glomerulonephritis
- Kidney stone

ABDOMINAL PAIN/APPENDICITIS *(continued from previous page)*

<u>Ovaries, Fallopian Tubes and Uterus</u>
- Dysmenorrhea (menstrual cramps) (recurrent)
- Rupture of ovarian follicle at ovulation (mittelschmerz)
- Pelvic inflammatory disease (PID)
- Complication of pregnancy (ectopic pregnancy/abortion)
- Sexual abuse

Extra-abdominal causes:
- Abdominal migraine
- Diabetic ketoacidosis
- Functional abdominal pain (emotional or psychosocial)
- Group a streptococcal pharyngitis ("strep throat")
- Hypoglycemia
- Lead poisoning
- Leukemia
- Lower lobe pneumonia
- Rheumatic fever

Common causes considered by age of students:
1. <u>Preschool</u>: constipation, gastroenteritis, viral infection, urinary tract infection, pneumonia, trauma, lactose intolerance, sickle cell episode
2. <u>School age</u>: gastroenteritis, viral infection, constipation, appendicitis, trauma, urinary tract infection, pneumonia, lactose intolerance, sickle cell pain episode
3. <u>Adolescent</u>: Early adolescence is prime time for occurrence of appendicitis, mittelschmerz (ovulation pain), pelvic inflammatory disease (PID), dysmenorrhea, complication of pregnancy

SIGNS AND SYMPTOMS:
Symptoms vary depending on the etiology of the pain. A good assessment will help to differentiate the cause of the abdominal pain.
- <u>Mildly ill</u>: pain interferes minimally with normal activities
- <u>Moderately ill</u>: interferes with normal routine or signs of infection or systemic illness
- <u>Severely ill</u>: signs of peritonitis or intestinal obstruction or mental change

ABDOMINAL PAIN/APPENDICITIS *(continued from previous page)*

ASSESSMENT:

History:
- Onset, location, duration, frequency, severity and pattern of the pain
- Associated symptoms such as fever, vomiting, diarrhea, red or dark red blood in stool, urinary symptoms, weight loss, jaundice, arthritis or cough and sore throat
- Precipitating factors including constipation, trauma, underlying diseases (sickle cell anemia), menstruation, medication and diet history

Physical examination:
- Check temperature; assess circulation and hydration status
- Note signs of emergency surgical conditions:
  - peritonitis: includes guarding and rigidity of the abdominal muscles, rebound tenderness, decreased bowel sound, abdominal distention or shock
  - intestinal obstruction: distention, decreased bowel sounds and persistent vomiting
  - appendicitis:
    - fever 99°-102° F (oral)
    - nausea, vomiting
    - anorexia
    - vague diffuse epigastric or periumbilical pain, over several hours pain becomes more intense and shifts to right lower quadrant , rebound tenderness, release of pressure on left lower quadrant of abdomen elicits pain in right lower quadrant of abdomen (Rovsing sign)
    - decreased bowel sounds
    - prefers to lie on left side/right knee flexed
    - **If suspect appendix, perform auscultation, percussion, followed by palpation**
  - complication of pregnancy (female with history of delayed menstrual period) includes lower abdominal pain, pallor or shock, abnormal vaginal bleeding

- Assess location and severity of the pain:

Potential medical conditions according to pain location (list is not inclusive):
  - Diffuse abdominal pain: associated with diabetic ketoacidosis, food poisoning, gastroenteritis, intestinal obstruction, pancreatic disease, peritonitis, pharyngitis and sickle cell anemia
  - Epigastric pain: associated with duodenal/gastric/peptic ulcers, esophagitis, gastritis, gastroenteritis, GERD/hiatal hernia, myocardial infarction, irritable bowel disease, liver conditions and ulcerative colitis

ABDOMINAL PAIN/APPENDICITIS *(continued from previous page)*

- o <u>Right lower quadrant:</u> associated with appendicitis, ectopic pregnancy, gastroenteritis, inguinal hernia, irritable bowel syndrome (IBS), kidney stone, ovarian conditions, pelvic inflammatory disease and testicular torsion
- o <u>Right upper quadrant:</u> associated with acute pancreatitis, gallbladder conditions, kidney stone, duodenal ulcer, liver conditions and lower lobe pneumonia
- o <u>Left upper quadrant:</u> associated with bowel obstruction, constipation, IBS, kidney stone, left lower lobe pneumonia, leukemia, pyelonephritis, splenic conditions and ulcerative colitis
- o <u>Left lower quadrant:</u> associated with constipation, ectopic pregnancy, inguinal hernia, irritable bowel syndrome (IBS), kidney stone, ovarian conditions, pelvic inflammatory disease, sigmoid colon and testicular torsion
- o <u>Suprapubic region:</u> associated with dysmenorrhea, endometriosis, pelvic inflammatory disease, sexually transmitted disease, and urinary tract infection/ bladder infections

MANAGEMENT/TREATMENT:
1. If signs of appendicitis (the most common serious condition) or moderate-severe illness notify the parent/guardian immediately and refer to the student's healthcare provider.
2. If mild, may rest for 15-30 minutes. If symptoms persist, refer for evaluation. If symptoms subside, return student to class.
3. No food or drink by mouth. May sip small amount of plain water.

FOLLOW-UP:
- If student returns to classroom, re-evaluate within 2-4 hours.
- If student requires surgery, upon the student's return, follow healthcare provider's instructions regarding athletic or PE participation.

ABDOMINAL PAIN/APPENDICITIS *(continued from previous page)*

References

American Academy of Pediatrics. (2015). *Appendicitis in teens*. Retrieved from
    https://www.healthychildren.org/English/health-issues/conditions/abdominal/Pages/Appendicitis-in-Teens.aspx

Cosby, M., Miller, N.B., & Youngman, K. (2013). Acute measures for emergent problems. In J. Selekman (Ed.), *School nursing: A comprehensive text* (2nd ed.) (pp.516-577). Philadelphia, PA: F. A. Davis.

Cunha, J.P. (2014). Appendicitis. *EMedicine health*. Retrieved from
    http://www.emedicinehealth.com/appendicitis/article_em.htm

Hung, M., Lin, L.H., & Chen, D. F. (2012). Clinical manifestations in children with ruptured appendicitis. *Pediatric Emergency Care, 5,*433-35. doi: 10.1097/PEC.0b013e3182531ace

Mayo Clinic. (2014). *Appendicitis.* Retrieved from
    http://www.mayoclinic.org/diseases-conditions/appendicitis/basics/definition/con-20023582

The Merck Manual. (2014). *Acute abdominal pain.* Retrieved from http://www.merck.com/mmpe/sec02/ch011/ch011b.html

Minkes, R., & Cuffari, C. (2015). Pediatric appendicitis clinical presentation. *Medscape.* Retrieved from
    http://emedicine.medscape.com/article/926795-clinical#b3

ABRASIONS

DEFINITION/ETIOLOGY:
An abrasion is a denuded area of skin (epidermis) resulting from a scrape on a hard or rough surface. Abrasions can occur on any part of the body, but most often occur on bony areas, such as the hands, forearms, elbows, knees, shins, and face. Abrasions often result from falls or friction accidents.

SIGNS AND SYMPTOMS:
- Most abrasions are superficial.
- There is usually minimal bleeding and may ooze serosanguinous fluid. The amount of bleeding is greater when deeper layers of skin are scraped off.
- Abrasions can contain particles of dirt.

MANAGEMENT/TREATMENT:
1. Wash gently under running tap water with plain soap to remove foreign material. If feasible, allow a running stream of lukewarm water to pour over the wound.
2. During wash, if necessary, try to remove debris by gently rubbing with 4x4 gauze pads.
3. Do not scrub a wound imbedded with dirt. Instead, refer to healthcare provider.
4. Assess Tetanus immunization status.
5. Do not use povidone-iodine, Dakin's solution and hydrogen peroxide for cleansing wounds. These solutions can damage normal tissue and hinder neodermal development necessary for healing. Only use antibiotic creams and any topical medication if individualized or standing orders are on file.
6. Small abrasions may be left open to the air.
7. Cover larger abrasions with a sterile, non-adherent bandage.
8. After partial thickness abrasions are cleaned, a moist wound dressing can be applied within two hours of injury. This dressing can be a hydrogel or hydrocolloid dressing and can be any of a variety of brand-name products. This dressing must stay in place at least forty-eight hours and up to seven days to enhance optimal wound healing. Moist wound dressings allow rapid resurfacing or re-epithelialization of wound surfaces and allow for migration of proteins necessary for wound healing.
9. Notify parent/guardian if abrasion is not minor and enter on injury report.

ABRASIONS *(continued from previous page)*

FOLLOW-UP:
- Instruct the parent/guardian and student that the dressing is to remain in place for seven days or until wound is healed. Wrap the dressing with plastic for bathing. The student may be given an extra dressing to take home in the event that his/her dressing falls off or is damaged and needs replaced.
- The student should have a daily wound and dressing recheck; replace dressing as needed.
- A registered nurse should re-evaluate the partial thickness abrasion after seven days using the Bates-Jensen Wound Assessment Tool. If re-epithelialization has occurred at day 7, no further dressing or evaluation is needed.
- Refer the student to his/her healthcare provider if after seven days, the laceration or abrasion is not healing.
- Repeat cleansing at least daily, more often if necessary to keep wound clean.
- This should be done at home, but school nurse may need to monitor or guide.

POTENTIAL COMPLICATIONS:
1. Infection:
    - Pus on abrasion itself, usually located under crusts.
    - Cellulitis: spreading redness immediately around the abrasion.
    - Lymphangitis: red streaks radiating out from abrasion. (Sometimes this is mistakenly referred to as blood poisoning. It is actually an infection of the lymph channels.)
    - Regional lymph nodes enlarged; if abrasion on arm, nodes will be in axilla; if on leg, nodes will be in groin.
2. Scarring:
    - Minor abrasions: scar very superficial, usually regains pigmentation and blends with surrounding skin.
    - Deep abrasions: scar usually deeper and permanent. (May require later management for cosmetic reasons).

NOTES:
- If no improvement in ONE day, refer to healthcare provider.
- For lymphangitis, refer to healthcare provider immediately.
- Nurse practitioners or other nurses with prescriptive authority may order amoxicillin or other antibiotics.

ABRASIONS *(continued from previous page)*

References

Ball, J., Binder, R., & Cowen, K. (Eds.). (2015). Alterations in skin integrity. *Principles of Pediatric Nursing: Caring for Children (6th ed.)* Upper Saddle River, NJ: Pearson Education, Inc.

Harris, C., Bates-Jensen, B., Parslow, N., Raizman, R., Singh, M., & Ketchen, R.J. (Eds.) (2010). Bates-Jensen wound assessment tool: pictorial guide validation project. *Journal of Wound, Ostomy & Continence Nursing, 37*(3), 253-9. doi: 10.1097/WON.0b013e3181d73aab

Houser, J. (2011). Evidence-based practice in healthcare. In J. Houser, S. Oman (Eds.), *Evidence-based practice an implementation guide for healthcare organizations,* (p. 7). Sudbury, MA: Jones & Bartlett Learning.

Medicinenet. (2015). *Cuts, scrapes (abrasions), and puncture wounds*. Retrieved from http://www.medicinenet.com/cuts_scrapes_and_puncture_wounds/article.htm

Merck Manual. *Abrasions*. (2013). Retrieved from http://www.merckmanuals.com/professional/injuries_poisoning/lacerations/lacerations.html?qt=abrasions&alt=sh#v1110280

Sanford Health/ Healthwise. (2010). *Scrapes*. Retrieved from http://www.sanfordhealth.org/HealthInformation/Healthwise/Topic/srape#hw101236

ADRENAL INSUFFICIENCY

DEFINITION/ETIOLOGY:
Adrenal insufficiency is an endocrine disorder that occurs when the adrenal glands do not produce a sufficient amount of the hormone cortisol. Adrenal insufficiency can also affect the production of the hormone aldosterone. Cortisol and aldosterone are crucial for the body to regulate blood pressure, metabolism, heart contractibility and sodium balance. Cortisol also regulates the body's response to stress. Lack of cortisol production affects the body's ability to appropriately respond to physiological stressors. Onset of adrenal insufficiency is usually gradual.

There are over 60 known causes for adrenal insufficiency. Adrenal insufficiency is classified as either primary or secondary.

Primary adrenal insufficiency (commonly referred to as Addison's disease) occurs when the adrenal glands are compromised and do not produce the hormone cortisol. Addison's disease is caused by an autoimmune response in approximately 80% of cases.

Secondary adrenal insufficiency occurs when the pituitary gland is diseased and unable to produce the hormone adrenocorticotropin (ACTH). ACTH stimulates the adrenal gland to produce the hormone cortisol. Impaired production of ACTH causes a decrease in the production of cortisol thereby triggering shrinkage of the adrenal glands. Secondary adrenal insufficiency is more common than primary adrenal insufficiency.

SIGNS AND SYMPTOMS:
Symptoms are the same for primary and secondary adrenal insufficiency unless specifically noted:
- Muscle and joint pain
- Nausea and vomiting
- Diarrhea
- Hypotension
- Loss of appetite
- Hypoglycemia (unexplained)
- Generalized weakness
- Growth delay
- Chronic fatigue

11

ADRENAL INSUFFICIENCY *(continued from previous page)*

Late Symptoms:
- Weight loss
- Bronze pigmentation to skin (occurs only with primary adrenal insufficiency)
- Salt cravings

MANAGEMENT/TREATMENT:
Adrenal insufficiency results in a lack of essential hormones, and therefore treatment focuses on replacing these vital hormones. Individuals with adrenal insufficiency are glucocorticoid dependent and must take cortisol daily. Cortisol is taken orally once or twice a day. If necessary, aldosterone is replaced orally once a day. The student may also need to follow a high sodium diet and/or have salty snacks at school.

FOLLOW-UP:
1. Monitor for necessary medication dosage changes. Medication dosages often need to be adjusted to meet client needs during times of stress. Once the stressor is over, medication dosages typically return to pre-illness (pre-injury) levels.
2. Encourage student to wear medical alert identification.

POTENTIAL COMPLICATIONS:

> **Adrenal Crisis is a serious complication of adrenal insufficiency. An adrenal crisis is a sudden, severe worsening of adrenal insufficiency symptoms. This can occur when an individual with adrenal insufficiency experiences a traumatic physical or emotional stressor.**

An adrenal crisis is life-threatening. Symptoms of an adrenal crisis include:
- Dizziness/lightheaded
- Sudden, muscle pain (can be severe – often occurs in low back, abdomen or legs)
- Severe nausea and vomiting
- Severe abdominal pain
- Confusion
- Hypotension
- Neurological deficits (headache/confusion/seizure)
- Shock like symptoms
- Loss of consciousness
- Death (if left untreated)

ADRENAL INSUFFICIENCY *(continued from previous page)*

Rapid physical deterioration can occur. **If a person with adrenal insufficiency exhibits these symptoms act immediately!**
1. Administer prescribed Solu-Cortef IM.
2. Call 911.
3. Provide appropriate first aid care.
4. Notify parent/guardian.

NOTES:
Children with adrenal insufficiency may experience short-term memory difficulties and/or learning disabilities. Evaluate for need of Section 504 or Special Education services.

References

Mayo Clinic. (2012). *Addison's disease.* Retrieved from http://www.mayoclinic.org/diseases-conditions/addisons-disease/basics/causes/con-20021340

Merck Manual. (2014). *Secondary adrenal insufficiency.* Retrieved from http://www.merckmanuals.com/professional/endocrine-and-metabolic-disorders/adrenal-disorders/secondary-adrenal-insufficiency

National Endocrine and Metabolic Diseases. (2014). *Adrenal insufficiency and Addison's disease.* Retrieved from http://www.niddk.nih.gov/health-information/health-topics/endocrine/adrenal-insufficiency-addisons-disease/Pages/fact-sheet.aspx#prepare

U.S. National Library of Medicine. (2013). *Acute adrenal crisis.* Retrieved from https://www.nlm.nih.gov/medlineplus/ency/article/000357.htm

ALLERGIES

See also Anaphylaxis, Food Allergies, Poison Ivy/Oak, Rashes

DEFINITION/ETIOLOGY:

The immune system reacts to a foreign substance that is not generally harmful (examples – certain foods, latex, pollen, insect stings/bites, medications or pet dander).

SIGNS AND SYMPTOMS:

Symptoms vary and depend on the persons' specific allergy. Allergy symptoms range from mild to life threatening.

Allergic Dermatitis	• Rash (papules/vesicles) at site of contact • Pruritus • May have areas of excoriation from scratching • Thickened dry skin that may ooze
Allergic Rhinitis	• Allergic shiners – bluish discoloration and edema below eyes • Clear nasal discharge • Sneezing • Itchy, watery and/or swollen eyes
Atopic Dermatitis (type of eczema)	• Thickened, cracked, or scaly patches of skin • Patches red to brownish-gray in color • Itchy skin • Extremely dry skin may ooze
Medication Allergy (penicillin, sulfa, anticonvulsants, iodine and insulin are the most common cause of medication allergies)	• Hives • Rash • Pruritus • Difficulty breathing/wheezing • Anaphylaxis

ALLERGIES *(continued from previous page)*

MANAGEMENT/TREATMENT:

General treatment
1. Avoidance of allergen
2. Medications (as prescribed) to reduce symptoms
3. Immunotherapy (allergy shots)
4. Emergency epinephrine

The following medications may be prescribed by the healthcare provider:

Allergic Dermatitis
1. Corticosteroids creams/ointments – to ease itching
2. Corticosteroid (oral) – reduces inflammation, immune response and itching
3. Antihistamines – to relieve severe itching
4. Antibiotics – if lesions are infected from scratching

Allergic Rhinitis
1. Antihistamines - relieves sneezing, runny nose, itching, and watery eyes
2. Nasal corticosteroid sprays – start working quickly but may take several weeks to obtain the full effect of the medication
3. Decongestants – reduce symptoms of nasal congestion
4. Leukotriene inhibitor (i.e. Singulair®) to relieve seasonal allergy symptoms
5. Immunotherapy

Atopic Dermatitis
1. **Oral corticosteroids – may be prescribed short-term to treat severe cases**.
2. Corticosteroid creams or ointments to ease scaling of skin and itching.
3. Antihistamines to relieve severe itching.
4. Antibiotics to treat bacterial skin infections from scratching.
5. Immunomodulators – reduces atopic dermatitis flare-ups. These medications are approved for children over the age of two. The FDA recommends that these medications be used only when other treatment options have failed.

Medication Allergy
1. **Discontinue medication that caused allergic response immediately.**
2. Antihistamines to relieve mild symptoms of rash/hives/itching.
3. Bronchodilators to relieve wheezing.
4. Corticosteroids - reduce inflammation associated with allergic reaction.
5. Epinephrine for severe allergic reaction.

ALLERGIES *(continued from previous page)*

FOLLOW-UP:
- Refer to specialist if symptoms do not respond to treatment.
- Educate as to the importance of avoiding known allergens.
- For severe allergies – provide information regarding the importance of wearing a Medical Alert necklace/bracelet.
- Identify coexisting medical conditions such as asthma – commonly associated with allergic rhinitis and atopic dermatitis.

POTENTIAL COMPLICATIONS:
General
- Skin infections from frequent scratching
- Another allergy
- Anaphylaxis (severe allergic reaction)
- Death

Allergic rhinitis
- Sinusitis
- Otitis Media

NOTES:

An Individualized Healthcare Plan <u>AND</u> an Individualized Emergency Plan should be prepared for every child with a serious known food, substance or insect allergy potential. Appropriate school staff (including bus personnel and cafeteria and playground personnel) should receive in-service preparation for dealing with a general allergic reaction and with child specific needs. Staff training in the use of injected epinephrine should be conducted according to state and district laws and policies.

Many states have adopted legislation that allows schools provide undesignated epinephrine auto injectors.

ALLERGIES *(continued from previous page)*

Allergy Resources for School Personnel
American Academy of Allergy and Asthma and Immunology (AAAAI)
1-800-822-ASMA
www.aaaai.org
Professional and patient education resources on the website

Food Allergy and Anaphylaxis Network (FAAN)
4744 Holly Ave.
Fairfax, VA 22030-5647
1-800-929-4040
www.foodallergy.org
www.fankids.org
School guidelines (including school bus and field trips) and teaching materials.

Asthma and Allergy Foundation of America
1233 20th St NW, Ste 402
Washington, DC 20036
800-7-ASTHMA
www.aafa.org
Resources and free student Asthma Action Cards

References

Food Allergy and Anaphylaxis Network. (2015). *Types of allergic reactions/managing food allergies.* Retrieved from
    www.foodallergy.org

Mayo Clinic. (2014). *Allergies.* Retrieved from http://www.mayoclinic.org/diseases-conditions/allergies/basics/definition/
    con-20034030

Hogate, S., Giel, J., Selekman, J. (2013). Allergy. In J. Selekman (Ed.), *School nursing: A comprehensive text* (2nd ed.)
    (pp. 784-816). Philadelphia, PA: F.A. Davis.

LATEX ALLERGY

DEFINITION/ETIOLOGY (*see also Allergies and Anaphylaxis*):
Latex allergy is a reaction to certain proteins found in natural rubber latex, a product manufactured from a milky fluid that comes from the rubber tree. Natural rubber latex is different from synthetic rubber made from chemicals. Synthetic rubber products, including "latex" house paints, are not made with natural latex and do not trigger allergic reactions in people who are allergic to natural rubber latex products. The more frequently exposed a person is to latex either by direct contact or inhalation (e.g., staff administering daily care requiring use of gloves, persons with spina bifida who use latex catheters), the more likely they are to develop sensitivity.

A latex allergy may cause allergic reactions ranging from sneezing or a runny nose to anaphylaxis, a potentially life-threatening condition.

Type IV-Delayed (due to chemicals used in processing latex):
- Itchy, red, mildly swollen skin rash on sites which touched latex
- Typically appearing 48-96 hours after contact
- Blisters appear in severe cases

Type I-Immediate (due to proteins which are part of the natural latex):
- Involves parts of the body that did not touch latex
- Hives on any part of the body
- "Hay fever-like" nasal stuffiness, sneezing, runny nose, itchy nose, eyes or roof of the mouth
- Wheezing, coughing and shortness of breath - *an emergency*
- Anaphylaxis - a life threatening blockage of the airway and shock

MANAGEMENT/TREATMENT
Treatment is individualized but management essentially involves avoidance of the offending source that causes the reaction. **Students with known latex allergies should have an individualized emergency plan. Additionally, a policy should be established for action for unknown allergies.**
1. *Delayed reactions*: short-term, over-the-counter or prescribed steroid topical cream or ointment usually relieve rash.
2. *Hives or "hay fever"- like signs*: over-the-counter antihistamines or decongestants provide relief. If no relief seek advice from healthcare provider.
3. *Wheezing, coughing or shortness of breath*: this may indicate severe reaction or anaphylaxis. **Seek urgent medical advice**. Anti-inflammatory and bronchodilator medications for reactive airway may be prescribed.

LATEX ALLERGY *(continued from previous page)*

4. *Anaphylaxis*: epinephrine (e.g., Epi-Pen®, Auvi-Q®, AdrenaClick® and generic auto injectors) injected as quickly as possible, followed by immediate call to 911 for transport to emergency facility.

FOLLOW UP:

- Educate persons to avoid contact and exposure to items containing latex (gloves, hairbrushes, bandages, balloons, rubber bands, erasers, etc.). A list of common healthcare and daily items containing latex and alternative products is available through the Latex Allergy Support Group at http://www.lasg.org.uk/information/.
- Persons with a latex allergy may need to avoid certain foods: avocado, banana, kiwi, water chestnut, tomato, apple, carrot, celery, melons, papaya, and potato. There are other foods with a low degree of association to latex allergies.
- Develop an Individualized Healthcare Plan for a student with a latex allergy that includes specific actions to prevent exposure, staff training, and the emergency action plan.
- Schools should provide latex free gloves for staff that use them in their daily job performance.

Resources

1. NASN's Anaphylaxis Toolkit at http://www.nasn.org/ToolsResources/FoodAllergyandAnaphylaxis

2. FARE (Food Allery Research and Education at http://www.foodallergy.org/

3. Allergyhome.org. Specific information for schools at http://www.allergyhome.org/schools/

References

American College of Asthma, Allergy and Immunology. (2014). *Latex allergy*. Retrieved from http://acaai.org/allergies/types/skin-allergies/latex-allergy

American Latex Allergy Association. (n.d.) *About latex allergy*. Retrieved from http://www.latexallergyresources.org/about-latex-allergy

Centers for Disease Control and Prevention. (2014). Latex allergy a prevention guide. Retrieved from http://www.cdc.gov/niosh/docs/98-113/

Mayo Clinic. (2014). *Latex allergy*. Retrieved from http://www.mayoclinic.org/diseases-conditions/latex-allergy/basics/definition/con-20024233

Selekman, J., Bochenek, J., & Lukens, M. (2013). Children with chronic conditions. In J. Selekman (2nd Ed.), *School nursing: A comprehensive text* (2nd ed.) (pp. 792, 1031). Philadelphia, PA: F.A. Davis.

ANAPHYLAXIS

> *IMPORTANT:*
> - *Students with a known allergic reaction should have an individualized healthcare plan (see sample below) in place and all staff (including bus drivers) must be aware of the emergency plan and how to initiate it.*
> - *Determine how epinephrine will be available to the student at all times (on person, in classroom(s)/cafeteria, when on bus or school sponsored event).*
> - *Point to consider: Some schools have obtained Standing Orders/or a physician directed nursing protocol for epinephrine from a school physician/healthcare provider and non-patient specific stock epinephrine in the health room. Many states have laws, which require schools to stock epinephrine in schools.*

OVERVIEW/DEFINITION:

Anaphylaxis is a severe, potentially life-threatening allergic reaction. It may occur in adults or children not previously known to be allergic or hypersensitive. The reaction ranges from mild, self-limited symptoms to rapid death. Symptoms of a reaction can occur within seconds to minutes after exposure.

Extreme sensitivity to one or more of the following can cause anaphylaxis:
- Insect sting, usually bee, wasp or fire ants
- Medication or immunizations, usually by injection
- Food such as peanuts, tree nuts, shellfish, cow's milk or egg (most common triggers in children adolescents and young adults)
- Industrial or office chemicals or their vapors
- Latex rubber

Most allergic reactions are not severe enough to cause anaphylaxis. Anaphylaxis can have a sudden onset. The severity of the reaction depends on how sensitive, amount ingested and route of exposure. Symptoms that begin within 15 minutes after exposure to trigger agent usually result in the more severe type of anaphylactic reaction, but reactions can occur hours after an exposure.

CAUTION: The severity of the symptoms can change quickly.

ANAPHYLAXIS *(continued from previous page)*

SYMPTOMS OF ANAPHYLAXIS INCLUDE:

Mouth	Itching, swelling of lips and or tongue, tingling (burning) sensation in mouth or around lips or drooling
Throat	Swelling of the tongue and throat, difficulty swallowing, itching, tightness/closure, hoarseness, changes in quality of voice
Skin	Itching, hives, redness, swelling
Gut	Abdominal pain/cramping, nausea/vomiting, diarrhea
Lungs	Respiratory difficulty, shortness of breath, cough, shallow respirations, wheezing, stridor
Heart	Weak pulse, heart palpitations, drop in blood pressure, dizziness, light-headedness, loss of consciousness

Only a few symptoms may be present. **All of the above symptoms can potentially lead to a life-threatening situation. Provide prompt medical attention.**

ANTICIPATED CONCERNS/PROBLEMS
- Every minute counts with anaphylaxis. Delay in treatment is associated with fatalities.
  - Cardiac arrest
  - Respiratory arrest
  - Shock
  - Coma
  - Death
- Respiratory difficulty and changes in quality of voice are symptoms of laryngeal edema and may signal closure of the airway. Laryngospasm (closure of the vocal cords blocking air intake) can occur as part of anaphylaxis or by itself without any of the above symptoms. **Call 911 immediately.** Sudden standing or sitting after receiving the epinephrine injection can lead to empty ventricle syndrome, which can be fatal.
- Eighty to ninety percent of anaphylactic reactions include skin signs and when they are absent, anaphylaxis is harder to recognize.
- Symptoms of an anaphylactic reaction may vary in multiple episodes in the same person. Medications, age-related factors, and co-existent diseases, may contribute to severe or fatal anaphylaxis.
- Co-factors such as infections, exercise, emotional stress, and premenstrual status may possible amplify anaphylaxis.

ANAPHYLAXIS *(continued from previous page)*

MANAGEMENT/TREATMENT: Follow student's individualized emergency care plan. Administer medication as ordered. Plan should include medical orders and staff responsibilities for emergency care.

Recommended Dosages

Immediate Injection of adrenalin 1:1000 SQ		Immediate administration of Epi-pen
Age 3-5	0.15cc	33-66 lbs. 0.15 (epi-pen jr.)
Age 6-8	0.25cc	>66 lbs. 0.3　(epi-pen)
Age 9-18	0.3cc	

Immediate call to 911 and transport to nearest medical facility despite initial improvement after first epinephrine injection, biphasic reactions often occur. The following information should be sent with the EMS:

— Allergen to which patient is reacting, if known.
— Signs and symptoms of distress.
— Emergency measures instituted.
— Patient response to emergency measures.
— Time of all activities, including giving adrenalin.
— Epinephrine auto injector if given.
— Contact/emergency information.

1. **If student is still at school in 15-20 minutes, repeat dose of epinephrine according to healthcare provider orders.**
2. Monitor vital signs including blood pressure continuously.
3. Place person on their back or other comfortable position with their legs elevated. Do not allow person to sit up.
4. Cover with blankets, if necessary, to keep warm; do not allow blankets to interfere with handling or observation.
5. Refer all cases to healthcare provider.

ANAPHYLAXIS *(continued from previous page)*

FOLLOW-UP:
- Review the student's individualized emergency plan to make sure there are no changes required based on this incident.
- If this is the first known incident of an allergic reaction, ensure that an individualized emergency plan (see sample below) is developed and make sure all staff (including bus drivers) are aware of the emergency plan and how to initiate it.
- Provide health education with family, student, and school staff regarding further exposure to sensitizing agent.
- Emphasize wearing Medic Alert tag or bracelets (www.medicalert.org).
- Ask about desensitization procedure by healthcare provider.
- Have parent/guardian replace epinephrine if expired or administered.
- Record as "Medical Alert" on student's record.

NOTES:
- Your district should have a written procedural guideline in place for anaphylaxis. Post this guideline in the health room.
- An emergency care plan must be in place and mock drills practiced regularly
- Prevention – avoid known allergens.
- Do not store injectable epinephrine devices in a frequently opened drawer as repeated motion may cause premature release and injury when handled.
- Do not store injectable epinephrine in car glove box/bus or where it can become overheated.
- Consider sending epinephrine home during school breaks depending on temperature of building when school is not in session.
- Do not use epinephrine that is cloudy or discolored.
- Do not store epinephrine in refrigerator. Normal **room temperature** is best. Dispose of used auto-injector according to OSHA guidelines.

ANAPHYLAXIS *(continued from previous page)*

RESOURCES:

- NASN's Anaphylaxis **Planning Algorithm** can be found at http://nasn.org/ToolsResources/FoodAllergyandAnaphylaxis/AnaphylaxisPlanningAlgorithm
- Tools to train school nurses and staff include and can be found at http://www.ncbi.nlm.nih.gov/pmc/articles/PMC3500036/

  - Charts that include Clinical Criteria for Diagnosing Anaphylaxis
  - Patient Risk Factors for Severe or Fatal Anaphylaxis and Co-Factors that Amplify Anaphylaxis
  - Anaphylaxis Mechanisms and Triggers
  - Clinical Criteria for the Diagnosis of Anaphylaxis, and Symptoms and Signs of Anaphylaxis)

References

Mayo Clinic. (2013). *Anaphylaxis*. Retrieved from http://www.mayoclinic.com/health/anaphylaxis/DS00009

Selekman, J. & Gray, C. (2013). Allergy. In J. Selekman (Ed.), *School nursing: A comprehensive text (2nd ed.)* (pp. 787-790). Philadelphia, PA: F.A. Davis.

Simons, F., Ardussol, L., Bilo, B., Gamal, Y., Ledford, D., Ring, J., Sanchez-Borges, M., Senna, G., Sheikn, A., Thong, B., & World Health Organization. (2011). World allergy organization guidelines for the assessment and management of anaphylaxis. *The World Allergy Organization Journal, 4*(2), pp.13-37. Retrieved from http://www.ncbi.nlm.nih.gov/pmc/articles/PMC3500036/

ANAPHYLAXIS *(continued from previous page)*

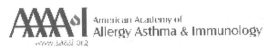

Anaphylaxis Emergency Action Plan

Patient Name: _____ Age: _____

Allergies: _____

Asthma ☐ Yes *(high risk for severe reaction)* ☐ No

Additional health problems besides anaphylaxis: _____

_____

Concurrent medications: _____

_____

Symptoms of Anaphylaxis

MOUTH	itching, swelling of lips and/or tongue
THROAT*	itching, tightness/closure, hoarseness
SKIN	itching, hives, redness, swelling
GUT	vomiting, diarrhea, cramps
LUNG*	shortness of breath, cough, wheeze
HEART*	weak pulse, dizziness, passing out

Only a few symptoms may be present. Severity of symptoms can change quickly.
*Some symptoms can be life-threatening. ACT FAST!

Emergency Action Steps - DO NOT HESITATE TO GIVE EPINEPHRINE!

1. Inject epinephrine in thigh using (check one): ☐ Auvi-Q (0.15 mg)   ☐ Auvi-Q (0.3 mg)

    ☐ EpiPen Jr (0.15 mg) ☐ EpiPen (0.3 mg)

    ☐ Other (0.15 mg)   ☐ Other (0.3 mg)

Specify others: _____

IMPORTANT: ASTHMA INHALERS AND/OR ANTIHISTAMINES CAN'T BE DEPENDED ON IN ANAPHYLAXIS.

2. Call 911 or rescue squad (before calling contact)

3. Emergency contact #1: home_____ work_____ cell_____

    Emergency contact #2: home_____ work_____ cell_____

    Emergency contact #3: home_____ work_____ cell_____

Comments: _____

_____

_____

_____

_____

Doctor's Signature/Date/Phone Number

_____

Parent's Signature (for individuals under age 18 yrs)/Date

This Information is for general purposes and is not intended to replace the advice of a qualified health professional. For more information, visit
www.aaaai.org. © 2013 American Academy of Allergy, Asthma & Immunology   4/2013

ANAPHYLAXIS *(continued from previous page)*

⊕ FARE — FOOD ALLERGY & ANAPHYLAXIS EMERGENCY CARE PLAN

Food Allergy Research & Education

Name: _____ D.O.B.: _____

Allergy to: _____

PLACE PICTURE HERE

Weight: _____ lbs. Asthma: [   ] Yes (higher risk for a severe reaction)   [   ] No

NOTE: Do not depend on antihistamines or inhalers (bronchodilators) to treat a severe reaction. USE EPINEPHRINE.

Extremely reactive to the following foods: _____

THEREFORE:

[   ] If checked, give epinephrine immediately for ANY symptoms if the allergen was likely eaten.

[   ] If checked, give epinephrine immediately if the allergen was definitely eaten, even if no symptoms are noted.

FOR **ANY** OF THE FOLLOWING:

SEVERE SYMPTOMS

LUNG
Short of breath, wheezing, repetitive cough

HEART
Pale, blue, faint, weak pulse, dizzy

THROAT
Tight, hoarse, trouble breathing/ swallowing

MOUTH
Significant swelling of the tongue and/or lips

SKIN
Many hives over body, widespread redness

GUT
Repetitive vomiting, severe diarrhea

OTHER
Feeling something bad is about to happen, anxiety, confusion

OR A COMBINATION of symptoms from different body areas.

1. **INJECT EPINEPHRINE IMMEDIATELY.**
2. **Call 911.** Tell them the child is having anaphylaxis and may need epinephrine when they arrive.

- Consider giving additional medications following epinephrine:
  » Antihistamine
  » Inhaler (bronchodilator) if wheezing
- Lay the person flat, raise legs and keep warm. If breathing is difficult or they are vomiting, let them sit up or lie on their side.
- If symptoms do not improve, or symptoms return, more doses of epinephrine can be given about 5 minutes or more after the last dose.
- Alert emergency contacts.
- Transport them to ER even if symptoms resolve. Person should remain in ER for at least 4 hours because symptoms may return.

MILD SYMPTOMS

NOSE
Itchy/runny nose, sneezing

MOUTH
Itchy mouth

SKIN
A few hives, mild itch

GUT
Mild nausea/ discomfort

FOR **MILD SYMPTOMS** FROM **MORE THAN ONE** SYSTEM AREA, GIVE EPINEPHRINE.

FOR **MILD SYMPTOMS** FROM **A SINGLE SYSTEM** AREA, FOLLOW THE DIRECTIONS BELOW:

1. Antihistamines may be given, if ordered by a healthcare provider.
2. Stay with the person; alert emergency contacts.
3. Watch closely for changes. If symptoms worsen, give epinephrine.

MEDICATIONS/DOSES

Epinephrine Brand: _____

Epinephrine Dose: [   ] 0.15 mg IM   [   ] 0.3 mg IM

Antihistamine Brand or Generic: _____

Antihistamine Dose: _____

Other (e.g., inhaler-bronchodilator if wheezing): _____

_____

PARENT/GUARDIAN AUTHORIZATION SIGNATURE   DATE   PHYSICIAN/HCP AUTHORIZATION SIGNATURE   DATE

FORM PROVIDED COURTESY OF FOOD ALLERGY RESEARCH & EDUCATION (FARE) (WWW.FOODALLERGY.ORG) 5/2014

ANAPHYLAXIS *(continued from previous page)*

⊕ FARE
Food Allergy Research & Education

PLAN DE ATENCIÓN DE EMERGENCIA EN CASO DE ALERGIA A ALIMENTOS Y ANAFILAXIA

Nombre: _____ Fecha de nacimiento: _____

Alergia a: _____

Peso: _____ libras Asma: [ ] Sí (mayor riesgo de reacción grave) [ ] No

COLOQUE LA IMAGEN AQUÍ

NOTA: No dependa de agentes antihistamínicos ni inhaladores (broncodilatadores) para tratar una reacción grave. USE EPINEFRINA.

Extremadamente reactivo a los siguientes alimentos: _____

ENTONCES:

[ ] Si esta opción está marcada, administre epinefrina inmediatamente en caso de que se presente CUALQUIER síntoma si existe la posibilidad de que se haya ingerido el alérgeno.

[ ] Si esta opción está marcada, administre epinefrina inmediatamente si definitivamente se ingirió el alérgeno, incluso si no hay síntomas.

PARA **CUALQUIERA** DE LOS SIGUIENTES:

SÍNTOMAS **GRAVES**

PULMONES
Falta de aire, sibilancia, tos reiterada

CORAZÓN
Palidez, color azulado, desmayos, pulso débil, mareo

GARGANTA
Oclusión, voz ronca, dificultad para respirar/tragar

BOCA
Hinchazón significativa de la lengua y/o los labios

PIEL
Muchas ronchas en el cuerpo, enrojecimiento generalizado

INTESTINO
Vómitos reiterados o diarrea grave

OTRA ÁREA
Sensación de que algo malo sucederá, ansiedad, confusión

O UNA COMBINACIÓN de síntomas de diferentes áreas del cuerpo.

⇩ ⇩ ⇩

1. **INYECTE EPINEFRINA INMEDIATAMENTE.**
2. **Llame al 911.** Comuníqueles que el niño presenta un cuadro de anafilaxia y puede necesitar epinefrina a su llegada.
- Considere administrar más medicamentos luego de la epinefrina:
  - » Agentes antihistamínicos.
  - » Inhalador (broncodilatador) si hay sibilancia.
- Recueste al niño, levántele las piernas y manténgalo abrigado. Si tiene problemas para respirar o vomita, hágalo sentarse o recostarse sobre un lado.
- Si los síntomas no mejoran, o regresan, pueden administrarse más dosis de epinefrina aproximadamente 5 minutos o más después de la última dosis.
- Avise a los contactos de emergencia.
- Lleve al niño a la sala de emergencias incluso si los síntomas desaparecen. El niño debe permanecer en la sala de emergencias durante más de 4 horas porque los síntomas podrían volver a manifestarse.

SÍNTOMAS **LEVES**

NARIZ
Picazón/secreción nasal, estornudos

BOCA
Picazón bucal

PIEL
Algunas ronchas, picazón leve

INTESTINO
Náuseas leves/molestias

PARA **SÍNTOMAS LEVES** DE **MÁS DE UNA** DE LAS DIFERENTES ÁREAS DEL CUERPO, ADMINISTRE EPINEFRINA.

PARA **SÍNTOMAS LEVES** DE **UNA ÚNICA ÁREA** DEL CUERPO, SIGA LAS INDICACIONES A CONTINUACIÓN:

1. Se pueden administrar antihistamínicos, si así lo indica el médico.
2. Quédese con el niño; avise a los contactos de emergencia.
3. Observe detenidamente para detectar cambios. Si los síntomas empeoran, administre epinefrina.

MEDICAMENTOS/DOSIS

Marca de epinefrina: _____

Dosis de epinefrina: [ ] 0.15 mg por vía intramuscular
[ ] 0.3 mg por vía intramuscular

Agente antihistamínico de marca o agente antihistamínico genérico: _____

Dosis del agente antihistamínico: _____

Otro (p. ej., broncodilatador inhalable si hay sibilancia): _____

FIRMA DE AUTORIZACIÓN DEL PADRE/MADRE/TUTOR LEGAL   FECHA   FIRMA DE AUTORIZACIÓN DEL MÉDICO/PROVEEDOR DE ATENCIÓN MÉDICA   FECHA

FORMULARIO PROPORCIONADO COMO CORTESÍA DE FOOD ALLERGY RESEARCH & EDUCATION (FARE) (WWW.FOODALLERGY.ORG) 4/2014

ASTHMA AND ASTHMA EMERGENCIES

OVERVIEW/DEFINITION:

Asthma is a chronic inflammatory disease of the airways. It is best understood as the clinical result of two linked processes, airway inflammation and bronchial hyper-reactivity. While bronchial hyper-reactivity is often genetically determined, it may be induced by viral infection. Airway inflammation is often triggered by allergies or viral illness. Environmental exposure to known allergens, or cigarette smoke at home may aggravate symptoms and lead to more persistent and significant airways hyper-reactivity.

Asthma is the most common "medical" cause of chronic school absenteeism and may present in a number of distinct fashions:

- Episodes of wheezing and shortness of breath related to exposure to an allergen, such as cats, dust, outdoor pollens or mold
- Prolonged and often refractory cough and wheeze with shortness of breath related to acute respiratory viral illness
- Shortness of breath, cough or wheeze triggered by exercise or cold-air that takes more than just a minute or two from which to recover

Asthma symptoms vary from person to person. Symptoms range from minor wheezing to life-threatening asthma attacks. In most children without active symptoms, physical examination is very normal.

Early signs and symptoms of asthma may include:

- Nighttime cough
- Chronic fatigue
- Bags under eyes
- Irritability

Persistent cough or shortness of breath may be the only signs of active asthma. Wheezing is often but not always heard. Reduced peak flows from baseline helps separate asthma from other conditions such as bronchitis or poor physical conditioning. A greater than 20% improvement in peak flow rates after albuterol administration is seen in asthma too.

Common signs and symptoms of asthma:

- Shortness of breath
- Tightness (or pain) in chest
- Wheezing
- Coughing
- Difficulty sleeping due to coughing, wheezing and/or shortness of breath

ASTHMA AND ASTHMA EMERGENCIES *(continued from previous page)*

Children with a *severe asthma attack* often evidence observable signs:
- Sitting upright, leaning forward, using neck muscles to assist inspiration; nasal flaring may be present
- Abnormal breath sounds (decreased/wheezing)
- Prolonged expiration, sometimes with pursed lips
- High pitched cough; irregular high pitched wheeze
- Poor air movement; rapid shallow breathing
- Tachycardia (pulse>120)
- Speaking in very short sentences
- Blue lips or fingernails
- Inability to record a peak flow

> **The presence of signs or symptoms suggestive of a severe asthma attack in a child is considered a medical emergency and immediate treatment commenced.**

ANTICIPATED CONCERNS/PROBLEMS:
- Complications can range from secondary infections to more serious respiratory arrest
- Permanent narrowing of the bronchial tubes
- Unresponsiveness to medications
- Side effects from long-term use of some asthma medications
- Severe asthma attack resulting in increased emergency room visits and hospitalizations

IMMEDIATE DANGER SIGNS:
- Struggling to breath – may be hunched over
- Abnormal breath sounds – absent/decreased/wheezing
- Retractions – intercostals, substernal, suprasternal
- Nasal flaring
- Using accessory muscles
- Bluish discoloration (cyanosis) around lips or nailbeds
- Tachycardia
- Tachypnea
- Difficulty walking
- Difficulty carrying on a conversation
- Little relief from bronchodilator – not responding to medication
- *Severely restless*
- *Decreased level of consciousness*
- Symptoms worsening

ASTHMA AND ASTHMA EMERGENCIES *(continued from previous page)*

MANAGEMENT/ TREATMENT:

Treat acute symptoms of asthma with as-needed rescue short-acting bronchodilators as prescribed. Albuterol sulfate *(Proventil®, Ventolin®, Xopenex®)* is the most commonly prescribed metered dose inhaled rescue bronchodilator. It may also be given in tablet, extended release tablet, syrup, or nebulized with the means of an air compressor driven hand-held nebulizer.

Rules of Two®[1] serve as an easy asthma assessment tool to indicate when further medical therapy is needed, and are derived from the content of the NHLBI* *Guidelines for the Diagnosis and Management of Asthma.* Answering "yes" to one of the *Rules of Two®* suggests that anti-inflammatory therapy using an inhaled corticosteroid (such as Flovent® Diskus, Flonase®, AeroBid®, QVAR® or Pulmicort®) should be added to as-needed bronchodilators as prescribed. This is especially true in evaluating the asthmatic child who is taking only rescue medication for control.

Rules of Two® ask:
- ✓ Do you need a quick-relief inhaler (rescue) bronchodilator for asthma symptoms more than two times/week?
- ✓ Do you awaken with asthma symptoms at night more than two times/month?
- ✓ Do you refill a canister of rescue bronchodilator more than two times/year?

In low doses, inhaled corticosteroids have been shown to reduce mortality, hospitalizations, emergency asthma flares, exercise and allergen triggering, nighttime awakenings from asthma and total cost of care.

If anti-inflammatory therapy is already being utilized, then additional therapy with either a long acting bronchodilator *(Serevent®, Foradil®, Performist®)* or leukotriene modifier *(Accolate®, Singulair®, Zyflo®)* may be appropriate. Occasionally theophyllines may be added as long-acting bronchodilators. A combination medication containing both a long-acting beta agonist and a corticosteroid *(Advair®, Symbicort®, Dulera®)* may be another option for better asthma control.

Management should also include avoiding asthma triggers. Specific inquiry into asthma triggers is important and should include symptoms related to exposure to pets, dust, foods, medication (such as aspirin or ibuprofen) or cigarette smoke. Studies have shown that

---

[1] *Rules of Two®* is a registered service mark of Baylor Health Care System, Dallas, Texas.

ASTHMA AND ASTHMA EMERGENCIES *(continued from previous page)*

reducing exposure to specific allergens or irritants (such as cigarette smoke) improves asthma symptoms and reduces the amount of medication necessary for good control. *An acute asthma attack is a medical emergency that should be treated promptly and effectively.*

General guidelines for dealing with an asthma attack include:
1. Implement child's Asthma Action Plan.
2. Administer inhaled or nebulized bronchodilator (usually albuterol) as per Action Plan.
3. Allow the child to assume a comfortable posture in a quiet setting.
4. Measure peak flow, if possible, to document severity and response to therapy.
5. Record pulse and respiratory rate.
6. Monitor – do not leave student alone.
7. Notify parent/guardian.

> **A child who does not completely and quickly respond to bronchodilator therapy and with normalization of peak flows should not return to class.**

1. **Seek immediate emergency care – *CALL 911 IMMEDIATELY.***
2. ***Transport to nearest hospital for emergency care.***
3. ***Notify Parent/guardian.***

UNTIL EMS ARRIVES:
- Continue to follow healthcare provider's orders.
- Allow the child to assume a comfortable posture in a quiet setting.
- Monitor vital signs.
- Keep student calm.
- Provide reassurance.
- Do not leave student alone.

Potential complications of a severe asthma attack include:
- Respiratory failure
- Death

NOTE:
- This information is not meant to be substituted for the professional advice / guidance of a healthcare provider.

ASTHMA AND ASTHMA EMERGENCIES *(continued from previous page)*

FOLLOW-UP:
- Monitor effectiveness of pharmacological therapy.
- Monitor student inhaler technique. Provide reinforcement as needed.
- Educate student/staff on asthma basics and how to manage an asthma emergency.
- Educate student/staff on how to properly care for inhaler:
  - Clean inhaler mouthpiece weekly – remove canister from jacket and wash jacket with soap and water.
  - Follow HFA priming instructions.

Prime HFA bronchodilator inhalers per pharmaceutical directions

HFA Bronchodilator	Priming Instructions
ProAir®	3 sprays (1st use; after 2 weeks non-use)
Proventil®	4 sprays (1st use; after 2 weeks non-use)
Ventolin®	4 sprays (1st use; after 2 weeks non-use) [Prime – 1 spray if MDI dropped and 1 spray after washing]
Xopenex®	4 sprays (1st use; after 3 days non-use)

NOTES:

Every child identified with asthma should have a written **Asthma Action Plan** approved by the child's healthcare provider and available in the school nurse's office.

ASTHMA AND ASTHMA EMERGENCIES *(continued from previous page)*

The goal of asthma management is <u>prevention</u>:

1. Education regarding avoiding known allergies or irritants and the need to use medications as directed is important.
2. Yearly influenza vaccine may be recommended.
3. In some circumstances, children may be allowed to self-carry short-acting rescue inhaled bronchodilators on their person for use before exercise or with asthma symptoms. This decision should be the joint agreement between the school nurse, parent and child's healthcare provider and should be supported by school policy and/or state regulations.
4. Educate student/staff on the importance of avoiding extreme weather conditions. Student may need to stay indoors when:
   - ✓ It is extremely windy
   - ✓ Pollen count is high
   - ✓ Outdoor temperature is <32^0 F (including wind chill factor). Encourage student to cover mouth and nose with a scarf or mask during cold weather!
   - ✓ Outdoor temperature is > 90^0F (including heat index)
5. The school nurse may consider offering a school based asthma education program such as the American Lung Association's "Open Airways for Schools" program to students with asthma. The Open Airways program consist of six 40 minute lessons covering topics such as:
   - Asthma basics
   - Recognizing asthma symptoms
   - Identifying and avoiding asthma triggers
   - Learning how to manage an asthma episode
   - Learning how to manage asthma while at school

<u>Note on inhalers:</u> Albuterol inhalers should have a dose counter. You cannot get an accurate estimate of how much active ingredient is in a canister by floating it in water (and you risk damaging the valve). Counters also help indicate if a person is overusing the inhaler and needs a different controller medication plan.

ASTHMA AND ASTHMA EMERGENCIES *(continued from previous page)*

Resources

Centers for Disease Control and Prevention: Asthma – School and Childcare Providers
http://www.cdc.gov/asthma/schools.html

National Association of School Nurses Asthma Resources
http://www.nasn.org/ToolsResources/Asthma

References

American Lung Association. (2015). *About OAS*. Retrieved from http://www.lung.org/lung-disease/asthma/in-schools/open-airways/about-oas.html

Baylor Health Care System. (2015). *Asthma toolbox*. Retrieved from http://www.baylorhealth.com/PhysiciansLocations/Dallas/SpecialtiesServices/Asthma/Pages/AsthmaToolbox.aspx

Centers for Disease Control and Prevention (CDC). (2013). *Asthma and schools*. Retrieved from http://www.cdc.gov/healthyyouth/asthma/

Ficca, M. & Moore, C. (2013). Asthma. In J. Selekman (Ed.), *School nursing: A comprehensive text* (2nd ed.) (pp.677-704). Philadelphia, PA: F. A. Davis.

Mayo Clinic. (2014). *Asthma attack*. Retrieved from http://www.mayoclinic.com/health/asthma-attack/DS01068/DSECTION=symptoms

MedlinePlus. U.S. National Library of Medicine. (2015). *Signs of an asthma attack*. Retrieved from www.nlm.nih.gov/medlineplus/asthma.html

Merck Manual. (2015). *Asthma*. Retrieved from http://www.merckmanuals.com/professional/pulmonary_disorders/asthma_and_related_disorders/asthma.html?qt=asthma&alt=sh

National Heart, Lung and Blood Institute. (2014). *What is asthma?* Retrieved from http://www.nhlbi.nih.gov/health/dci/Diseases/Asthma/Asthma_WhatIs.html

Thompson, J. (2014). *New HFA reliever inhalers for asthma – things you should know*. Retrieved from http://www.healthcentral.com/allergy/c/3989/19952/hfa-asthmathings

Ventolin HFA. (2015). *How to use ventolin-HFA*. Retrieved from http://www.ventolin.com/about-ventolin-hfa/how-to-use.html

ATTENTION DEFICIT HYPERACTIVITY DISORDER

DEFINITION/ETIOLOGY:
The American Psychiatric Association defines attention deficit hyperactivity disorder (ADHD) as "characterized by a pattern of behavior, present in multiple settings (e.g., school and home), that can result in performance issues in social, educational, or work settings." ADHD is a neurobehavioral disorder that is characterized by inattention, hyperactivity and/or impulsive behaviors that may include behaviors like failure to pay close attention to details, difficulty organizing tasks, and activities, excessive talking, fidgeting, or an inability to remain seated in appropriate situations. The patterns of behavior need to be observed in more than one setting. Children with ADHD differ in their symptoms, causes, prognosis, and responses to treatment. Some children are thought to have attention deficit without hyperactivity. These students may perform poorly in school despite normal intellect because they cannot sit still, attend, or complete a task. They are often rejected by their peers. Boys are affected more than girls. Symptoms appear by age 3 years but often the condition is not medically diagnosed until school age. ADHD should be considered a chronic illness.

SIGNS AND SYMPTOMS:

DIAGNOSTIC CRITERIA:
The DSM-5 (2013) sets diagnostic criteria for ADHD. Children must have at least six symptoms from either (or both) the inattention group of criteria and the hyperactivity and impulsivity criteria, while older adolescents and adults (over age 17 years) must present with five. Using DSM-5, several of the individual's ADHD symptoms must be present prior to age 12 years.

The DSM-5 lists the following symptoms of inattention. The symptoms must have persisted for at least six months to a degree that is maladaptive and inconsistent with developmental level.

ATTENTION DEFICIT HYPERACTIVITY DISORDER *(continued from previous page)*

Inattention
- Often fails to give close attention to details or makes careless mistakes in schoolwork, work, or other activities.
- Often has difficulty sustaining attention in tasks or play activities.
- Often does not seem to listen when spoken to directly.
- Often does not follow through on instructions and fails to finish schoolwork or chores (not due to oppositional behavior or failure to understand instructions).
- Often has difficulty organizing tasks and activities.
- Often avoids, dislikes, or is reluctant to engage in tasks that require sustained mental effort (such as schoolwork or homework).
- Often loses things necessary for tasks or activities (e.g., toys, school assignments, pencils, books, or tools).
- Is often easily distracted by extraneous stimuli.
- Is often forgetful in daily activities.

The following symptoms of hyperactivity-impulsivity are listed by the DSM-5 and must have persisted for at least 6 months to a degree that is maladaptive and inconsistent with developmental level.

Hyperactivity
- Often fidgets with hands or feet or squirms in seat.
- Often leaves seat in classroom or in other situations in which remaining seated is expected.
- Often runs about or climbs excessively in situations in which it is inappropriate (adolescents or adults may only feel restless).
- Often has difficulty playing or engaging in leisure activities quietly.
- Is often "on the go" or often acts as if "driven by a motor".
- Often talks excessively.

Impulsivity
- Often blurts out answers.
- Often has difficulty waiting for a turn.
- Often interrupts or intrudes on others.

  - ✓ Some hyperactive-impulsive or inattentive symptoms that caused impairment were present before age 12 years.

ATTENTION DEFICIT HYPERACTIVITY DISORDER *(continued from previous page)*

✓ Some impairment from the symptoms is present in two or more structured settings (e.g., at school and at home).

✓ There must be clear evidence of clinically significant impairment in social, academic, OR occupational functioning.

DIAGNOSTIC PROCEDURES
1. Observations may be conducted:
   - At home, in several locations and circumstances (e.g. meal time, outdoor play, performance of homework and household chores)
   - At healthcare provider's office
   - At school - classroom, cafeteria, and playground
   - At church, restaurants and family gatherings
2. Rating scales: many available
3. Behaviors must cause functional impairment
4. Diagnosis of exclusion
5. Provide all data to healthcare provider upon referral

MANAGEMENT/TREATMENT:
While there is no cure for ADHD, it can be successfully managed. Treatment management may include medication and educational and behavioral interventions.
- **Educational:** modification of lesson plans, teacher instruction, special class placement. Many strategies are available in educational manuals, such as decreasing environmental stimuli, providing structure, and assisting with organization. Student may need a Section 504 plan.
- **Psychological/behavioral:** counseling, (group, individual and family), behavior modification.
- **Medication:** Stimulants are commonly used to treat AHDH. Dosage is not based on body weight; rather dosages are calculated on achieving desired effect with minimal side effects.

ATTENTION DEFICIT HYPERACTIVITY DISORDER *(continued from previous page)*

Types of Medication
Methylphenidate (Ritalin®)
Methylphenidate (sustained release or once daily forms)
Concerta® ER (extended release)
Metadate CD
Metadate ER (extended release)
Methylin
Ritalin SR (sustained release)
Daytrana® transdermal patch
DextroAmphetamines
Dexedrine®
Dexedrine® spansules
DextroStat®
Adderall® (mixture)
Methamphetamine (Desoxyn®)
Dexmethylphenidate (Focalin®)
Lisdexamfetamine dimesylate (Vyvanse®)
Atomoxetine (Strattera®) which works on norepinephrine
Pemoline (Cylert®)

High blood pressure medication for ADD / ADHD — Certain blood pressure medications can be used to treat ADD / ADHD. Options include clonidine (Catapres®) and guanfacine (Tenex®). They are especially beneficial for those with tics or Tourette's Syndrome. While these medications can be effective for hyperactivity, impulsivity, and aggression, they are less helpful when it comes to attention problems.

FOLLOW-UP:
Stimulants (Ritalin, etc.) can cause loss of appetite: control by taking medication with or after meal. Monitor growth: height and weight three times each school year (e.g. September, January, and May).

ATTENTION DEFICIT HYPERACTIVITY DISORDER *(continued from previous page)*

POTENTIAL COMPLICATIONS:
Monitor for adverse effects of medications. The following are the most common adverse effects. For a complete list, see Physician's Desk Reference® or other drug resource.
- Risk of liver toxicity
- Abdominal pain
- Jitteriness, nervousness, anxiety, irritability
- Sleeplessness if taken after 4-5 P.M.
- New onset tic

NOTES:
Families require support and education regarding the diagnosis and management of this condition.

MEDICATION REMINDER
Healthcare provider must individualize dose for each child.
- All have side effects and must be monitored closely, especially early in therapy.
- Do not insist that child be put on medication.
- If child is prescribed medication, try to obtain child's assent. All psychoactive medications work better if they are taken willingly by child with parental cooperation.
- It may be necessary to continue medication into adolescence and adult years.
- Children and teens should not take medication without supervision.

ASSOCIATED DISORDERS (Co-morbid conditions)
While ADHD does not cause psychological problems, children with ADHD are more likely to have co-morbid conditions. The most common associated disorders seen with ADHD include oppositional defiant disorder, conduct disorder and learning disabilities.

CONDUCT DISORDER
A repetitive and persistent pattern of behavior in which the basic rights of others or major age-appropriate societal norms or rules are violated, as manifested by the presence of three or more of the following criteria in the past 12 months, with at least one criterion present in the past 6 months:
- Aggression to people and animals
- Destruction of property
- Deceitfulness or theft
- Serious violations of rules

ATTENTION DEFICIT HYPERACTIVITY DISORDER *(continued from previous page)*

OPPOSITIONAL DEFIANT DISORDER (ODD)

A pattern of negativistic, hostile, and defiant behavior lasting at least 6 months, during which four or more of the components are present.

Note: Consider a criterion met only if the behavior occurs more frequently than is typically observed in individuals of comparable age and development level.

The disturbance in behavior causes clinically significant impairment in social, academic, or occupational functioning. ODD may start during preschool years. Conduct disorder usually appears in older children (Adapted from DSM-5).

LEARNING DISABILITES

Learning disabilities are common in children with ADHD. Children with both ADHD and learning disabilities may need extra academic support in the classroom or even special education services.

References

American Academy of Pediatrics, Subcommittee on Attention-Deficit/Hyperactivity Disorder, Steering Committee on Quality Improvement and Management. (2011). ADHD: Clinical practice guideline for the diagnosis, evaluation, and treatment of Attention-Deficit/Hyperactivity Disorder in children and adolescents. *Pediatrics, 123*(5). Published online October 16, 2011. doi: 10.1542/peds.2011-2654. Retrieved from http://pediatrics.aappublications.org/content/early/2011/10/14/peds.2011-2654.full.pdf+html

American Psychiatric Association. (2013). Diagnostic and statistical manual of mental disorders (5th ed.). Washington D.C.: Author.

American Psychiatric Association. (2013). *Attention deficit hyperactivity disorder. Retrieved from* http://www.dsm5.org/Documents/ADHD%20Fact%20Sheet.pdf

Goldson, E., & Reynolds, A. (2014). Child development and behavior. In W. Hay, M. Levin, R. Deterding, & M. Abzug (Eds.), *Current diagnosis and treatment pediatrics* (22nd edition) (pp. 105-107). McGraw Hill Education, Inc.

Mayo Clinic. (2013). *Attention-deficit/hyperactivity disorder (ADHD) in children*. Retrieved from http://www.mayoclinic.com/helth/adhd/DS00275

National Institutes of Health. (2012). *Attention deficit hyperactivity disorder.* Retrieved from http://www.nimh.nih.gov/health/publications/attention-deficit-hyperactivity-disorder/index.shtml

Selekman, J. & Foley, M. (2013). Attention deficit/ hyperactivity disorder and learning disabilities. In J. Selekman (Ed.), *School nursing: A comprehensive text (2nd ed.) (*pp. 840-871). Philadelphia, PA: F.A. Davis.

AUTISM SPECTRUM DISORDER

DEFINITION/ETIOLOGY:

Autism Spectrum Disorder (ASD) falls under a group of complex neurodevelopmental disorders. According to the Diagnostic and Statistical Manual of Mental Disorders (DSM) – fifth edition (published by the American Psychiatric Association), **Asperger's Syndrome, Pervasive Developmental Disorder – Not Otherwise Specified and Childhood Disintegrative Disorder are no longer separate autistic diagnosis. All of these subcategories of autism are now incorporated into a single category; the (ASD) diagnosis.** Prevalence varies according to race, gender and ethnic group.

The exact etiology of autism is unknown. Given the varied severity and symptoms of autism, the etiology is most likely multifactorial. Potential causes include:

- Children with medical conditions such as congenital rubella syndrome, phenylketonuria, tuberous sclerosis, Tourette syndrome, RETT syndrome, epilepsy or fragile X syndrome have a higher risk of being diagnosed with ASD.
- Genetic predisposition – based on sibling research studies, there is also a genetic tendency; families that have one child diagnosed with ASD have a higher occurrence of autism in subsequent children.
- Brain structure abnormalities – some children diagnosed with ASD have enlarged ventricles, abnormalities of the cerebellar vermis and of the brain stem nuclei.
- Gender – boys are approximately 4 times more likely to be diagnosed with autism.
- Environmental – while suspected, there is no proof of an environmental connection to ASD.

SIGNS AND SYMPTOMS:

Autism symptoms typically appear within the first three years of life. Symptoms vary from person to person. Diagnostic evaluation involves a multidisciplinary approach. Potential team members include trained healthcare providers (developmental pediatrician/neurologist) and psychiatrist/psychologist who administer specific autistic behavioral testing/evaluations. Diagnosis criteria is based on social communication/interaction and restricted/repetitive behaviors. These symptoms must interfere with functional abilities.

AUTISM SPECTRUM DISORDER *(continued from previous page)*

Social communication/interaction symptoms (deficits must be met in each category)
- Impaired social interaction/emotional interaction
  - Difficulty reciprocating social and emotion interactions with others
  - Difficulty making friends
  - Does not display physical affection
  - May reject physical affection
  - Prefer not to be held or touched by others
  - Absence of social play
  - Difficulty verbalizing needs
- Difficulty with nonverbal communication
  - Tend to avoid eye contact (poor eye contact)
  - Inability to understand facial expressions, gestures and tone of voice
- Unable to maintain relationships
  - Lack empathy for others
  - Difficulty playing with others

Restrictive/repetitive movements (2 of the 4 symptoms must be met)
- Repetitive speech (ECHOLALIA)/motor movements (rocking back and forth, hand flapping)
- Strict adherence to routines/rituals – resistant to change
- Highly restricted interest – these interests are often obsessive and may be limited to specific topics/activities (lining up cars, etc.)
- Hypo/hyper reactive to sensory input
- Self-abusive behaviors (head banging)

MANAGEMENT/TREATMENT:
There is no cure for autism. ASD can be diagnosed by experienced professionals in children as young as 2 years of age. Refer children with suspected autism diagnosis for evaluation. Early detection and interventions improves quality of life and overall outcomes. Interventions must be based on student need. Interventions may include:
- Speech therapy
- Physical therapy
- Occupational therapy
- Behavioral therapy – social work services
- Family therapy – to promote social interaction
- Special education services

AUTISM SPECTRUM DISORDER *(continued from previous page)*

- Pharmacological therapy – antipsychotic medication for aggressive and harmful behaviors, ADHD medications to help treat impulsive and hyperactive behaviors, antidepressant for anxiety, etc.

FOLLOW-UP:
Tend to lose skills that they once possessed. Ongoing evaluation of interventions to determine effectiveness is necessary. Monitor for potential medication side effects. Some medications can interact, causing dangerous side effects. Report suspected side effects to parent/healthcare provider.

POTENTIAL COMPLICATIONS:
Comorbidities may include:
- ADHD
- Pica
- Seizure disorder – more than 20 % of individuals with autism develop seizure disorder by adulthood
- Sleep disorders
- Gastrointestinal issues

NOTES:
- Controversy remains on whether a link exists between autism and certain childhood vaccines; specifically the measles, mumps and rubella vaccine (MMR). Educate parent/guardian that no reliable study has shown a link between autism and the MMR vaccine and the potential complications of contracting a vaccine preventable disease such as rubeola, mumps, rubella and/or pertussis.
- Some parents/guardians seek alternative therapy in the treatment of autism including chelation therapy. Chelation therapy is thought to remove mercury and heavy metals from the body and is considered dangerous; there have been deaths associated with chelation therapy as an alternative therapy for autism. As needed, educate parents/guardians on the dangers of chelation therapy.
- Dietary interventions – parents/guardians may choose vitamin supplements, gluten-free and a casein-free diet in the treatment of ASD; more research is needed regarding how effective dietary interventions are in addressing ASD. Refer parents/guardians with questions related to dietary interventions to a registered dietician with an expertise in ASD.

AUTISM SPECTRUM DISORDER *(continued from previous page)*

RESOURCES
Autism Society of America
http://www.autism-society.org/
1(800) 328-8476

Autism Speaks
http://www.autismspeaks.org/what-autism/symptoms

Centers for Disease Control and Prevention (CDC)
http://www.cdc.gov/ncbddd/autism/facts.html
1(800) 232-4636

Early Childhood Technical Assistance Center (ECTA)
http://www.ectacenter.org/contact/ptccoord.asp
919-962-2001

National Institute of Neurological Disorders and Stroke
http://www.ninds.nih.gov/disorders/autism/detail_autism.htm

References

American Academy of Pediatrics. (2014). *Autism prevalence now 1 in 68, varies.* Retrieved from http://aapnews.aappublications.org/content/early/2014/03/27/aapnews.20140327-1.full

American Psychiatric Association. (2013). *Diagnostic and statistical manual of mental disorders* (5th ed.). Arlington, VA: American Psychiatric Publishing.

Centers for Disease Control and Prevention (CDC). (2015). *Autism spectrum disorders.* Retrieved from http://www.cdc.gov/ncbddd/autism/facts.html

Hyman, S. (2013). New DSM-5 includes changes to autism criteria. *AAP News.* Retrieved from http://aapnews.aappublications.org/content/early/2013/06/04/aapnews.20130604-1

Mayo Clinic. (2014). *Autism.* Retrieved from http://www.mayoclinic.com/health/autism/DS00348

Merck Manual. (2013). *Autism spectrum disorder.* Retrieved from http://www.merckmanuals.com/professional/pediatrics/learning_and_developmental_disorders/autism_spectrum_disorders_asd.html?qt=autism&alt=sh

National Institute of Neurological Disorders and Stroke. (2015). *Autism fact sheets.* Retrieved from http://www.ninds.nih.gov/disorders/autism/detail_autism.htm

Selekman, J. Diefenbeck, C., & Guthrie, S. (2013). Mental health concerns. In J. Selekman (Ed.), *School nursing: A comprehensive text* (2nd ed.) (pp. 927-969). Philadelphia, PA: F. A. Davis.

BACK AND NECK INJURY

DEFINITION/ETIOLOGY:

The etiology of back and neck injury is multifactorial. Severe injuries may occur from a traumatic blow to the back or neck that fractures, dislocates, or compresses a vertebrae. Most injuries are sprains and strains. Back and neck injuries may result from motor vehicle accidents and playground injuries. Youth are at increased risk of injury because they often participate in risky behaviors and physical activities/sports. Severe injuries may occur to athletes (football, soccer, gymnastics, etc.) trampoline jumpers, horseback riders, divers who hit bottom, etc. Neck injuries can occur when the neck is forcefully flexed, and the chin strikes the chest.

SIGNS AND SYMPTOMS:

Symptoms depend on the location of the injury. Symptoms can affect the neck, arms, legs, back and shoulders. Symptoms may include:
- Pain made worse by pressure or movement
- Pain may radiate into arm or leg
- Nerve involvement: weakness, tingling, numbness, or inability to move arm or leg

Signs of a serious injury include:
- **Extreme pain in neck or back**
- **Abnormal positioning of neck or back**
- **Loss of sensation**
- **Loss of bowel and bladder function**
- **Difficulty walking**
- **Lacks control over extremities**
- **Paralysis**
- **Difficulty breathing**
- **Shock**
- **Loss of consciousness**

When damage to the spinal cord is suspected, DO NOT MOVE STUDENT until assessment is done by emergency medical personnel.

BACK AND NECK INJURY *(continued from previous page)*

MANAGEMENT/TREATMENT:

Treatment depends on the extent of the injury.

1. If you suspect a neck injury or back injury do not move, bend, or rotate neck or spinal column of student. Permanent complications such as paralysis could result.

2. ***Assess airway, breathing, and circulation – if airway is compromised, and CPR is necessary, use jaw thrust maneuver instead of head tilt. Call 911 immediately.***

3. Perform comprehensive neurological assessment. If you suspect a serious injury, immobilize student until assessment by emergency medical personnel is completed.

4. Assess student's ability to move extremities slowly, and only a small amount. Test response to stimuli such as a finger touch or pin prick. Determine strength by checking hand grasp.

5. If severe neck or back injury is suspected or if pain, sensory impairment, or weakness persists, have student remain lying down and **call emergency ambulance for additional evaluation.**

6. If sensation is intact, pain is minimal to absent, and student is able to move all extremities normally, allow student to slowly sit up and then walk.

7. If all neurological signs are normal and student is able to move all extremities freely, ice may be applied to relieve pain.

8. Notify parent/guardian.

9. Refer to healthcare provider for further follow-up and treatment if necessary.

10. If prescribed, administer pain/anti-inflammatory medications as ordered. Monitor for medication side effects.

11. Complete injury/incident report.

FOLLOW UP:

- Student with minor injuries who remains at school should be observed several times during school day.

- Notify PE teacher of injury and potential accommodations.

BACK AND NECK INJURY *(continued from previous page)*

POTENTIAL COMPLICATIONS (serious injuries):
- Chronic pain
- Fecal and bladder incontinence
- Permanent paralysis

NOTES:

BACK PACKS AND BACK PAIN

The amount of weight carried by children in their backpacks is an important issue that deserves serious consideration. Loading of the spine is a risk factor for low back pain not only in adults but also in children; the load that children most commonly carry is their school backpack. **A backpack limit of 10-20% of ideal body weight for students is recommended** (obese children already carry an additional built-in burden which should not be used in calculating 15% of body weight). The backpack should have two wide (at least 2") shoulder straps and a waist or chest strap to distribute the load. Although back pain in children is likely to be multifactorial, heavy backpacks are probably an important contributing cause. Some schools have policies on the use of backpacks and rolling cases.

While increasing numbers of children are developing back pain, it is difficult to assign the cause of this increase to heavy backpack use alone. Students may also have back or neck pain due to postural lordosis, spondylolysis, and/or Scheuermann's kyphosis.

References

American Academy of Pediatrics. (2015). *Backpack safety.* Retrieved from http://www.healthychildren.org/English/safety-prevention/at-play/pages/Backpack-Safety.aspx?nfstatus=401&nftoken=00000000-0000-0000-0000-000000000000&nfstatusdescription=ERROR%3a+No+local+token

American College of Emergency Physicians. (n.d.). *Neck or back injury.* Retrieved from http://www.emergencycareforyou.org/Emergency-101/Emergencies-A-Z/Neck-or-Back-Injury/

Cosby, M., Miller, N. & Youngman, K. (2013). Acute measures for emergent problems. In J. Selekman (Ed.), *School nursing: A comprehensive text* (2nd ed.) (pp.516-577). Philadelphia, PA: F. A. Davis.

Mayo Clinic. (2012). *Spinal injuries: First aid.* Retrieved from http://www.mayoclinic.com/health/first-aid-spinal-injury/FA00010

Mayo Clinic. (2014). *Spinal cord injuries.* Retrieved from http://www.mayoclinic.org/diseases-conditions/spinal-cord-injury/basics/symptoms/con-20023837

MedlinePlus. U.S. National Library of Health. (2015). *Back injuries.* Retrieved from http://www.nlm.nih.gov/medlineplus/backinjuries.html

Merck Manual. (2013). *Evaluation of neck and back pain.* Retrieved from http://www.merckmanuals.com/professional/musculoskeletal-and-connective-tissue-disorders/neck-and-back-pain/evaluation-of-neck-and-back-pain

BED BUGS

DEFINITION/ETIOLOGY:

Bed bugs (*Cimex lectularius*) are small, reddish brown, wingless, flat, parasitic insects that bite humans and animals while they sleep. They can go without feeding for up to six months. They are not known to transmit or spread disease and should not be considered a medical or public health hazard.

Bedbugs were eradicated at one time in most developed countries because of the use of DDT, a pesticide that is no longer used and is banned because of its toxicity. The discontinuation of DDT use and the increase of international travel are thought to have led to bedbugs becoming a problem again.

Bed bug infestations usually occur around or near the areas where people sleep, e.g. beds, bed frames, mattress seams, box springs, behind wallpaper, or any other clutter or objects around a bed. The insects can travel anywhere from 8 to 100 feet but are found to live usually within 8 feet of where people sleep. Bedbugs hide in luggage and clothing, crawl and hitchhike so they can be transported easily. They may be brought to school in book bags and clothing.

SIGNS AND SYMPTOMS:
- Itchy bites, sometimes in a row
- Bites usually found on face, arms, legs, neck
- Bites may have a red dot in the middle of a raised bump
- Bite marks may take as long as 14 days to develop
- Some people have no reaction to bedbug bites
- Some people may experience an allergic reaction that results in severe itching, blisters or hives
- Difficult to distinguish bed bug bites from other insect bites

MANAGEMENT/TREATMENT:
- **<u>No exclusion is necessary</u>**
- Avoid scratching
- Relief for itching may include:
  - antiseptic creams or lotions
  - prescribed steroid creams
  - antihistamines (such as Benadryl®)

BED BUGS *(continued from previous page)*

POTENTIAL COMPLICATIONS:
- Scratching may lead to secondary infection
- Boils
- Cellulitis
- Allergic symptoms (e.g. swelling/pain at the bite site)
- Anaphylaxis (on rare occasions)

FOLLOW UP:
Family may need to contact their landlord or contact a professional exterminator to eliminate any home infestation. Exterminators may use a combination of pesticides and nonchemical treatments.
Nonchemical treatments may include:
- **Vacuuming**
- **Washing clothes in hot water.** Washing clothes and other items in water at least 120°F (49°C) can kill bedbugs.
- **Using clothes dryer.** Placing wet or dry items in a clothes dryer set at high heat for 30–60 minutes will kill bedbugs and their eggs.

For School Buildings
- Limit items that travel back and forth between home and school.
- Limit clutter.
- Clean cubbies/ lockers routinely (seasonally).
- Vacuum rugs frequently. Dispose of vacuum cleaner bags/filters in tightly sealed plastic bag.
- Avoid fabric-covered furniture, pillows in schools.
- Provide space between coat hooks and backpacks.
- Keep "Lost and Found" clothing, backpacks, etc. in closeable plastic storage bins.
- Involve facilities maintenance and pest management staff to address any bed bug infestation in schools.

NOTES:
The school nurse can be extremely helpful in helping families and staff from overreacting to this nuisance condition. Education is very important, reminding people that bed bugs do not discriminate, and infestations is not a reflection of cleanliness. Bed bugs do not infest the person; they infest the living area and require extermination.

Having a plan/guideline that includes how the school will physically address prevention and elimination of bed bugs and how families will be notified is helpful.

BED BUGS *(continued from previous page)*

Resources:

Environmental Protection Agency (www.epa.gov/bedbugs);
IdentifyUs (https://identify.us.com/idmybug/bed-bugs/)

References

American Academy of Pediatrics. (2015). *Bedbugs*. Retrieved from https://www.healthychildren.org/English/health-issues/conditions/from-insects-animals/Pages/Bedbug-Bites.aspx

American Academy of Pediatrics. (2013). Bedbugs. In S. Aronson, & T. Shope (Eds.), *Managing infectious diseases in child care and schools (2nd ed.)* (pp. 69-70). Elk Grove Village, IL: American Academy of Pediatrics.

Center for Disease Control and Prevention. (2013). *Bed bugs FAQs*. Retrieved from www.cdc.gov/parasites/bedbugs/faqs.html

Doerr, S. (2015). *Bedbugs*. Retrieved from http://www.emedicinehealth.com/bedbugs/article_em.htm

Mayo Clinic. (2015*). Bed bugs*. Retrieved from http://www.mayoclinic.org/diseases-conditions/bedbugs/basics/definition/con-20026119

BIPOLAR DISORDER

DEFINITION/ETIOLOGY:
Bipolar disorder (previously called manic-depressive disorder) is a mental disorder characterized by extreme changes in energy and affect, mood swings, periods of unusual highs (mania) and lows (depression). The exact etiology is unknown. However, genetics and environment have been linked to bipolar disorder. Onset usually occurs in mid-to-late adolescence, though there are cases in children. Children and adolescents diagnosed as bipolar are typically unpredictably explosive, moody, and aggressive toward themselves and others. Their mood cycles are mixed and unpredictable, which is very different from the adult presentation of bipolar disorder which has cycles of mania (euphoric behavior) followed by periods of depression. In children and adolescents mania is not usually a period of extreme happiness but seen as aggressive, explosive, and a violent episode. The behavioral outburst can be very dangerous (e.g. hitting, kicking, biting, destroying property, hurting animals, using weapons, etc.) and can last until the child or adolescent is too exhausted to continue. Bipolar disorder is a life-long illness but in most cases, can be controlled with medications and psychological counseling.

SIGNS AND SYMPTOMS:
Symptoms vary from person to person. Symptoms may include:

Manic stage
- Euphoria
- Flight of ideas
- Feelings of grandiose
- Agitation/irritation
- Aggressive behaviors
- Inflated self-esteem
- Risky behaviors
- Substance/alcohol abuse
- Talking fast
- Decreased need for sleep

Depressive stage:
- Withdrawn
- Sadness/feelings of hopelessness
- Irritability
- Anxiety
- Fatigue
- Difficulty concentrating
- Chronic pain with unknown cause
- Suicidal thoughts

Children and adolescents may demonstrate symptoms of intense rage, aggressive and impulsive behaviors. These symptoms can be misdiagnosed as Obsessive Compulsive Disorder and/or ADHD.

BIPOLAR DISORDER *(continued from previous page)*

MANAGEMENT/TREATMENT:
1. Primary treatment includes daily medication and psychotherapy.
2. If indicated, administer medication per healthcare provider's orders.
3. Potential medication treatment includes:

Drug	Examples of medications	Comments
Lithium®	Lithium- prevents extreme highs and lows, stabilizes mood; may need to take lithium for several weeks before feeling better; healthcare provider will order regular blood test to monitor lithium levels	• Monitor for side effects – dry mouth, gastrointestinal issues; **beware of lithium toxicity** – gastrointestinal issues, dizziness, weakness, slurred speech, seizures, nystagmus, coma; follow up with healthcare provider immediately if lithium toxicity is suspected • Risk of lithium toxicity increases with dehydration; therefore, maintain hydration
Antipsychotics	Used to treat acute mania. Examples include risperidone, olanzapine, ziprasidone, chlorpromazine, aripiprazole, paliperidone, and quetiapine.	Monitor for side effects which may include weight gain, sedation and neurological symptoms
Anticonvulsants	Used to stabilize mood. Examples include carbamazepine, divalproex and lamotrigine	Monitor for potential side effects – weight gain, dizziness, drowsiness

FOLLOW UP:
- Be aware that some adolescents are non-adherent to drug regimens (often due to side effects such as weight gain).
- Educate parent/guardian and student that bipolar disorder is a lifelong illness that requires lifelong treatment.
- Monitor for medication side effects.

BIPOLAR DISORDER *(continued from previous page)*

POTENTIAL COMPLICATIONS:
- Poor school attendance/performance
- Difficulty maintaining relationships
- Suicide

References

American Academy of Child Adolescent Psychiatry (AACAP). (2013*). Bipolar disorder resource center*. Retrieved from https://www.aacap.org/AACAP/Families_and_Youth/Resource_Centers/Bipolar_Disorder_Resource_Center/Home.aspx

American Psychiatric Association. (2015). *Help with bipolar disease.* Retrieved from http://www.psychiatry.org/bipolar-disorder

American Psychiatric Association. (2013). Diagnostic and statistical manual of mental disorders: DSM-5 (5th ed.). Washington, DC: Author.

Mayo Clinic. (2015). *Bipolar disorder.* Retrieved from http://www.mayoclinic.com/health/bipolar-disorder/DS00356

Merck Manual. (2014). *Bipolar disorders in children and adolescents.* Retrieved from http://www.merckmanuals.com/professional/pediatrics/mental_disorders_in_children_and_adolescents/bipolar_disorder_in_children_and_adolescents.html?qt=bipolar disorder&alt=sh

Selekman, J. Diefenbeck, C., & Guthrie, S. (2013). Mental health concerns. In J. Selekman (Ed.), *School nursing: A comprehensive text* (2*nd ed.)* (pp. 927-969). Philadelphia, PA: F. A. Davis.

BITES: Animal and Human (if skin is broken)

DEFINITION/ETIOLOGY:
Soft tissue injuries resulting from animal or human bites and include a puncture wound or crushing injury combined with lacerations. Commonly, such injuries are to the head, face, and neck.

SIGNS AND SYMPTOMS:
- Pain and bleeding
- Punctures and/or lacerations are usually jagged; pieces of tissue may be torn away in severe bites

MANAGEMENT/TREATMENT:
1. Stop bleeding by applying firm pressure with clean, dry gauze or cloth.
2. Wash and irrigate with copious amounts of soap and water.
3. Apply loose dressing.
4. Topical antibiotics may be applied if approved.
5. Refer all but most minor bites (skin not broken) to healthcare provider.
6. Record date of last tetanus.

FOLLOW-UP:
Prevention of Infection
- Dog bites likely to be open, jagged lacerations that can be thoroughly irrigated, have a low infection rate, and usually require no prophylactic antibiotics.
- Cat bites are usually deep puncture wounds and have a high infection rate. They often require prophylactic antibiotics.
- **Human bites *that break the skin* have the greatest potential for infection. Also, consider transmission of Hepatitis B to both parties** (consult current AAP Redbook for guidance or follow school district policy).

Prevention of Tetanus
Verify immunization status with student's healthcare provider. If not possible, follow these general guidelines:
- If no previous active immunization with tetanus toxoid, encourage tetanus immune globulin and begin series of tetanus toxoid.
- If active immunization is 10 years ago or longer: Booster of tetanus toxoid (adult Td).
- If active immunization within the past five years: Mild bite—no booster. Severe bite—booster adult Td.
- Severe, neglected, old (over 24 hours) or dirty bites—Adult Td, unless person has had one in the previous 12 months.

BITES: Animal and Human *(continued from previous page)*

POTENTIAL COMPLICATIONS:

Animal bites

- Early cellulitis - *Pasteurella multocida*
- Secondary infection – *Staphyloccoccus aureus*
- Rabies

Human Bites

- Cellulitis
- Infection

NOTES:

- Follow procedure for notifying animal control of animal bites.
- While it is theoretically possible for any mammal to develop rabies, rodents have not been implicated in transmitting the disease; therefore, a child bitten by a squirrel, rat, mouse, gerbil, hamster, or rabbit is not considered to be in danger, but a healthcare provider should be consulted.
- Common carriers of rabies are dogs, cats, foxes, skunks, and raccoons. Bats carry rabies but only bite if handled. Children who touch a dead or sick bat are at small risk, but a healthcare provider and public health department should be notified (airborne infection from bat guano is only a theoretical possibility).
- Unprovoked bites (especially from a dog) raise greater suspicion than if animal is provoked or teased. The biting animal must be confined and observed 10 days—notify the health department or police. If the animal cannot be apprehended, then a series of rabies vaccine injections may need to be given.
- Isolate all students from area where bite occurred (if on school property) until animal control/police arrive.
- Bites on fingers and face are more dangerous.

References

American Academy of Pediatrics. (2013). Bites (human and animal). In S.S. Aronson & T.R. Shope (Eds.), *Managing infectious diseases in child care and schools, a quick reference guide (3rd ed.)* (pp. 71-72). Elk Grove Village, IL: Author.

Barrett, J., & Revis, D.R. (2015). *Human bites*. Retrieved from http://emedicine.medscape.com/article/768978-overview

Brehm, C. (2013). Common injuries. In C. Burns, M. Brady, A. Dunn, N.B. Starr, C. Blosser (Eds.), *Pediatric primary care (5th ed.)* (pp. 1017-1091). Philadelphia, PA: Saunders Elsevier.

Garth, A. P., Harris, N. S., & Spanierman, C.S. (2015). *Animal bites in emergency medicine*. Retrieved from http://emedicine.medscape.com/article/768875-overview

Hockenberry, M., Baker, R., and Mondozzi, M. (2013). The child with hematalogic or immunologic dysfunction. In M. Hockenberry (Ed.), *Wong's essentials of pediatric nursing* (9th ed.) (pp.1017-1021). St. Louis, MO: Mosby Elsevier.

Mayo Clinic. (2014). *Rabies, prevention*. Retrieved from http://www.mayoclinic.com/diseases-conditions/rabies/basics/prevention/.CON20019900

Medline Plus, U.S. National Library of Medicine. (2015). *Rabies*. Retrieved from http://www.nlm.nih.gov/medlineplus/rabies.html#cat11

BLISTERS

DEFINITION/ETIOLOGY:
A blister is a round or oval bubble of fluid under the skin that may or may not be painful or itchy depending on the cause. The cause is varied:
- Irritation (friction/shoes; repetitive activity/rowing, shoveling)
- Burns from intense heat (sunburn, hot liquids or appliances, etc.)
- Exposure to cold (frostbite)
- Contact dermatitis (poison ivy, oak and sumac, detergents, chemicals)
- Allergies (e.g. medications, food)
- Infection (impetigo, eczema, ringworm, herpes, varicella [chicken pox])

SIGNS AND SYMPTOMS:
- Blisters from irritation and burns are red and often painful, particularly if the blister is on a weight bearing part of the body (foot) or in an area that is frequently used (hand).
- Contact dermatitis and allergic skin responses have redness and are itchy.
- Blisters present with some infections are called vesicles. Depending on the source of the infection, these vesicles can be red, itchy, and/or painful.

MANAGEMENT/TREATMENT:
- Treatment is largely symptomatic.
- Leave skin covering the blister intact. If the blister is broken, skin integrity is compromised leaving an entry for bacteria. Cover the broken blister with a sterile dressing and attempt to avoid activity that requires further friction or pressure on the affected area.
- Monitor for signs of infection.

POTENTIAL COMPLICATIONS:
- Infection after blister skins over or blister ruptures.
- Signs of infection include increasing redness, edema, area warm to touch, area becomes increasingly more painful, or purulent drainage is present.

FOLLOW UP:
Monitor for signs of infection and refer to healthcare provider if redness increases, edema present, area warm to touch, area becomes increasingly more painful, or purulent drainage is present.

BLISTERS *(continued from previous page)*

NOTES:
Prevention Education

- Proper fitting shoes, socks, clothing, and equipment for walking, running and participation in athletic/sports activities.
- If an area of redness appears, stop the activity.
- Observe sun-safety cautions and use sunscreen.
- Dress appropriately for winter weather and know the signs of frostbite.
- Be able to identify poison ivy, oak, and sumac.
- Read instructions accompanying tools, equipment, and appliances. Pay particular attention to safety.

References

Medline Plus, US National Library of Medicine. (2013). *Vesicles.* Retrieved from http://www.nlm.nih.gov/medlineplus/ency/article/003939.htm

The Merck Manual. *Sunburn.* (2014). Retrieved from http://www.merckmanuals.com/professional/dermatologic_disorders/reactions_to_sunlight/sunburn.html?qt=sunburn&alt=sh

Web MD. (2015). *Understanding blisters -- the basics.* Retrieved from http://www.webmd.com/skin-problems-and-treatments/guide/understanding-blisters-basics

BURNS

DEFINITION/ETIOLOGY: Lesions caused by extreme heat or other cauterizing agents

First-degree or superficial burns: Superficial – only affects the top layer of skin (epidermis).

Second degree or partial-thickness burns: Involves the epidermis and extends into the dermis.

Third degree or full-thickness burns: Full thickness of skin is destroyed and involves the epidermis, dermis, and fat layer. Usually destroys the sweat glands, hair follicles, and nerve endings as well.

Fourth degree burns: Full thickness through all layers of skin into the muscle and bone.

Minor burns: Less than 10% of the body surface area (BSA) for partial thickness burns or less than 2% for full thickness burns. Partial or full thickness burns of the hands, feet, face, eyes, ears and perineum are considered major.

SIGNS AND SYMPTOMS:
1. **Superficial burns**
   - Begins with pain and redness as in minimal sunburn – no blisters.
   - Later, slight to no peeling of skin.
2. **Partial-thickness burns**
   - Begins with pain, redness, and blisters as in moderate to severe sunburn.
   - Later, skin peels in large pieces, scarring only if secondary infection ensues.
3. **Full thickness burns**
   - Begins with little or no pain (nerves are gone), with red, black, or white discoloration.
   - Some unbroken blisters may be present.
   - Third degree burns always scar and often need skin graft.

MANAGEMENT/TREATMENT:
1. **General**
   a. For superficial and partial-thickness burns: Rapidly immerse burn in cool water. This not only helps stop the pain but it also stops destruction of tissue. There is a correlation between how fast the area is cooled and how fast it heals.
   b. Wash gently but thoroughly with antiseptic soap, pat dry with sterile pad.
   c. Avoid Vaseline®, butter, antibiotic or other greasy ointments.
   d. Avoid tight, air-excluding bandages.
   e. Check date of latest tetanus booster.
   f. Complete injury report.

BURNS *(continued from previous page)*

2. **Superficial burns**
   a. Cool compress or submerge in cool water (not ice).
   b. No further treatment necessary.
3. **Partial-thickness burns**
   a. Cool compress.
   b. Wash gently with antiseptic soap and dry.
   c. DO NOT break blister.
   d. Apply non-sticking dressing that does not exclude air.
   e. Notify parent.
4. **Full-thickness burns**
   a. Cover with clean or sterile dressing or sheet.
   b. Evacuate to emergency room or healthcare provider's office.
5. **Chemical burn**
   a. Flush with copious amounts of cool water for 15 minutes.
6. **Chemical or electrical burns: refer in all cases for further medical treatment.**

FOLLOW-UP:
- Change dressing daily (if this is not done at home) until danger of infection has passed.
- Observe for secondary infection.
- Teach student and parent/guardian to clean the affected area gently twice a day with soap and water and keep the area clean.
- Teach student and parent/guardian signs and symptoms of infection and the need to see the healthcare provider if they occur.
- Refer to healthcare provider for any developing signs of infection or if no improvement after FIRST day of treatment.
- Observe for scarring, especially on flexor areas of arms, legs, and neck.
- Children with facial scarring need emotional support on return to school. Prepare classmates/peers.

POTENTIAL COMPLICATIONS:
- Minor burns are typically superficial and do not cause complications.
- Moderate to severe burns can cause serious complications due to tissue damage and extensive fluid loss. Complications include dehydration, infection, shock, muscle and tissue damage, chemical imbalances, etc.

BURNS *(continued from previous page)*

NOTES:
- Facial burns: refer to healthcare provider in all cases.
- Send date of last tetanus booster with all healthcare provider referrals.
- Be alert to possible child abuse, self-tattoo, or deliberate injury.
- Record shape/size of burns as well as document history of event.
- Do not use ice on burns as it can cause further damage
- Children with burns greater than 10% of body surface area should be admitted to the hospital.

Teach children safety rules such as **stop, drop, and roll** if their clothing catches on fire so they can help extinguish the flame and prevent getting burned more extensively.

Burns are a common cause of accidental death in children. It also may be associated with child abuse. Areas of prevention include:

- Hot liquids should be placed away from counter edges with the handles facing backwards.
- Water heater thermostats should be kept less than 120° F (49° C).
- Irons and electrical cords should be kept out of reach of children.
- Barriers should be used around fireplaces.

References

Bowden, V., & Greenberb, C. (Eds.). *(2013).* The child with altered skin integrity. In V. Bowden, & C. Greenberb (Eds.), *Children and their families: The continuum of care (*3rd ed.) (p.p. 1348-1349). Philadelphia PA: Lippincott Williams and Wilkins.

Morelli, J.G., & Prok, L.D. (2014). Skin. In W. Hay, M. Levin, R. Deterding, & M. Abzug (Eds.), *Current diagnosis and treatment pediatrics* (22nd edition) (pp. 426-425). McGraw Hill Education, Inc.

Mayo Clinic. (2015). *Burns: First aid.* Retrieved from http://www.mayoclinic.com/health/first-aid-burns/FA00022

CARDIAC CONDITIONS – LIFE THREATENING
(HYPERTROPHIC CARDIOMYOPATHY and LONG QT INTERVAL [LQTS])

DEFINITION/ETIOLOGY:
Sudden death in children and adolescents is rare. About 25% of cases occur during sports. Most children/adolescents with sudden cardiac death (SCD) have underlying heart disease, with hypertrophic cardiomyopathy and long QT syndrome (LQTS) being among the most common life threatening cardiac conditions. Other conditions that may contribute to sudden cardiac death include congenital aortic stenosis, myocarditis, abnormal development of cardiac arterial vessels, and aortic dissection.

Hypertrophic cardiomyopathy (HCM) is the most common cause of SCD in the United States in people 30 years old or younger. HCM often presents itself in mid to late adolescence, and usually presents without warning clinical signs or symptoms. Diagnosis is confirmed echocardiography however an electrocardiogram may show left ventricular hypertrophy or T-wave abnormalities. HCM is an autosomal dominant congenital disorder typically characterized by asymmetric septal hypertrophy and marked disarray of ventricular muscle fibers, which contribute to the risk of arrhythmias even in patients with minimal hypertrophy and no evident left ventricular outflow tract obstruction.

Risk factors:
- septal thickness ≥30 mm
- family history of sudden cardiac death

SIGNS AND SYMPTOMS:
- non-sustained ventricular tachycardia (VT) (which is VT that lasts <30 seconds)
- syncope
- hypotensive response to exercise

CARDIAC CONDITIONS – LIFE THREATENING (continued from previous page)

LONG QT INTERVAL (LQTS)

Long QT syndrome (LQTS) is a rare inherited cardiac disorder that occurs in about one in 2500–3500 individuals. LQTS results from a delay in repolarization of the heart muscle following a ventricular contraction leading to a ventricular arrhythmia (ventricular tachycardia and/or fibrillation). Diagnosis is difficult because only in a percentage of cases a prolonged QT interval is noted on during an electrocardiogram (ECG/ EKG). These episodes may lead to palpitations, fainting, and sudden death due to ventricular fibrillation. For symptomatic patients, the presenting symptom is usually syncope, which is due to the form of ventricular tachycardia. The syncope may occur with specific triggers, such as stress, swimming, and loud auditory stimuli, or it may occur when the child is relatively bradycardic, as during rest or sleep.

Risk factors:
- female sex
- family history of congenital long QT syndrome
- pre-existing cardiovascular disease
- electrolyte imbalance
- concurrent administration of interacting drugs
- anorexia nervosa

SIGNS AND SYMPTOMS:

Many people with long QT syndrome have no signs or symptoms. Signs and symptoms may include:
- fainting
- dizziness
- seizures
- sudden death

MANAGEMENT/TREATMENT:

Diagnosing LQTS is not an easy diagnosis to make because the majority of people with LQTS have no signs or symptoms. Patients diagnosed with LQTS are advised to avoid drugs that would further prolong the QT interval. Treatment is usually the administration of arrhythmia medications (such as beta blockers) which prevents severe symptoms and sudden death in most cases. In severe cases, a implantable cardioverter-defibrillator (ICD) may be indicated.

CARDIAC CONDITIONS – LIFE THREATENING *(continued from previous page)*

All signs and symptoms need to be taken seriously. Children/adolescents need to be referred to the healthcare provider (HCP) for follow up and possible cardiologist referral. The school nurse may want to request a healthcare provider note to ensure that student has been appropriately followed up by a healthcare provider.

FOLLOW-UP:
It is critical that the school nurse has clear orders from the student's HCP as well as their parent or guardian regarding the plan of care for the student with any life threatening cardiac conditions. The plan must include medications, signs and symptoms to watch for, physical activity or any other restrictions, and any plans that need to be implemented in the event of an emergency.

All sports activities need to be stopped until the student has been cleared to participate by their HCP. Emergency preparedness is essential with trained staff in cardiopulmonary resuscitation and automatic external defibrillators. School physicals, especially sports physical examination polices need to be adhered to.

POTENTIAL COMPLICATIONS:
1. Sudden Death

References

Cosby, M., Blake Miller, N. & Youngman, K. (2013). Acute measures for emergent problems. In J. Selekman (Ed.), *School nursing: A comprehensive text (2nd ed.)* (pp.516-577). Philadelphia, PA: F.A. Davis.

Gajewski, K. K., & Saul, J. P. (2010). Sudden cardiac death in children and adolescents (excluding Sudden Infant Death Syndrome). *Annual Pediatric Cardiology*, 3(2), 107–112. Retrieved from http://www.ncbi.nlm.nih.gov/pmc/articles/PMC3017912/

Sreekanth, S., & Raghavan, M. (2014). *Pediatric Long QT Syndrome. Medscape.* Retrieved from http://emedicine.medscape.com/article/891571-overview

Thompson, A., & Galletta, G. (2010). Pediatric cardiovascular disorders. In R. Aghababian (Ed.), *Essentials of emergency medicine* (pp. 510-527). Sudbury, MA: Jones & Bartlett Learning.

Van Hare, G. F. (2016). Syncope. In R.M. Kliegman, B.S. Stanton, J. St. Geme, & N.F. Schor (eds.), *Textbook of pediatrics: Expert consult (20th ed.)* (p. 514). Philadelphia, PA: Elsevier.

CELIAC DISEASE

DEFINITION/ETIOLOGY:

Celiac disease is an autoimmune response to eating gluten. Gluten is a protein found in wheat and related grains, such as barley and rye. When a person with celiac disease eats gluten the body's immune system reacts by causing inflammation of the intestinal villa in the small colon. The small villa absorbs nutrients from food in the gastrointestinal (GI) system. Damage to the villa prevents absorption of necessary nutrients leading to malnutrition.

Celiac disease is more common in Caucasian, females. Celiac disease also has genetic tendencies with about 50% of individuals with celiac disease reporting that they have a family member who also has the disorder.

SIGNS AND SYMPTOMS:

Signs and symptoms vary from person to person. Some individuals with Celiac disease are asymptomatic – leading to undiagnosed cases of Celiac disease. Individuals with Celiac disease may present with gastrointestinal symptoms including:
- chronic diarrhea (30% persons with celiac disease);
- bloating;
- flatulence;
- constipation (20% persons with celiac disease);
- abdominal pain;
- nutritional deficiency;
- nausea, vomiting;
- foul-smelling (pale) stool; and
- weight loss (after eating gluten-containing products).

It is important to note that not everyone with Celiac disease experience GI symptoms. Other symptoms may include:
- irritability;
- iron deficiency anemia;
- osteopenia/osteoporosis; and/or
- itching/blistering dermatitis (called – dermatitis herpetiformis – rash usually appears elbows, knees, buttocks and back).

Symptoms also vary depending on age. School age children may experience growth and development delays secondary to poor nutritional absorption, delayed puberty, and damage to dental enamel of secondary teeth.

CELIAC DISEASE *(continued from previous page)*

MANAGEMENT/TREATMENT:

There is no cure for Celiac disease. It is a lifelong disorder. Management includes strict avoidance to gluten (e.g., wheat, barley and rye). Typically once gluten is removed from the diet, symptoms start to improve within a few days. It can take several months to years for complete healing of the intestinal villa to occur. The healthcare provider may recommend daily vitamin supplements due to poor nutrient absorption.

If no improvement in symptoms after starting gluten-free diet, look for hidden sources of gluten.

- Gluten can be found in products such as lip balm, cosmetics, hair and oral hygiene products.
- Check with pharmacist to see if gluten is in prescribed prescription and/or over the counter medications, vitamins and nutritional supplements that student may be taking to manage condition.

FOLLOW-UP:

- Educate students/parent/staff on necessity of strict gluten avoidance.
- Consult with school Registered Dietician to ensure necessary dietary accommodations are made in school meals.
- Only use non-food items for manipulatives in classroom projects.
- Avoid using modeling dough (e.g. Play-Doh) for art or classroom projects.
- To facilitate the avoidance of accidental exposure, include information on student's medical condition in teacher's sub folder.

POTENTIAL COMPLICATIONS:

- Malnutrition
- Osteoporosis
- Liver disease
- Neurological conditions
- Infertility
- Lactose intolerance
- Intestinal cancers (intestinal lymphoma and bowel cancer)

NOTES:

Monitor for other autoimmune disorders such as autoimmune thyroid disease, Type 1 diabetes, Addison's disease, Sjogren's syndrome, multiple sclerosis and rheumatoid arthritis.

CELIAC DISEASE *(continued from previous page)*

References

Celiac Disease Foundation. (2015). *Celiac disease foundation.* Retrieved from https://celiac.org/celiac-disease/what-is-celiac-disease/

Mayo Clinic. (2013). *Celiac disease.* Retrieved from http://www.mayoclinic.org/diseases-conditions/celiac-disease/basics/definition/con-20030410

Merck Manual. (2015). *Celiac Disease.* Retrieved from http://www.merckmanuals.com/professional/SearchResults?query=celiac+disease

National Institute of Diabetes and Digestive and Kidney Diseases. (2015). *Celiac disease.* Retrieved from http://www.niddk.nih.gov/health-information/health-topics/digestive-diseases/celiac-disease/Pages/facts.aspx

CHEST PAIN

DEFINITION/ETIOLOGY:
Chest pain is a common complaint in the health office and accounts for 6 in 1000 visits to urban emergency departments and urgent care clinics (Darst, Collins, & Miyamoto, 2014). Pediatric chest pain can be classified as cardiac or non-cardiac. Non-cardiac is the most prevalent cause of chest pain in school-aged children and adolescents. Chest pain can originate from any structure in the chest - lungs, ribs, chest wall, diaphragm, joints between sternum and ribs, and heart. It can be caused from injury, infection, respiratory conditions, referred pain from the abdomen, or irritation. The pain may also be the result of stress or anxiety.

Chest pain from the heart is rare (unless child is known to have heart defect or disease). While the pain may be a symptom of serious disease, most chest pain is benign or self-limiting.

SIGNS AND SYMPTOMS:
Signs and symptoms will vary widely with cause and the person's age and personality. For many people, the heart is the most identifiable organ in the chest so they describe discomfort by saying their "heart hurts". It is important to remember this may be a figure of speech and not to over react. The determination of the cause of pain is a diagnostic decision and the term "heart pain" should be assessed similarly to other types of pain, focusing on associated signs and symptoms and severity and conveying that information to a diagnostician.

MANAGEMENT/TREATMENT:
1. Conduct an assessment
   - It is important to take a careful history; make close observation as person describes symptoms. Determine if history of recent injury, presence of underlying health condition (asthma, heart defect or cardiovascular history, recent illness, sickle cell disease, history of genetic disorder).
   - Determine onset of symptoms (acute, gradual, growing worse).
   - Length of time with symptoms?
   - Any association with activity (including at rest, only after activity, on inspiration, after coughing, etc.)?
   - What makes it better?
   - What makes it worse?
   - Determine type of pain - constant, intermittent, sharp, dull, radiating, etc.

67

CHEST PAIN *(continued from previous page)*

- Are there associated respiratory symptoms?
- Assess skin condition (indicative of oxygen exchange).
- Assess psychological demeanor (calm, anxious, dramatic), history of increased stress.
- History of huffing, smoking or other drug use.
- Perform a general physical assessment including vital signs and note any irregularities.

2. The person who has pain of acute onset that:
   a. interferes with breathing and /or sleep,
   b. is precipitated by exercise, or
   c. is associated with alteration of vital signs and dizziness, palpitations, syncope, or fever should be evaluated by their healthcare provider. Symptomatic individuals should not be allowed to drive alone.

3. EMS should be contacted if an individual is more seriously compromised, particularly with symptoms of cyanosis, difficulty breathing, and decreased level of consciousness. Activate EMS if open chest wound or signs and symptoms of pneumothorax (rapid/shallow respiration, painful respiration, cyanosis, and hypotension).

COMMON ILLNESSES THAT CAUSE CHEST PAIN

Costochondritis

A condition where there is inflammation in the cartilage between the sternum and ribs. It may be caused by a viral illness or by frequent coughing. The pain will occur with inhalation. The majority of people will have tenderness over the costochondral joint (depression on side of sternum where rib joins sternum). May be treated with OTC anti-inflammatories.

Musculoskeletal Injury/Pain

The most common cause of pediatric chest pain. Children frequently strain chest wall muscles while wrestling, carrying heavy books, or exercising. Direct trauma to the chest may result in a mild contusion of the chest wall or, with more significant force, a rib fracture, hemothorax, or pneumothorax. If pain can be reproduced through direct palpation of the chest wall, it is almost always musculoskeletal in nature. In most cases, there is a straightforward history of trauma and the diagnosis is clear.

CHEST PAIN *(continued from previous page)*

Respiratory Conditions

Children who have severe, persistent cough, asthma, bronchitis, pleurisy or pneumonia may complain of chest pain due to overuse of chest wall muscles. Some children may complain of chest pain with exercise due to exercise-induced asthma. Pulmonary embolism should be considered in adolescent girls taking oral contraceptives.

Psychogenic Disturbances

Stress or anxiety can precipitate chest pain in both boys and girls. Often the stress that results in somatic complaints is not readily apparent and not all of these children present with hyperventilation or an anxious appearance. However, if the child has had a recent major stressful event, such as separation from friends, divorce in the family, or school failure that correlates temporally with the onset of the chest pain, it is reasonable to conclude that the symptoms are related to the event.

Gastrointestinal Disorders

Conditions such as reflux esophagitis often cause chest pain in young children and adolescents. The pain is described classically as burning, substernal in location, and worsened by reclining or eating spicy foods. Be aware that students with eating disorders such as purging may have pain secondary to esophageal trauma related to the purging. The timing of the pain in relation to eating may suggest a gastrointestinal cause.

Miscellaneous Causes

Some young children will complain of chest pain following ingestion of a coin or other foreign body that lodges in the esophagus. Generally, the child or parent/guardian gives a clear history of recent foreign body ingestion.

Some instances of chest pain are related to an underlying disease. A careful history and physical exam will often sort these out. For instance, sickle cell disease may lead to vaso-occlusive crises or acute chest syndrome. Marfan syndrome may result in chest pain and fatal dissection of an abdominal aortic aneurysm. Collagen vascular disorders may lead to pleural effusions. Shingles may result in severe chest pain that precedes or occurs simultaneously with the classic rash.

CHEST PAIN *(continued from previous page)*

References

American Heart Association. (2015). *Commonly asked questions about children and heart disease.* Retrieved from http://www.heart.org/HEARTORG/Conditions/More/CardiovascularConditionsofChildhood/Commonly-Asked-Questions-About-Children-and-Heart-Disease_UCM_311917_Article.jsp

Ball, J., Binder, R., & Cowen, K. (Eds.). (2012). Alterations in respiratory function. *Principles of Pediatric Nursing: Caring for Children (5th ed.)* (pp. 594-595). Upper Saddle River, NJ: Pearson Education, Inc.

Darst, J.R., Collins, K.K., & Miyamoto, S.D. (2014). Cardiovascular diseases. In Hay, W.W., Deterding, R.R., Levin, M.J. & Abzug, M.J. (Eds.*), Current diagnosis and treatment pediatrics* (22nd ed.) (pp.636-638). New York, NY: McGraw Hill Education, Inc.

John, R. & Chewey, L. (2013). Common complaints. In J. Selekman (Ed.), *School nursing: A comprehensive text* (pp. 608-610). Philadelphia, PA: F.A. Davis.

CHILDHOOD CANCER

Childhood cancer is the leading cause of death from disease in children. On a positive note, it is still a rare disease, and has a survival rate of 80% (defined as surviving 5 years after diagnosis). Because children are growing, childhood cancer is unlike cancer seen in adults. Adult cancers tend to be slow in growth, but childhood cancers grow quickly, and a child may become ill in a short period of time. Childhood cancers predominate in the areas of the body that exhibit rapid growth such as the blood, lymphatic system, central nervous system, and bones.

DEFINITION/ETIOLOGY:

Cancer is defined as cell growth out of control. The rapid growth results in immature, abnormal cells that invade surrounding tissue. The etiology of childhood cancer varies from adult cancers. Adult cancers tend to be epithelial in nature, while childhood cancers often stem from nonepithelial or embryonal cells.

Numerous types of cancers are seen in children. Following is a brief overview of the most common cancers seen in children.

Leukemia	Leukemia is the most commonly diagnosed childhood cancer. Leukemia is characterized by an abnormal amount of white blood cells (WBC) in the body. It is considered a cancer of the bone marrow and blood. As the WBC's proliferate, the cells they produce are immature. The increasing production of WBC's affects normal production of red blood cells and platelets. Abnormal WBC's are called blast cells. The common types of leukemia in children are acute lymphoblastic leukemia (ALL) and acute myeloid leukemia (AML). Typical symptoms include lethargy, bruising and other abnormal bleeding, bone and joint pain, weakness and weight loss. (See Leukemia for further information, if needed.)
Brain tumor	Second most common cancer in children. The overall prognosis is dependent on the size, type, and location of the tumor. Neurological symptoms such as headache, blurred vision, dizziness, change in gait or fine motor skills, nausea, and vomiting are often seen. School staff may note a change in school performance and/or concentration. Typically, occurring tumors include astrocytoma, glioma, medulloblastoma, and ependymoma.
Neuroblastoma	Tumors that form along the sympathetic nervous system chain. They are often found above the kidneys in the adrenal glands, but can start anywhere.
Bone tumors	Tend to occur in older children and in the teenage years. **Osteosarcoma-** usually affects the large bones of the arms and legs. **Ewing's sarcoma-** can occur anywhere but most likely found in spine, ribs or pelvis.

CHILDHOOD CANCER *(continued from previous page)*

Lymphoma	These malignant diseases affect the lymph system and tissues. The two main types of lymphoma are Hodgkin lymphoma (also known as Hodgkin disease) and Non-Hodgkin lymphoma.
Retinoblastoma	Originates in the retina of the eye. Dependent on the size of the tumor, it may be necessary to remove the entire eye. This tumor is often discovered during well child exams, and is rarely seen in children over the age of six.
Wilm's tumor	Also known as nephroblastoma. Wilm's tumor is the most common kidney cancer. Symptoms include swelling or lump in the abdomen. Other symptoms such as poor appetite, fever, pain, or nausea may be present. **Nursing alert: DO NOT** palpate the abdomen if this tumor is suspected.

SIGNS AND SYMPTOMS (General):
- Keep in mind that symptoms may have a relatively fast onset, secondary to the rapidly growing cells in children
- Pain
- Loss of appetite
- Weight loss
- Anemia
- Increased susceptibility to infection
- Bruising
- Prolonged bleeding
- Neurological disturbances: change in behavior, change in gait, headache, dizziness, blurred or double vision
- Symptoms are related to the location of the cancer

MANAGEMENT/TREATMENT:
1. Treatment is based on the type of cancer and may include surgery, radiation, and/or chemotherapy.
2. In some cases, a bone marrow transplant may be indicated for treatment.
3. In addition to treating the cancer, the effects of the tumor on the body (i.e. pain) and any side effects from treatment must be managed.
4. Be aware that 80% of patients use some type of complementary treatment in addition to conventional care.
5. Cancer therapy is complex and is usually managed by a pediatric oncologist.

CHILDHOOD CANCER *(continued from previous page)*

MANAGEMENT/TREATMENT: *(continued)*

6. In most cases, the oncology team develops an individualized treatment plan for the child that may be followed for several years.
7. Side effects from treatment include increased susceptibility to infection, bleeding/bruising, hair loss, loss of appetite, nausea, vomiting.
8. Students may attend school while receiving treatment.

FOLLOW-UP:

1. Potential for infection
   a. Monitor for signs and symptoms of infection.
   b. Notify parent/guardian if temperature > 99.9°.
   c. Notify parent/guardian of any exposure to communicable diseases.
   d. Educate student, staff and class on handwashing techniques.
   e. Provide health promotion information.

2. Bleeding
   a. Educate staff regarding potential for abnormal bleeding and situations to report to the school nurse.
   b. Monitor for petichiae, nosebleeds, bleeding gums or prolonged bleeding.
   c. Contact parent/guardian for nosebleeds lasting longer than 10 minutes.

3. Pain
   a. Contact parent/guardian with any new complaints of pain or severe pain.
   b. Partner with oncology team for chronic pain management.
   c. Administer analgesics only if ordered specifically for the student, even if standing orders available.

4. Gastro-intestinal side effects (nausea, vomiting, constipation, diarrhea)
   a. Educate staff on potential GI side effects and importance of notifying school nurse.
   b. Maintain adequate hydration.
   c. Accommodate for frequent, small meals throughout the day if necessary.
   d. Provide opportunities for rest as needed.
   e. Notify parent/guardian if vomiting persists.

CHILDHOOD CANCER *(continued from previous page)*

FOLLOW-UP: *(continued)*

5. Alteration in coping
   a. Assess for stress and coping abilities.
   b. Provide resource information to families.
   c. Hair loss, surgical scars, and effects of long-term corticosteroids can contribute to altered body image. Monitor for body image disturbances through observation, discussion, and collaboration with parents and school staff.
   d. Art can be a therapeutic form of expression and stress management for the child.
   e. Provide support to siblings and make appropriate referrals as needed.

POTENTIAL COMPLICATIONS:

It is important for the school nurse to be aware of late effects of treatment in survivors of childhood cancers. Potential adverse outcomes include decreased growth and development, developmental delays, cognitive disorders, heart or lung disease, infertility and development of secondary cancers.

Interventions for the school nurse:

1. Monitor growth.
2. Monitor development and refer student if regression is noted.
3. Provide psycho-social support and referrals as need.
4. Educate staff on potential complications.
5. Plan for school re-entry.
6. Refer for social skills training, vocational rehabilitation, cognitive remediation therapy as needed.

SCHOOL RE-ENTRY:

It is often recommended that the student remain in school part-time to maintain a sense of normalcy and to continue with established peer relationships. Homebound or hospital-based instruction should be instituted when the student is unable to attend school. Prior to the student returning to school:

- Schedule a meeting with parent/ guardian, school staff such as school nurse, counselor, teacher, school psychologist, principal, healthcare provider.
- Establish guidelines for care while child is at school, along with a plan for any potential emergencies.
- Create an Individualized Healthcare Plan.
- Update parent/guardian emergency contact numbers.

CHILDHOOD CANCER *(continued from previous page)*

SCHOOL RE-ENTRY: *(continued)*
- With parent/guardian permission, consider a presentation to the class prior to student returning to school. Often a provider from the child's cancer treatment team is willing to assist with transitioning the student back to school.
- Continue to monitor student after the child returns to school, re-evaluate and revise plan as needed.

IMPLICATIONS FOR LEARNING:
- Treatment and follow-up appointments will affect attendance.
- Side effects from cancer and treatment impacts learning and performance.
- Learning problems may emerge years after treatment is completed.
- Common problems seen after treatment:
  - Attention disorders
  - Cognitive deficits
  - Difficulty remembering and processing information
  - Difficulty "keeping up"
  - Delayed processing
  - Difficulty with reading
  - Difficulty with handwriting
  - Difficulty with new material
  - Lower grades than previous to treatment
  - Alterations in executive functioning
  - Behavioral disorders
  - Trouble reading social cues

It may be necessary to institute an Individualized Education Plan (IEP) or Section 504 Plan to provide the necessary academic accommodations and supports.

NOTE: There may be cases when not all treatment options have been successful. The shift in care will become palliative. Often these students wish to continue to attend school. Accommodations can be made to make the child comfortable and have optimal quality of life while at school.

See **Do Not Attempt Resuscitation (DNAR)** for further information, if needed.

CHILDHOOD CANCER *(continued from previous page)*

Resources

1. **American Cancer Society-** Website contains an abundance of information and resources. http://www.cancer.org/treatment/childrenandcancer/ whenyourchildhascancer/children-diagnosed-with-cancer-returning-to-school

2. **Candlelighters Childhood Cancer Foundation-** Provides information on cognitive effects in survivors along with advocacy information. www.candlelighters.org

3. **Learning and Living with Cancer-** https://www.mskcc.org/sites/default/files/ node/1228/documents/learning-livingwcancer-pdf.pdf

4. **Lionfighters-**Tips for returning to school in easy to read format. *http://lionfighters.childrensomaha.org/3-back-to-school-tips-for-childhood-cancer-patients-and-survivors/*

5. **MedlinePlus-** Cancer in Children. Links for additional information. Many parent resources also available in Spanish. https://www.nlm.nih.gov/medlineplus/ cancerinchildren.html

6. **Welcoming the Child with Cancer Back to School-** An excellent downloadable guide for educators. Includes medical information, tips for transitioning back to school, peer support guidelines, and discusses grief and loss. Available at: http://impactofspecialneeds.weebly.com/uploads/3/4/1/9/3419723/ onco_educators_guide.pdf

7. **Young people with cancer: A guide for parents-**http://www.cancer.gov/publications/ patient-education/children-with-cancer.pdf

CHILDHOOD CANCER *(continued from previous page)*

References

American Cancer Society. (2015). *Children diagnosed with cancer: Returning to school*. Retrieved from http://www.cancer.org/treatment/childrenandcancer/whenyourchildhascancer/children-diagnosed-with-cancer-returning-to-school

American Cancer Society. (2015). *Cancer in children*. Retrieved from http://www.cancer.org/cancer/cancerinchildren/detailedguide/index

Ball, J., Binder, R., & Cowen, K. (Eds.). (2012). The child with cancer. *Principles of Pediatric Nursing: Caring for Children (5th ed.)* (pp. 706-751). Upper Saddle River, NJ: Pearson Education, Inc.

Castellino, S., Ullrich, N., Whelen, M. & Lange, B. (2014). Developing interventions for cancer-related cognitive dysfunction in childhood cancer survivors. *Journal of National Cancer Institute, 106 (8)*. doi:10.1093/jnci/dju186

Selekman, J., Bochenek, J., & Lukens, M. (2013). Alterations in cellular health: The student with cancer. In J. Selekman (Ed.), *School nursing: A comprehensive text* (2nd ed.) (pp. 724-732). Philadelphia, PA: F.A. Davis.

CYTOMEGALOVIRUS (CMV)

DEFINITION/ETIOLOGY:

Cytomegalovirus (CMV) is one of a group of highly host-specific herpes viruses (herpes 1 & 2, Epstein Barr and varicella/shingles). The virus cycles between stages of an active infection and dormancy and an infected person can "shed" the virus at any time. Depending upon the age and the immune status of the host, CMV can cause a variety of clinical syndromes, collectively known as cytomegalic inclusion disease, although the majority of infections are very mild or subclinical. Young children are often infected from the saliva of playmates and older people by sexual partners. CMV can be transmitted through body fluids including urine, blood, saliva, secretions (e.g. breast milk, tears, semen, and vaginal fluids), blood transfusion products, transplanted organs and during the birthing process.

CLINICAL MANIFESTATIONS:

1. Congenital CMV *(Fetus/Newborn)*: may cause intrauterine death or severely affect newborn (microcephaly, poor temperature control, hearing loss, vision impairment, chronic liver disease, developmental disabilities, intellectual disabilities, pneumonia, seizures etc.). Symptoms may develop months after birth.

2. Acquired CMV *(Infant/Toddler)*: milder infections may be asymptomatic with excretion of virus in the urine.

3. Older Children/Adults: CMV is present in the environment; about 40% of adults have antibodies against the organism; blood transfusions and organ transplants can convey infection; immunosuppressed and pregnant individuals are at particular risk.

SIGNS AND SYMPTOMS :

- Generally none except in the severely affected newborn; those who survive will usually be served in Special Education due to cognitive impairment and other developmental disabilities.
- An infectious mononucleosis-like syndrome can occur in older children and young adults (fever, sore throat, fatigue, jaundice, and swollen glands).
- Symptoms may be seen in people with compromised immunity
- Diagnosis is made by rising antibody titer in blood, or isolation of virus from the urine.

CYTOMEGALOVIRUS (CMV) *(continued from previous page)*

MANAGEMENT/TREATMENT:
1. Acute disease is rarely diagnosed in school-age children.
2. Special education and other school personnel who handle diapers should always use "standard precautions".
3. Quarantine is unnecessary but pregnant teachers should not change diapers of children known to be shedding the virus.
4. No vaccine is available.
5. Specific treatment with I.V. antiviral drugs is generally reserved for individuals who are immunosuppressed.
6. CMV has a predilection for the retina with the possible development of retinitis.

FOLLOW UP:
- Some children will have serial urine cultures to determine when they stop shedding.
- Educate staff that **pregnant women and immunosuppressed individuals are the only ones at significant risk.**

POTENTIAL COMPLICATIONS:
Most babies born with CMV never develop symptoms or disabilities. However, when babies do have symptoms, some resolve while others can be permanent. Examples of potential complications of CMV include:

Temporary Symptoms
- Liver problems
- Spleen problems
- Jaundice (yellow skin and eyes)
- Purple skin splotches
- Lung problems
- Small size at birth
- Seizures
- Pneumonia
- Intestinal complications
- Mononucleosis

Permanent Symptoms or Disabilities
- Hearing loss
- Vision loss
- Mental disability
- Small head (microcephaly)
- Lack of coordination
- Seizures
- Death

CYTOMEGALOVIRUS (CMV) *(continued from previous page)*

Children with compromised immunity may present with an illness similar to infectious mononucleosis and other organs may be affected. Symptoms may include:
- Fever
- Pneumonia
- Diarrhea
- Ulcers in the digestive tract, possible causing bleeding
- Hepatitis
- Encephalitis
- Behavioral changes
- Seizures
- Coma
- Visual impairment and blindness

Most people infected with CMV experience few if any symptoms. Some adults may present with symptoms similar to mononucleosis (fatigue, fever and muscle aches).

PREVENTION:
- Standard Precautions (for infection)
- Handwashing
- Avoid contact with infectious body fluids
- Avoid contact with tears and saliva of infected child
- Avoid sharing food, eating utensils and drinking from the same glass
- Do not put a child's pacifier in your mouth
- Do not use someone else's toothbrush
- Do not touch inside of mouth, nose or eye after contact with body fluids of an infection person

NOTES:
- After neonatal infection, virus may be excreted for 5-6 years (children 7 and older rarely pose a threat); CMV is excreted (urine, saliva) by a large number of children in day care centers, which may represent a community reservoir.
- If the mother has a primary CMV infection during pregnancy, the risk of transmitting the disease is high. However, if CMV is reactivated during pregnancy the risk of transmission to the fetus is low.
- If congenital CMV is suspected, it is important to test the infant within 3 weeks otherwise it is considered acquired CMV.

CYTOMEGALOVIRUS (CMV) *(continued from previous page)*

- CMV should be considers If an infant become severely ill shortly after birth.
- If CMV is found in breast milk, breast-feeding is not discouraged as usually no signs, symptoms or disease occur.
- Approximately 50% to 80% of women have the virus by the age of 40.
- Once CMV is in the body, it remains present for life. If healthy, CMV is often dormant and goes undiagnosed.
- CMV does not reactivate unless individual is immunosuppressed.
- No cure is available for CMV but antiviral medication is available to slow down the infection for those at risk.

Resource

Centers for Disease Control and Prevention. (2015). Guide to Infection Prevention for Outpatient Settings: Minimum Expectations for Safe Care. http://www.cdc.gov/HAI/settings/outpatient/outpatient-care-gl-standared-precautions.html

References

American Academy of Pediatrics. (2013). Cytomegalovirus. In S. Aronson, & T. Shope (Eds.), *Managing infectious diseases in child care and schools* (2nd ed.) (p.81). Elk Grove Village, IL: American Academy of Pediatrics.

Centers for Disease Control. (2010). *Cytomegalovirus (CMV) and congenital CMV infection*. Retrieved from http://www.cdc.gov/cmv/overview.html

Levin, M.J., & Weinberg, A. (2014). Infections: Viral & rickettsial. In W. Hay, M. Levin, R. Deterding, & M. Abzug (Eds.), *Current diagnosis and treatment pediatrics* (22nd edition) (pp. 1250-1253). McGraw Hill Education, Inc.

Mayo Clinic. (2014). *Cytomegalovirus (CMV) infection*. Retrieved from http://www.mayoclinic.com/health/cmv/DS00938

Mayo Clinic. (2014). Cytomegalovirus (CMV) infection. Retrieved from http://www.mayoclinic.org/diseases-conditions/cmv/basics/symptoms/con-20029514

National Institute of Neurological Disorders and Stroke. (2011). *NINDS neurological consequences of cytomegalovirus infection information page*. Retrieved from http://www.ninds.nih.gov/disorders/cytomegalic/cytomegalic.htm

CONCUSSION/HEAD INJURY

DEFINITION/ETIOLOGY:

Concussion

A concussion is a type of traumatic brain injury (TBI) that affects children, adolescents and young adults . Children and teens take longer to recover than adults. It is caused by a blow, bump or jolt to the head. The impact generally causes the brain to move back and forth in the head. The CDC estimates that approximately 1.6-3.8 million sports/recreation related concussions happen each year and many occur without loss of consciousness. All concussions are serious and recognition and proper response when they first occur can help aid recovery and prevent further injury. Subsequent or repeated concussions can have lifelong complications or even death. Although 90% of concussions resolve within 10 days (Alessi, 2014), students who experience a concussion may exhibit cognitive and emotional issues that can impact the learning process and requires a collaborative approach in which the school nurse plays a vital role in supporting the student and educating the school team on potential implications in the school setting.

Other head injuries include:
- **Trauma to scalp:** laceration, bruise, abrasion
- **Trauma to bony skull:** fracture
- **Trauma to brain:** contusion, laceration, hematoma

SIGNS AND SYMPTOMS:
1. **Concussion**
    a. **Physical**
        - Headache
        - Nausea or vomiting
        - Dizziness
        - Fatigue, feeling "foggy"
        - Blurry or double vision
        - Sensitivity to light
        - Vomiting
        - Unequal size of pupils
        - Unusually rapid or slow pulse rate

CONCUSSION/HEAD INJURY *(continued from previous page)*

   b. **Cognitive**
   - Difficulty concentrating
   - Difficulty remembering
   - Feeling slowed down
   - Difficulty thinking clearly
   c. **Emotional**
   - Irritable
   - Sad
   - Nervous

2. **Scalp injury:**
   - Abrasion
   - Laceration: more bleeding than similar cut on other parts of the body because the skin over the scalp has a larger blood supply.
   - Bruise: causes mildly painful swelling (synonyms: pump-knot, goose-egg). Edges may feel depressed, but it is not to be mistaken for the depressed skull fracture described below.
   - In all these conditions, there is no disturbance of consciousness unless there is accompanying injury to the brain.

3. **Skull fracture:**
   - Non-displaced linear fracture: no symptoms except pain unless the base (bottom) of the skull is fractured (X-ray required for diagnosis) .
   - Basal skull fracture: usually associated with severe injury which almost always produces disturbance of consciousness or leakage of blood or spinal fluid from the mouth, nose, or ear.
   - Depressed skull fracture: due to a fragment or larger piece of bone pressing down on the brain as a result of trauma. Usually it cannot be felt by palpation and requires an X-ray for diagnosis.

CONCUSSION/HEAD INJURY *(continued from previous page)*

Red Flags: Students should seek guidance from their healthcare provider or be sent to the emergency room if they suddenly experience any of the following:

Seizures
Neck pain
Extreme drowsiness
Repeated vomiting
Slurred speech
Increasing confusion
Weakness or numbness
Unusual behavior change
Loss of consciousness

MANAGEMENT/TREATMENT:
Concussion:

- Any student expected of having a concussion or head injury should be removed from play immediately and sent for medical evaluation.
- Students should not participate in any high risk activity such as contact sports, bike riding and Physical Education (PE) class while experiencing the symptoms of a concussion.
- Students and parents/guardians should be educated on the signs and symptoms of a concussion and be instructed on the importance of not hiding their injury.
- Students should return to their normal activities gradually. Only when student's symptoms have reduced significantly, in consultation with their healthcare provider, should they gradually return to activities. If symptoms worsen or return, activities should be lessened and students should be encouraged to contact their healthcare provider.
- Students should get plenty of rest and avoid high risk, high intensity activities until symptoms resolve.
- When returning to school students may need accommodations such as a shortened school day, less testing, rest periods during the day, reduced computer use and classroom screen time (e.g. use of SMART boards and tablets), restrictions on physical education and/or recess or moderations to the workload.
- Prior to returning to sports students should take part in a "return to play" protocol that gradually allows the student to increase activities while monitoring for symptoms.

CONCUSSION/HEAD INJURY *(continued from previous page)*

Scalp injury:
- Abrasion: wash with plain soap. Apply pressure with 4x4 gauze or other clean cloth until bleeding stops. Dressing is usually not necessary.
- Laceration: same as abrasion but apply pressure longer to make sure bleeding stops (see *Laceration Guideline*).
- Bruise: apply cold pack to relieve pain. DO NOT apply pressure. Prognosis excellent if no sign of brain injury.

Skull fracture:
- If skull fracture suspected, refer to healthcare provider.
- Linear fracture: Limitation of activity as directed by healthcare provider.
- Basal fracture: refer to medical facility.
- Depressed skull: if fragment is significantly depressed to encroach on brain, surgery may be required to elevate bony segment.

POTENTIAL COMPLICATIONS (SERIOUS):
- Epidural/subdural hematoma
- Intracranial hemorrhage
- Cervical spinal injury
- Skull fracture
- Cerebrospinal fluid leak

Notes
- Students with chronic conditions such as migraines or ADHD may take longer to recover from a concussion. Students with depression and/or anxiety may also have trouble dealing with the complications of a concussion.
- Neurocognitive testing to access concentration, memory and processing speed may be done to help assess the impact of the concussion.
- Children and adolescents should avoid computer use (at home and at school) , texting and video games while symptoms persist.
- After a concussion a collaborative approach to the student's needs in school is needed. Guidance counselors, teachers, nurses and support staff must be educated on the complications of concussions and the impact on learning.
- Students who have experienced concussion symptoms over a longer period of time that is expected may benefit from an individualized healthcare plan (IHP) or Section 504 accommodation plan.

CONCUSSION/HEAD INJURY *(continued from previous page)*

References

Alessi, A. (2014, September). *Return to learn then return to play*. Presentation at the Concussion Conference, The Gaylord Center for Concussion Care hosted by Quinnipiac University, Hamden, CT.

Center for Disease Control. (2015). *Heads up: Brain injuries in your practice*. Retrieved from http://www.cdc.gov/concussion/HeadsUp/physicians_tool_kit.html

Mayo Clinic. (2014). *Concussion*. Retrieved from http://www.mayoclinic.com/health/concussion/DS00320

CONJUNCTIVITIS (Pink Eye)

DEFINITION/ETIOLOGY:
Inflammation and/or infection of the conjunctiva (mucous membrane lining the eye), caused by allergens, irritants (e.g., foreign object, dust, smoke), bacterial (staphylococcal, streptococcal, haemophilus) or viral (usually adenovirus, but also herpes simplex) infections. Both bacterial and viral conjunctivitis are contagious.

SIGNS AND SYMPTOMS:
- Redness of sclera
- Discharge: purulent or watery
  - Purulent drainage may cause blurred vision
- Itchiness: student rubs eye(s)
- Eyelids may be red and/or swollen
- Crusts in inner corner of eyes, especially on waking from sleep

Physical Findings That Help Differentiate Etiology:

Allergic	• Itchy eyes. Eyes may feel gritty. • Occurs in response to agent causing allergic reaction. • Discharge remains watery; bilateral. • No contagious period. • May occur with the common cold.
Bacterial	• The common meaning of "pink eye": purulent drainage (thick, yellow to green-yellow) and more crusting during sleep causing matting of the eyelashes. • Often beginning unilaterally and progressing to bilateral. Is spread to others by hand, contaminated eye mascara, etc. • This is contagious but less easily transmitted to others than viral. • Contagious period ends when medication begins and symptoms are no longer present. Approximately 50% of cases resolve without treatment in 1 – 2 weeks. • May occur with the common cold.
Viral	• Usually less severe, watery discharge but may be thick and white to pale yellow. • Photophobia. • Self-limiting. Lasts 3-5 days. • Most often bilateral. • Highly contagious but does not require antibiotics. • May occur with the common cold. • Contagious period continues while symptoms are present.
Chemical	• Usually appears shortly after contact with irritating substance. • No contagious period.

CONJUNCTIVITIS (Pink Eye) *(continued from previous page)*

MANAGEMENT/TREATMENT (with specific care based on likely cause or medical diagnosis):

1. Exclusion from school: The registered nurse may not exclude those whose conjunctivitis is mild or associated with a cold or allergy. School policy should direct other personnel to exclude ALL cases for medical evaluation. Healthcare provider may prescribe antibiotic drops or ointment. Students return to school when they have been under treatment 24 to 48 hours unless close interaction with others can be avoided.
2. Discourage home treatment with cold ointment or steroid drops.
3. Over-the-counter drops may be used for comfort of mild allergic or viral conjunctivitis. Healthcare provider may order topical anti-inflammatory drops for significant allergic conjunctivitis.
4. Cool compress for temporary relief.
5. Check visual acuity; it should be normal or unchanged from the student's usual acuity.
6. Check fingers and nose for impetigo.
7. Review handwashing and other measures to prevent spread of infection.
8. Refer any case with subconjunctival hemorrhage.

FOLLOW UP:

- If healthcare provider orders medication, instruct to take for the entire prescribed time.
- Educate about handwashing and keeping fingers/hands away from eyes. Instruct the student to not share face washcloths and eye makeup.
- Discard unused eye makeup.

POTENTIAL COMPLICATIONS:

Conjunctivitis can be accompanied by an inflammation of the cornea which can affect vision.

CONJUNCTIVITIS (Pink Eye) *(continued from previous page)*

References

American Academy of Pediatrics. (2015). *Pinkeye (conjunctivitis).* Retrieved from https://www.healthychildren.org/English/health-issues/conditions/eyes/Pages/PinkEye-Conjunctivitis.aspx

American Academy of Pediatrics. (2013). Pinkeye (conjunctivitis). In S. Aronson, & T. Shope (Eds.), *Managing infectious diseases in child care and schools (2nd ed.)* (p. 133-134). Elk Grove Village, IL: American Academy of Pediatrics.

American Academy of Pediatrics, Committee on Infectious Diseases. (2015).Infections spread by direct contact. In D.W. Kimberlin, M. T. Brady, M.A. Jackson, & S.S. Long (Eds.), *Red Book: 2015 report of the committee on infectious diseases* (30th ed.) (pp. 156-157). Elk Grove Village, IL: American Academy of Pediatrics.

American Optometric Association (AOA). (2013). *Conjunctivitis.* Retrieved from http://www.aoa.org/patients-and-public/eye-and-vision-problems/glossary-of-eye-and-vision-conditions/conjunctivitis

Centers for Disease Control and Prevention. (2014). *Conjunctivitis: For clinicians.* Retrieved from http://www.cdc.gov/conjunctivitis/clinical.html

John, R. & Chewey. L. (2013). Common complaints. In J. Selekman (Ed.), *School nursing: A comprehensive text* (2nd ed.) (pp. 587-590). Philadelphia, PA: F.A. Davis.

Mayo Clinic. (2015). *Pink eye (conjunctivitis).* Retrieved from http://www.mayoclinic.com/health/pink-eye/DS00258

Merck Manual. (2014). *Overview of conjunctivitis.* Retrieved from http://www.merckmanuals.com/professional/eye-disorders/conjunctival-and-scleral-disorders/overview-of-conjunctivitis

CONSTIPATION (Idiopathic or Functional)

DEFINITION/ETIOLOGY:
Constipation is a very common gastrointestinal disorder that frequently becomes chronic. For most children constipation means two or less bowel movements a week, or hard, dry, and small bowel movements that are painful or difficult to pass.

Some children and young people with physical disabilities, such as cerebral palsy, Down syndrome or autism are more prone to idiopathic constipation as a result of impaired mobility.

Constipation is termed idiopathic or functional if it cannot be explained by any anatomical, physiological, radiological or histological abnormalities. The exact etiology is unknown but a number of factors may contribute to this condition including pain, fever, dehydration, dietary and fluid intake, toilet training, medicines and a family history of constipation. Withholding a bowel movement due to pain and the unavailability of a private restroom in school may create the psychological issues that also contribute to constipation. Toilet availability and busy schedules may also be a factor.

SIGNS AND SYMPTOMS:
Signs and symptoms include:
- infrequent bowel activity
- excessive and foul smelling flatulence
- foul smelling stools
- irregular stool texture
- passing occasional enormous stools or frequent small pellets
- volitional withholding or straining to stop passage of stools (retentive posturing or changing positions)
- soiling or overflow
- abdominal pains
- distension or discomfort
- poor appetite
- lack of energy
- unhappy, angry or irritable mood
- general malaise

CONSTIPATION (Idiopathic or Functional) *(continued from previous page)*

SIGNS AND SYMPTOMS *(continued)*

Other signs and symptoms include:
- history of painful or hard bowel movements or constipation
- history of large diameter stools which may obstruct the toilet
- urinary incontinence
- improved appetite with the passage of stool
- waxing and waning of abdominal pain with the passage of stool
- anal pain
- bleeding associated with hard stools

Physical exam may verify signs of abdominal distension and the palpation of stool in the abdomen.

Signs and symptoms of an underlying disorder include:
- passing ribbon stools
- failure to thrive
- abdominal distension with vomiting
- history of constipation symptoms since birth
- failure to pass meconium within 48 hours after birth

MANAGEMENT/TREATMENT:

Constipation
- Education of family on physiology of soiling and treatment plan.
- Behavioral Interventions: Suited to the child or young person's stage of development should be negotiated and non-punitive. These could include:
  - Scheduled toileting and support to establish a regular bowel habit such as 20 minutes (may use a timer), after meals 2-3 times a day for 10 – 15 minutes.
  - Children should sit on toilet with feet flat on floor.
  - Discussion of a bowel diary, information on constipation, and use of encouragement and rewards systems can also be offered.
  - How the bowels work, symptoms that might indicate a serious underlying problem.
  - How to take their medication.
  - What to expect when taking laxatives.
  - How to "poop".

CONSTIPATION (Idiopathic or Functional) *(continued from previous page)*

MANAGEMENT/TREATMENT: *(continued)*

- ○ Criteria to recognize risk situations for relapse (such as worsening of any symptoms soiling, etc.).
- ○ The importance of continuing treatment may also be included in patient education.
- Increase water: <u>Recommended Water intake per day:</u> More water is suggested if physically active, exposed to hot environment and possibly obese.
  - ○ For children ages 1-3 years old: From food and drink: 1300ml; from water and drinks: 900 ml
  - ○ For children ages 4-8 years old: From food and drink: 1700ml; from water and drinks: 1200 ml
  - ○ For boys ages 9-13 years: From food and drink: 2400ml; from water and drinks 1800 ml
  - ○ For girls ages 9-13 years: From food and drink: 2100 ml; from water and drinks: 1600 ml
  - ○ For boys ages 14-18 years: From food and water: 3300 ml; from water and drinks: 2600 ml
  - ○ For girls ages 14-18 years: From food and water: 2300 ml; from water and drinks: 1800 ml
- Increase fiber.
  - ○ Daily grams of fiber intake are calculated using the child's age in years plus five up to the age of 20. Recommend including foods with a high fiber content (such as fruit, vegetables, high-fiber bread, baked beans and wholegrain breakfast cereals). Do not recommend unprocessed bran, which can cause bloating and flatulence and reduce the absorption of micronutrients.
- Increase physical activity.
  - ○ Tailor daily physical activity to the child or young person's stage of development and individual ability.
- Polyethylene glycol (Miralax® or PEG 3550) is considered the first line of treatment. A maintenance dose of polyethylene glycol is recommended and is adjusted according to clinical response.
  - ○ Polyethylene glycol can be habit forming. Take only as prescribed. Usually takes 2-4 days to have a bowel movement.

CONSTIPATION (Idiopathic or Functional) *(continued from previous page)*

MANAGEMENT/TREATMENT: *(continued)*

- o Treatment should continue for at least 2 months and symptoms should be resolved for one month before slow tapering of treatment or until toilet training is achieved.
- o Milk of magnesia, stimulant laxatives, mineral oil, or enemas may be used as second line or additional treatment.
- Provide demystification, explanation, and guidance for toilet training in children with a developmental age of at least four and parental guidance on toilet training.
- Provide anticipatory guidance children and young people may require laxative therapy for several years.

Fecal Impaction
- Assess all children and young people with idiopathic constipation for fecal impaction.
- Use a combination of history and physical examination to diagnose fecal impaction - look for overflow soiling and/or fecal mass palpable abdominally.
- The basic tenets of therapy include:
  - o evacuation of the colon
  - o elimination of pain with defecation
  - o establishing regular bowel habits
  - o Polyethylene glycol, mineral oil, magnesium hydroxide, and lactulose are effective and can be used for prolonged time periods without risk
  - o intermittent use of stimulant laxatives may be necessary in some children; however, routine usage of these agents in young children is not generally recommended
- An escalating dose of polyethylene glycol (PEG) is considered the first line of treatment.
- A stimulant laxative is added if polyethylene glycol does not lead to disimpaction after 2 weeks.
- Inform families that disimpaction treatment can initially increase symptoms of soiling and abdominal pain.
- If the history and/or physical examination show evidence of faltering growth, refer for testing.
- If either the history and/or the physical examination show evidence of possible maltreatment, treat for constipation and refer.

CONSTIPATION (Idiopathic or Functional) *(continued from previous page)*

FOLLOW-UP:
- Develop a Section 504 plan as needed.
- Accommodate privacy needs.
- Be supportive of the family and student during any further treatment by the healthcare provider by following the treatment plan and documenting bowel activities/accidents at school.
- Children and young people undergoing disimpaction should see a healthcare provider in one week.
- Follow up by the healthcare provider for acute constipation is based on the child or young person's response to treatment, measured by frequency, amount and consistency of stools.
- The healthcare provider may schedule the child to be seen be at 2 weeks, one month, three months, six months, and may reassess children frequently during maintenance treatment to ensure they do not reimpact again and assess issues in maintaining treatment such as taking medicine and toileting.
- The frequency of assessment by the healthcare provider should be tailored to the individual needs of the child and their families (this could range from daily contact to contact every few weeks).

POTENTIAL COMPLICATIONS:
- Intractable constipation
- Possible fecal incontinence
- Increase in abdominal pain with high level PEG therapy

NOTES:
- The National Clinical Practice Guidelines notes school nurses as a key support for children and families with a diagnosis of constipation.

CONSTIPATION (Idiopathic or Functional) *(continued from previous page)*

References

American Dietary Recommendations/Institute of Medicine. (2005). *Dietary reference intakes for water, potassium, sodium chloride and sulfate.* Washington DC: The National Academies Press. Retrieved from http://fnic.nal.usda.gov/dietary-guidance/dri-nutrient-reports/water-potassium-sodium-chloride-and-sulfate

Eicher, P. S., Vitello, L., Roche, W. J., Martorana, P., Kalderon, V., & Kalderon, A. (2007). Children and constipation: Poop is not a four letter word. *Exceptional Parent, 37*(12), 72-75.

Hooban, S. (2010). NICE's first guideline on idiopathic childhood constipation and its implications for nurses. *Nursing Times, 106*(47), 14-14 11p. Retrieved from http://www.nursingtimes.net/#

National Guideline (2010). *Constipation in children and young people. Diagnosis and management of idiopathic childhood constipation in primary and secondary care.* Retrieved from http://www.ncbi.nlm.nih.gov/books/NBK65365/

National Guideline (2015). *Evaluation and treatment of functional constipation in infants and children: evidence-based recommendations from ESPGHAN and NASPGHAN.* Retrieved from http://www.guideline.gov/content.aspx?id=49114&search=constipation

Pasanen, M. E. (2014). Evaluation and treatment of colonic symptoms. *Common Symptoms in the Ambulatory Setting, 98*(3), 529-547. doi.org/10.1016/j.mcna.2014.01.009

Prynn, P. (2011). Childhood constipation. *Practice Nurse, 41*(16), 11-16. Retrieved from http://www.practicenurse.co.uk/

Tappin, D., Nawaz, S., McKay, C., MacLaren, L., Griffiths, P., & Mohammed, T. A. (2013). Development of an early nurse led intervention to treat children referred to secondary paediatric care with constipation with or without soiling. *BMC Pediatrics, 13*, 193-193. doi: 10.1186/1471-2431-13-193

Tobias, N., Mason, D., Lutkenhoff, M., Stoops, M., & Ferguson, D. (2008). Management principles of organic causes of childhood constipation. *Journal of Pediatric Healthcare, 22*(1), 12-23 12p. doi10.1016/j.pedhc.2007.01.001

CONTACT LENS PROBLEMS

OVERVIEW:

Contact lenses are used as a substitute for glasses in most situations. They may also be used to treat certain eye diseases or for cosmetic purposes to change eye color. Children between the ages of 6-9 are prescribed contact lenses for medical reasons only.

LENS TYPES include soft lenses, rigid gas permeable lenses, extended wear lenses, disposable lenses, and specialty lenses. Decorative lenses are illegally sold in beauty salons, novelty stores and online. These lenses are non-fitted lenses and cover a larger part of the eye, putting the wearer at a higher risk for a severe complication. Decorative lenses, if desired should be prescribed by an eye care professional.

Most problems encountered from wearing contact lenses are from inexperienced wearers, improper wear or care, or delay in follow-up with the eye healthcare provider. These problems range from a lens being out of position, eye irritations such as dryness, a foreign body on or under lens, to more serious complications such as pink eye, corneal abrasion, infection, corneal ulcer, and permanent vision loss.

ANTICIPATED CONCERNS/PROBLEMS:

As a new contact lens wearer, it is not uncommon to have:
- Tearing upon insertion
- Scratchy feeling or like there is something in the eye
- Mild light sensitivity
- Slight headache especially if stronger prescription
- Distorted vision that may be caused from:
  - Lens that is not centered
  - Soft lens inside out
  - Wearing disposable lenses beyond the suggested time
  - Not wearing lenses for several days (cornea may lose adaptation)
  - Dirty lens

SIGNS AND SYMPTOMS OF AN EYE IRRITATION, INFECTION, OR SERIOUS COMPLICATION INCLUDE:

- Persistent pain
- Burning and tearing
- Redness that will not clear
- Hazy vision that continues an hour or more after lens removal
- Continued sensitivity to light
- Swelling of eye

CONTACT LENS PROBLEMS *(continued from previous page)*

MANAGEMENT/TREATMENT:
Seek care from eye healthcare professional if symptoms of an eye irritation or infection (above) occur.

Removing Displaced Lenses
- Blink several times to make sure lens is in the eye. Blinking may center the lens.
- Wash hands before touching the eye or lens.
- Use your finger to feel the lens through the eyelid.
- Look in the opposite direction of the lens (downward, upward, to the right or left) to visualize the lens.
- When the lens is visualized, use your finger to move the lens back on the cornea.
- Massaging the lens through eyelid may help move it back in place.
- If you are unable to remove the lens, seek care from an eye healthcare provider.

FOLLOW UP: (Teaching Tips)
- Wash your hands before touching your eye or handling lenses.
- Don't wear lenses longer than prescribed.
- Don't sleep in your lenses unless specifically fitted for that purpose.
- Don't use saliva as a cleaning agent. The risk of bacterial contamination is great.
- Do not use homemade solutions that are not sterile. Do not use distilled or tap water for any part of the cleaning regimen.
- Use only solutions recommended by fitter – some are not compatible with other lenses and/or may be allergenic to wearer.
- Experts consider the "rub and rinse" method to be the superior cleaning method.
- Don't get cosmetics, sprays, etc. on lenses.
- Finish with makeup before handling lenses.
- Don't reuse the solution in your lens case. Throw away and use a new case every three months or if you get an eye infection.
- Do not rinse lenses in hot water or store in a hot or unusually cold place; lens may warp.
- Used lenses stored for 30 days should not be worn without re-disinfecting.
- Frequent blinking is essential for all contacts to maintain moisture and a constant supply of oxygen to the corneas.
- Wearing non-prescription decorative lenses or circle lenses purchased online or in novelty shops can result in permanent eye damage.
- Smokers have a higher incidence of problems wearing contact lenses than non-smokers.

CONTACT LENS PROBLEMS *(continued from previous page)*

References

American Academy of Ophthalmology, Eye Smart. (2015). *Contact lenses for vision correction.* Retrieved from
http://www.geteyesmart.org/eyesmart/glasses-contacts-lasik/contact-lens.cfm

American Academy of Ophthalmology, Eye Smart. (2012). *Removing a displaced content lens.* Retrieved from
http://www.geteyesmart.org/eyesmart/ask/questions/stuck-contact-lens.cfm

Medline Plus. U.S. National Library of Medicine. (2014). *Corneal ulcers and treatment.* Retrieved from
http://www.nlm.nih.gov/medlineplus/ency/article/001032.htm#visualContent

United States Food and Drug and Administration, Medical Devices. (2015). *Contact lenses.* Retrieved from
http://www.fda.gov/MedicalDevices/ProductsandMedicalProcedures/HomeHealthandConsumer/ConsumerProducts/ContactLenses/default.htm

CROHN'S DISEASE

DEFINITION/ETIOLOGY:
Crohn's disease is a debilitating, chronic inflammatory bowel disease that causes intermittent inflammation in the lining of the digestive tract. Inflammation commonly occurs in the ileum of the small intestines and colon, but can occur in any area in the gastrointestinal tract. The exact cause of Crohn's disease is unknown. There is no known cure for Crohn's disease. It is characterized by periods of flare-ups and periods of remission. A person has a higher incidence of developing Crohn's disease if they have a relative with the disease.

SIGNS AND SYMPTOMS:
Symptoms range from mild to severe and differ from person to person. Symptoms may include:
- Abdominal pain/intestinal cramping
- Diarrhea (can be severe)
- Fatigue
- Low grade fever – secondary to inflammation and/or infection
- Canker sores
- Inflammation in the joints, skin, eyes and/or liver
- Weight loss
- Malnutrition
- Impaired growth and development
- Rectal bleeding (rare)

MANAGEMENT/TREATMENT:
The overall goal of treatment is to reduce inflammation in the intestines. Students with abdominal cramps and diarrhea may be prescribed anti-diarrheal and anti-spasmodic medications to relieve symptoms.

Other treatment options may include anti-inflammatory medications (such as 5 aminosalicyclic acid) and/or antibiotics to reduce inflammation. Individuals with severe symptoms may be prescribed corticosteroids to reduce symptoms. Corticosteroids are not meant for long-term treatment of Crohn's disease.

CROHN'S DISEASE *(continued from previous page)*

MANAGEMENT/TREATMENT: *(continued)*

Surgical intervention may be necessary if individual does not respond to medications. As many as 70% of clients with Crohn's disease may ultimately need surgery during their lifetime to alleviate symptoms. Surgery does not cure the disease. Surgery removes the area of intestine that is severely inflamed, symptomatic and is not responding to medications. Surgery is typically performed in clients with recurrent bowel obstructions, fistulas, and abscesses. The recurrence rate of Crohn's disease after surgery is > 70% at 1 year and > 85% at 3 years postoperatively.

POTENTIAL COMPLICATIONS:

- Malnutrition (poor intestinal absorption)
- Anemia
- Fistula (may become infected and form an abscess)
- Bowel obstruction
- Anal fissures
- Ulcers (mouth, genital and/or anal)
- Gallbladder/liver disease
- Osteoporosis (poor intestinal absorption/corticosteroids also increase the risk of developing osteoporosis)
- Increased risk of colon cancer

FOLLOW UP:

- Monitor for medication side effects.
- Diet may aggravate Crohn's disease. Refer to school nutrition services for potential school-based dietary accommodations. Individual may be on a low fat, low fiber diet (fiber may make symptoms worse). May also need to limit dairy products and avoid spicy foods and caffeine.
- Monitor for potential need of school-based social work services.
- Smoking aggravates symptoms. Educate student on need to avoid cigarette/cigar smoke.
- Homebound school services may be necessary for extended absences (more than 5 consecutive school days).

CROHN'S DISEASE *(continued from previous page)*

NOTES:

Evaluate for possible Section 504 accommodations. Possible accommodations may include:
- Free access to bathroom.
- Self-paced activity at school.
- Provide rest as needed throughout the academic day.
- Access to snacks/water throughout the school day.
- Extra change of clothes at school.
- Student will not be penalized for excessive tardiness or absenteeism due to medical condition.
- Academic accommodations during periods of flare-ups (extended test taking time, extended time to turn in assignments, second set of books for home use, etc.).

References

Centers for Disease Control and Prevention (CDC). (2014). *What is inflammatory bowel disease.* Retrieved from http://www.cdc.gov/ibd/what-is-ibd.htm

Mayo Clinic. (2014). *Crohn's disease.* Retrieved from http://www.mayoclinic.org/diseases-conditions/crohns-disease/basics/definition/CON-20032061

Merck Manual. (2012). *Crohn disease.* Retrieved from http://www.merckmanuals.com/professional/gastrointestinal-disorders/inflammatory-bowel-disease-ibd/crohn-disease

National Institute of Diabetes and Digestive and Kidney Diseases. (2013). *What I need to know about Crohn's disease.* Retrieved from http://www.niddk.nih.gov/health-information/health-topics/digestive-diseases/crohns-disease/Pages/ez.aspx

Selekman, J., Bochenek, J. & Lukens, M. (2013). Children with chronic conditions. In J. Selekman (Ed.), *School nursing: A comprehensive text (2nd ed.)* (pp.734-737). Philadelphia, PA: F.A. Davis.

CYSTIC FIBROSIS

DEFINITION/ETIOLOGY:
Cystic fibrosis (CF) is an autosomal recessive genetic disease caused by a mutation of the **Cystic Fibrosis Transmembrane Regulator** (CFTR) gene, altering the salt balance in body secretions. Cystic fibrosis affects mainly the exocrine glands, resulting in a thick, sticky mucous that compromises the organs, primarily the lungs and pancreas. The exocrine glands produce sweat, saliva, pancreatic digestive juice and respiratory tract mucous.

SIGNS AND SYMPTOMS:
Vary with the severity of the disease.
- Salty taste to the skin – increased amount of sodium and chloride in sweat
- Weight loss despite voracious appetite
- Frequent, foul-smelling, greasy stools
- Stools may be gray or clay colored
- Flatulence
- Abdominal pain
- Delayed growth
- Thick, sticky sputum
- Productive coughing
- Wheezing
- Frequent respiratory infections

MANAGEMENT/TREATMENT:
There is no cure for cystic fibrosis. Treatment is aimed at alleviating symptoms, primarily to keep the lungs as clear as possible.

1. Chest physical therapy to loosen thick mucus secretions
   a. Postural drainage
   b. Chest percussion
   c. Positive expiratory pressure therapy
   d. Mechanical devices such as Flutter/Vest devices

2. Medications
   a. Pancreatic enzymes to aid in digestion with each meal/snack
   b. Aerosolize drugs thins mucus making it easier to cough up
   c. Bronchodilators to open airways

CYSTIC FIBROSIS *(continued from previous page)*

    d. Vitamin supplements (secretions prevent body from absorbing fat soluble vitamins A, D, E and K)

    e. Antibiotics to treat respiratory infections, may need longer duration of treatment than normal

3. Maintain adequate nutrition
   a. High calorie/diet high in protein and fat
   b. May need nutritional supplements
   c. May need supplemental feedings per nasogastric tube, or Total Parenteral Nutrition (TPN)
   d. For long term nutritional support, a gastrostomy or jejunostomy tube may be placed

4. Physical activity as tolerated
   a. Allow student to set his or her own pace, accommodate for rest periods as needed.
   b. Encourage adequate hydration (especially during hot weather or after exercise – increased salt in sweat – may need supplemental salt).
   c. Physical activity loosens lung secretions.
   d. Improves overall physical condition of heart and lungs.

5. Psychosocial assessment
   a. May feel different from peers
   b. Need for special diet, medications, respiratory management
   c. Potential for bullying from others

FOLLOW-UP:
- Develop individualized healthcare plan identifying signs of airway distress and appropriate responses.
- Assist student with administration of pancreatic enzymes.
- Act as a liaison with CF care centers to coordinate care for school.
- Monitor nutritional status – measure height/weight a minimum of 2 times per year.
- Educate staff regarding chronic cough.
  - Not contagious
  - Should not suppress cough – clears secretions
  - Allow student to keep water bottle on desk
  - Allow bathroom privileges as needed for digestive problems

CYSTIC FIBROSIS *(continued from previous page)*

- ○ Preferential seating near door so student may leave classroom as needed for heavy coughing
- ○ Tissues/plastic bag at desk for productive cough

POTENTIAL COMPLICATIONS:
- Asthma can result from chronic inflammation of the bronchial tubes
- Chronic respiratory infections
  - ○ Pneumonia
  - ○ Bronchitis
  - ○ Chronic sinusitis
- Liver damage due to blocked bile duct
- Cystic fibrosis-related diabetes (CFRD)– features similar to Type 1 and Type 2 diabetes but considered a separate condition
- Depressed growth rate
- Osteoporosis and/or osteopenia secondary to compromised absorption of calcium and vitamin D
- Infertility – 98% in males
- Death – typically as a result of lung complications

NOTES:
Children with cystic fibrosis are more likely to suffer complications from an illness. Educate regarding the importance of healthy lifestyle behaviors:
- Appropriate handwashing
- Immunizations – pneumococcal and influenza
- Avoiding cigarette smoke
- Healthy eating habits
- If there is more than 1 student with cystic fibrosis in a school building, avoid assigning both students to the same classroom
- Avoid sitting within 6 feet of another student with CF secondary to prevent cross infection

Resources
Cystic Fibrosis Foundation http://www.cff.org/AboutCF/
Cystic Fibrosis Foundation, specific for school: http://www.cff.org/LivingWithCF/AtSchool/
National Lung Heart and Blood Institute
http://www.nhlbi.nih.gov/health/health-topics/topics/cf/

CYSTIC FIBROSIS *(continued from previous page)*

References

Ball, J., Binder, R., & Cowen, K. (Eds.). (2012). Alterations in respiratory function. *Principles of Pediatric Nursing: Caring for Children* (5th ed.) (p.p. 551-599). Upper Saddle River, NJ: Pearson Education, Inc.

Cystic Fibrosis Foundation. (n.d.). *About cystic fibrosis.* Retrieved from http://www.cff.org/AboutCF/

Cystic Fibrosis Foundation. (n.d.). *Living with CF at school.* Retrieved from http://www.cff.org/LivingWithCF/AtSchool/

Mayo Clinic. (2015). *Cystic fibrosis.* Retrieved from http://www.mayoclinic.com/health/cystic-fibrosis/DS00287

Merck Manual. (2014). *Cystic fibrosis.* Retrieved from http://www.merckmanuals.com/professional/pediatrics/cystic-fibrosis-cf/cystic-fibrosis#SymptomsAndSigns

National Lung, Heart Blood Institute. (2013).What is *cystic fibrosis?* Retrieved from http://www.nhlbi.nih.gov/health/health-topics/topics/cf/

Selekman, J., Bochenek, J., & Lukens, M. (2013). Cystic fibrosis. In J. Selekman (Ed.), *School nursing: A comprehensive text* *(2nd ed.)* (pp. 721-724). Philadelphia, PA: F.A. Davis.

DENTAL EMERGENCIES

DEFINITION/ETIOLOGY:

Nearly one half of children have a dental injury to a tooth during their childhood. Tooth and mouth injuries are generally not considered life threatening, but may require immediate dental and/or medical attention. Common causes of dental injuries are related to sport activities, falls, with or without something in the mouth, fights, and automobile accidents. Frequently, injury to a tooth or the oral cavity can be prevented or lessened by use of appropriate equipment or a mouth guard. Prevention education is critical as injuries to permanent teeth can have a lasting impact on a person's self-esteem and confidence.

SIGNS AND SYMPTOMS:
A healthcare provider should be contacted for the following:
- Avulsed tooth (knocked out due to trauma)
- Fractured, chipped or missing tooth (may have been swallowed)
- Luxated/dislocated tooth
- Fractured jaw (pain with opening and closing jaw)
- Infections and/or inflammation
- Sensitivity to pressure or hot/cold
- Bleeding that can't be stopped after 10 minutes
- Problems breathing or swallowing
- A large cut inside the mouth
- An object stuck in any part of the mouth (throat, tongue, cheek)

MANAGEMENT/TREATMENT:

AVULSED TOOTH

> If a knocked out tooth is handled correctly, there is a good possibility the dentist will be able to put the tooth placed back into the socket if the child is seen within 30 minutes. Approximately 85% of avulsed teeth placed in the socket within 5 minutes survive.

1. **Do not touch the root of the tooth.**
2. Do not change the tooth's protective coating by trying to clean it. At most, <u>gently</u> rinse off debris with cool water.
3. If possible, gently place the tooth back into its socket securing it with gauze or aluminum foil around the tooth. If unsuccessful, place the tooth in student's mouth between cheek and gum (providing the student is old enough). This natural environment is most protective to the tooth.

DENTAL EMERGENCIES *(continued from previous page)*

AVULSED TOOTH *(continued)*
4. If student is too young, wrap tooth in gauze and immerse in cold milk for transportation.
5. Commercial containers to carry tooth to the dentist are available, but expensive. These containers are convenient but have no proven advantage.
6. Call parent and the dentist to arrange an immediate visit.
7. Do not attempt to reinsert a primary tooth back in the socket. This might cause damage to the developing permanent tooth. Instead, the tooth should be taken to the dentist so that he or she can be sure the tooth was lost in its entirety and the root not broken.

*Maxillary central incisor is most frequently avulsed.

FRACTURED TOOTH
1. Rinse the mouth with warm water.
2. Call parent. Refer to dentist for follow-up treatment.
3. Save fragment/ large chip.
4. Place tooth fragment in water and send with the child to the dentist.
5. Apply cool compress to reduce facial swelling.
6. If possible, call dentist and describe extent of chip.
7. Cover jagged edge of tooth with gauze.
8. Apply cold compress or a washcloth with ice to the cheek to reduce pain and swelling.

LUXATED/DISLOCATED TOOTH
1. For permanent tooth, **time is of the essence**.
2. Reposition tooth gently.
3. Call parent and dentist for emergency visit.
4. Put gauze around tooth and have student hold it there during transportation to dentist.

DENTAL EMERGENCIES *(continued from previous page)*

FRACTURED JAW
1. Immobilize jaw placing a scarf, tie or towel under the chin. Tie the ends on top of the head.
2. Apply ice to reduce swelling.
3. Call parent and dentist.

PUNCTURE WOUNDS
1. Do not remove the embedded object in any part of the mouth.
2. Seek immediate medical care.
3. This injury may require referral to surgeon.

FOLLOW-UP:
Monitor for:
- Persistent pain.
- Sensitivity to hot and cold.
- Discoloration of tooth.
- Possible tetanus booster if less than 12 years old.
- Persistent bleeding - prolonged or recurrent, after dental injury or extraction of tooth:
  1. Place a sterile gauze pad on the extraction site and have the student gently bite on it for 30 minutes.
  2. Replace soaked gauze pads as necessary.
  3. Consult a dentist if bleeding persists over 1 hour; sooner if bleeding appears excessive. If bleeding is spontaneous without trauma, refer to healthcare provider.

POTENTIAL COMPLICATIONS:
- Dental pulp fracture
- Displaced tooth
- Embedded tooth fragments
- Discoloration of tooth
- Loss of tooth
- Possible root canal, crown in the future
- Wounds may heal with a scar that may affect swallowing and speech

DENTAL EMERGENCIES *(continued from previous page)*

OTHER DENTAL CONCERNS:

Toothache
- Rinse mouth with warm water.
- Floss teeth to remove food particles that may be trapped between teeth.
- All toothaches should be referred to a dentist; severity will dictate the time frame.

Protruding braces wire
- Protruding wire from a brace can be gently bent out of the way to relieve discomfort by using a tongue depressor or pencil eraser. If the wire cannot be bent easily, apply dental wax or place a small piece of gauze or cotton over the end to prevent irritation to cheek or gum. Do not try to remove any wire embedded in the cheeks, gum, or tongue. (Local orthodontists often donate care kits.)
- Obtain orthodontic care same day.

Red, swollen or sore gums
- Have student rinse mouth thoroughly with a warm salt-water solution (1/4 teaspoon of table salt to 4 oz. glass of water).
- Instruct student to repeat rinses every two hours, and after eating or tooth brushing, and before bedtime.
- If no improvement in 1-2 days, refer to healthcare provider or dentist.
- Check for abscesses below the tooth line.

NOTES:

When a facial or dental injury occurs at school, the school nurse, rather than a dentist, may be the first one contacted. Taking a quick, complete, injury specific history is essential. If the child has no life-threatening symptoms, briefly obtain any additional history that would influence advice, such as past medical history, whether the child has any special healthcare needs, and/or significant social information. Next, it becomes important to determine if the injury is primarily dental or medical. The head, neck, and oral cavity have a tremendous vascular supply; therefore, blood may obscure a significant injury or it may make a mild injury appear much worse that it is. If it is clear the injury is primarily dental, help the caregiver to access a child's dentist immediately.

DENTAL EMERGENCIES *(continued from previous page)*

Other considerations include:

1. Education on prevention of dental injuries
    a. Types and use of mouth guards.
    b. Do not put anything but food in the mouth.
    c. Sit while eating.
    d. Do not chew hard candy, popcorn kernels, ice, etc.
2. Special hygiene and diet instructions

COMMONLY ASKED DENTAL QUESTIONS:

1. **What should school nurses know about tooth development?**
   Most importantly, the permanent teeth form very close to the apices (roots) of the primary teeth. Any injury to a primary tooth has the potential to damage the permanent tooth below. Primary tooth injuries range in damage from as minor as a small spot on the crown of the tooth to as severe as aborting further development of the permanent tooth bud. Consequently, all primary tooth injuries need evaluation by a dentist. School nurses should also be aware of other things that can affect tooth development such as excessive fluoride, tetracyclines, congenital defects, metabolic diseases and high fever. These can have deleterious effects on the quality of dental hard tissues, especially the enamel.

2. **What about students with disabilities?**
   They seem to have special problems because of the systemic problems (cognitive impairment, poor muscle control, diminished reflexes, etc.) or because of the secondary effects of diet, medications or the because of difficulty in maintaining good oral hygiene. Referral to a pediatric dentist or another dentist who has had advanced training in working with patients with special needs is extremely important. After dental work, monitor the child closely to prevent chewing on anesthetized surfaces.

DENTAL EMERGENCIES *(continued from previous page)*

References

American Academy of Pediatric Dentistry. (2014). *Fast facts.* Retrieved from
    http://www.aapd.org/assets/1/7/FastFacts.pdf

American Dental Association. (2013). *Dental emergencies.* Retrieved from http://www.ada.org/370.aspx

Baginska, J., Wilczynska-Borawska, M. (2012). First aid algorithms in dental avulsion. *The Journal of School Nursing 28* (2),
    pp.90-94. doi: 10.1177/1059840511434515

McTigue, D. J. & Thompson, A. (2015). *Patient information: Mouth and dental injuries in children.* Retrieved from
    http://www.uptodate.com/contents/mouth-and-dental-injuries-in-children-beyond-the-basics?view=print

Mraz, M. & Selekman, J. (2013). Athlete health promotion. In J. Selekman (Ed.), *School nursing: A comprehensive text*
    (2nd ed.) (pp. 641 – 677). Philadelphia: F. A. Davis.

National Institute of Dental and Craniofacial Research. (2013). *Oral Conditions in children with special needs: A
    guide for health care providers.* Retrieved from http://www.nidcr.nih.gov/OralHealth/OralHealthInformation/
    ChildrensOralHealth/OralConditionsChildrenSpecialNeeds.htm

DEPRESSION

DEFINITION/ETIOLOGY:

Depression is an affective illness or mood disorder characterized by dysphoric moods (emotions such as sadness, irritability, mood swings, and hopelessness) and affect (sad facies) and self-devaluation (e.g., feeling worthless). Clinical depression is characterized by a combination of specific symptoms that persist *more than three weeks* and *cause functional problems* at home, school or in social relationships. Depression is a leading cause of school failure, especially in students with learning difficulties, and suicidal ideation.

CAUSES:

Primary or familial-genetic depression. About a third of depressed children have a biological parent who is affectively ill. Research suggests that the right parietotemporal cortex of the brain plays a role in depression. In depressed states, there is a relatively low level of the neurotransmitters serotonin and norepinephrine.

Secondary or symptomatic depression is a response to problems such as early childhood traumas, chronic health conditions, learned patterns of helpless thinking, learning disabilities, peer pressure, significant losses or having a family member commit suicide.

Comorbidity with other mental health disorders (anxiety, disruptive disorders, ADHD, substance abuse) is common in adolescents.

SIGNS AND SYMPTOMS:

Depression is expressed differently among age groups. Developmentally, preschoolers may have difficulty expressing feelings and emotions. Symptoms in preschool age children include regression of developmental milestones and nonorganic failure to thrive.

Children are more likely to have:
- Somatic complaints
- Separation anxiety
- Insomnia at night and fears
- Irritability

DEPRESSION *(continued from previous page)*

Adolescents exhibit both emotional and behavioral symptoms:

Emotional:

- Crying spells for no apparent reason
- Irritability
- Difficulty focusing or concentrating – decline in school performance
- Fatigue
- Feelings of helplessness, worthlessness, isolation
- Feeling sad or down
- Tremendous sensitivity to failure or rejection
- Loss of interest and pleasure in developmentally appropriate activities
- Socially withdrawn from friends and family
- Recurrent suicidal ideations

Behavioral:

- Appetite changes associated with weight gain or weight loss
- Agitation, disruptive behavior
- Decrease in school performance
- Insomnia or hypersomnia
- Somatic complaints – headaches, stomachaches, etc.
- Disheveled appearance
- Self-mutilation (cutting, burning, excessive piercing/tattooing)
- Extreme risk taking

MANAGEMENT/TREATMENT:

1. **If immediate danger is suspected, student must not be left alone while 911 or local emergency crisis number is called.**

2. **Therapy:**
   Young children may benefit the most from play therapy. Comprehensive treatment including both individual (cognitive behavioral therapy/interpersonal psychotherapy) and family therapy has been shown to be effective in treating depression in older children and adolescents. The focus is not on emotions, but on behaviors that influence feelings, e.g., "feels sad but act positive to help you feel better."

DEPRESSION *(continued from previous page)*

MANAGEMENT/TREATMENT: *(continued)*

3. **Medication:**
   Treatment may also include the use of antidepressant medication. These drugs affect neurotransmitters such as serotonin and norepinephrine in the brain. The choice of drug is related to age, weight, family history of illness and response to medication, and the nature of depression or its related conditions, e.g., bipolar disorder. Selective serotonin reuptake inhibitors (SSRI's) such as Prozac®, Zoloft® and Paxil® have fewer side effects than older antidepressants. Other classes of drugs include tricyclics and MAOI's (monoamine oxidase inhibitors).

   > **Antidepressants may increase the risk that a child/teen may have suicidal ideations. Closely watch children/teens who take antidepressants. Educate staff and parents/guardians regarding the warning signs of suicide (talking, writing, or drawing about death, giving belongings away, withdrawing from family and friends, etc.).**

4. **Electroconvulsive therapy (ECT)** may be used in adolescents when there is no improvement in symptoms with other therapies.

5. **School-home Communication**
   A team approach with consistent messages from adults at home and school that reassure the child/youth and do not allow him/her to drop routines and social interactions.

FOLLOW UP:
- Collaborate with community based providers
- Monitor for adverse effects from pharmacotherapy
- Section 504 plan for accommodations, if needed
- Emergency Action Plan for students who exhibit behaviors that are safety concerns
- Encourage exercise: clinical evidence links physical activity with mood improvement

DEPRESSION *(continued from previous page)*

POTENTIAL COMPLICATIONS:
- Alcohol/Substance Abuse
- Anxiety
- Family/relationship conflicts
- Involvement with the court system
- School problems
- Social isolation
- Self-mutilation
- Suicide

NOTES:

The school nurse may suspect depression with:
- Teacher referrals for inattention, falling asleep in class (due to inadequate sleep at night).
- Frequent student visits for tiredness, headache, stomachache, panic attack, and muscle aches.
- Vague vision problems.
- Referrals for school avoidance (school "phobia") or declining school performance.
- Informal observation of weight change, disheveled appearance, irritability with friends, dropping out of extracurricular activities.
- Consider depression as a significant factor in students with learning failures or discipline infractions, e.g., fights, especially among males.
- Anticipate depression as a response to chronic illness, significant losses or stress, abuse, neglect or exposure to violence.

The school nurse is the key school professional to:
- Report responses to medication and communicate any concerns for missed or excessive doses with the parent.
- Inform teachers of anticipated side effects, particularly to prevent misinterpreting student behavior as "under the influence of drugs ".
- Develop a care plan, in partnership with the school-home team, to respond constructively to somatic complaints (without minimizing significant illnesses or injuries) and reinforce positive behaviors, e.g., good attendance, engaging in school activities.

DEPRESSION *(continued from previous page)*

- Educate the student about the need for consistent medication use and to not take anyone else's medication.
- Educate staff and students (health education) to recognize that children of any age can experience and exhibit signs of depression.

Other:

- Screening in 12-18 year olds for major depression is recommended by the U.S. Prevention Task Force if support systems are in place for diagnosis, therapy and follow up.
- Some diseases such as hypothyroidism or anemia can cause symptoms that look like depression. The healthcare provider may order diagnostic tests to rule out these physical conditions.

Resources

1. Families for Depression Awareness. http://familyaware.org. Webinars, tip sheets.
2. National Association of School Nurses. http://www.nasn.org/MentalHealth. Helpful handouts including interventions and screening.
3. SAMHSA's NationalSAMHSA's National Registry of Evidenced Based Programs and Practices. http://nrepp.samhsa.gov/SearchResultsNew.aspx?s=b&q=depression

References

Bobo, N., Kimel, L., & Bleza, S. (2013). Mental health screening. In J. Selekman (Ed.), *School nursing: A comprehensive text (2ⁿᵈ ed.),* (p. 466). Philadelphia, PA: F.A. Davis.

Mayo Clinic. (2012). *Teen depression.* Retrieved from http://www.mayoclinic.org/diseases-conditions/teen-depression/basics/definition/con-20035222

National Institute of Mental Health. (2015). *Antidepressant medications for children and adolescents: Information for parents and caregivers.* Retrieved from: http://www.nimh.nih.gov/health/topics/child-and-adolescent-mental-health/antidepressant-medications-for-children-and-adolescents-information-for-parents-and-caregivers.shtml

National Institute of Mental Health. (2015). *Depression.* Retrieved from http://www.nimh.nih.gov/health/publications/depression/complete-index.shtml

Ratey, J., & Hagerman, E. (2008). *Spark: The revolutionary new science of exercise and the brain* (pp. 113-140). New York: Little, Brown.

Selekman, J., Diefenbeck, C., Guthrie, S. (2013) Mental health concerns. In J. Selekman (Ed.), *School nursing: A comprehensive text (2ⁿᵈ ed.),* (pp. 945-952). Philadelphia, PA: F.A. Davis.

United States Preventive Task Force. (2013). *Major depressive disorder in children and adolescents.* Retrieved from http://www.uspreventiveservicestaskforce.org/uspstf/uspschdepr.htm

DIABETES – TYPE 1

DEFINITION/ETIOLOGY:

Type 1 Diabetes, previously called juvenile or insulin-dependent diabetes, is an autoimmune disease in which there is destruction of the beta cells (insulin producing cells) of the pancreas and leads to absolute insulin deficiency. Insulin is a hormone that is necessary to convert food into energy for normal body functioning. Without insulin, food is converted into high glucose levels in the blood stream, depriving the brain and muscles of glucose needed to function. In the U.S., about 3 out of 1000 people develop type 1 diabetes.

Type 1 diabetes was thought to be of sudden onset, but research suggests that the autoimmune process progresses over time and presents rather suddenly with hyperglycemia when the declining number of beta-cells can no longer compensate. It is usually diagnosed during childhood and requires lifelong insulin replacement, by multiple daily injections with syringe/vial or pen/needle or continuous insulin infusion via an insulin pump.

Normal fasting blood glucose is 70-100 mg/dl. Due to frequent changing needs during times of rapid growth and development, a child may have higher glucose goals. High blood sugar levels in the blood can lead to Diabetic Ketoacidosis (DKA), breaking down of fat and muscle, resulting in production of ketone (acid) bodies, dehydration, cerebral edema, and potentially death. Low blood sugar levels in the blood can lead to loss of consciousness, brain damage, and potentially death.

The management strategies used to achieve and maintain normal blood sugar levels are individualized for each child. The advances in technology have provided more options for treatment than ever before.

COMORBID CONDITIONS:

Thyroid dysfunction
Celiac Disease
Vitamin B deficiency

DIABETES – TYPE 1 *(continued from previous page)*

SIGNS AND SYMPTOMS:

Hyperglycemia:
- Increased thirst
- Increased urination
- Increased hunger
- Unexplained weight loss
- Fatigue
- Slow healing wounds
- Vision changes

Hypoglycemia*:
- Shakiness
- Dizziness
- Pale skin
- Weakness
- Confusion
- Behavior change/irritability/emotional
- Loss of consciousness
- Seizure

*Some children do not demonstrate any outward symptoms of hypoglycemia or may have hypoglycemic unawareness (inability to recognize symptoms of low blood glucose).

MANAGEMENT/TREATMENT:

1. Monitor blood glucose levels with glucometer (may also have a continuous glucose monitoring system- CGM) per healthcare provider orders. Often testing is before snack, lunch, gym/sports and as needed for symptoms of hypoglycemia and hyperglycemia.

2. Insulin - delivery systems vary among children and dosages vary with each administration. Basal/Bolus regimen mostly mimics the normal pancreatic function. Dosing may be based on a sliding scale, carb to insulin ratio and sensitivity factors.

3. Exercise is important in maintaining stable blood glucose levels. Exercise is a risk factor for hypoglycemia that can occur during the activity, right after the activity and up to 48 hours after an activity. Exercise is not recommended when blood glucose is elevated and/or urine ketones are present due to increased risk of DKA; follow healthcare provider orders.

DIABETES – TYPE 1 *(continued from previous page)*

4. Healthy well balanced diet is recommended for all children. Insulin dosing is often related to total carbohydrate count of each meal and current blood sugar level. Be aware of nutrition changes that may affect the carbohydrate count to avoid overdosing of insulin (many schools are decreasing carbohydrates to improve nutrition).

5. Treatment of hypoglycemia follows "The Rule of 15"- 15 grams of carbohydrate and recheck in 15 minutes for mild hypoglycemia. Moderate episodes of hypoglycemia may require the use of glucose gel if alert, but unable to follow directions. Emergency glucagon administration for episodes of severe hypoglycemia and the child is unconscious or has a seizure. (See Diabetes Emergencies Guidelines).

6. Treatment of hyperglycemia per the child's emergency plan. Encourage drinking water. Urine or blood ketone testing as ordered by healthcare provider during episodes of hyperglycemia and illness. (See Diabetes Emergencies Guidelines).

General Management

Diabetes requires an individualized care and lifestyle plan balancing daily dietary intake, physical activity, insulin, and self-monitored blood glucose. Children can learn to use glucometers and be able to interpret results, self-administer insulin, determine insulin dosage, and ultimately self-manage Type 1 Diabetes. Age and developmental stage are factors in identifying tasks children can safely manage.

A lab test called Hemoglobin A1c (HbA1c) measures the past 3-4 months' fasting and post-meal (postprandial) blood glucose levels to indicate the effectiveness of blood glucose control. According to the American Diabetes Association, an A1c goal of <7.5% is recommended for all children under the age of 19 diagnosed with type 1 diabetes.

A team approach including students, families, healthcare providers, and school staff (food services, physical education, counseling staff, teachers, bus drivers and administration) led by the school nurse, can assist with risk reduction as well as disease management. The school nurse is the coordinator of care in school, but all staff that have responsibility for the student should have basic training to understand Type 1 diabetes and the needs of these students. Diabetes management training for school personnel is recommended to follow three levels of training.

DIABETES – TYPE 1 *(continued from previous page)*

- Level One training should be provided as basic information to all personnel.
- Level Two training is more in depth for those who have direct contact with the child during the school day.
- Level Three training is in-depth training for a small group of unlicensed personnel who will assist with specific diabetes management tasks in those states that allow the registered nurse to delegate such tasks (see your state Nurse Practice Act).

Healthcare provider orders provide the basis of the Diabetes Medical Management Plan (DMMP). From the DMMP, the school nurse develops an individualized healthcare plan (IHP) to guide management throughout the school day. An emergency care plan (ECP) is developed to help guide the management during episodes of hypo/hyperglycemia. These documents are necessary attachments to Section 504 and IEP accommodation plans recommended for all children with Type 1 Diabetes. The individualized healthcare plan should be adapted to the student's developmental level. As appropriate, the plan includes immediate access to diabetes supplies and permission to self-manage tasks in the classroom or least restrictive setting. The plan also addresses emergency evacuation/school lock-down instructions.

FOLLOW-UP:
- Routine blood glucose monitoring
- Monitor height, weight, and blood pressure
- Dietary goals – reinforce need for healthy eating habits
- Review carbohydrate counting
- Encourage routine exercise

POTENTIAL COMPLICATIONS:
Short term
- Hypoglycemia
- Hyperglycemia
- Diabetic ketoacidosis (DKA)

Long term
- Cardiovascular disease
- Neuropathy
- Retinopathy
- Gastroparesis
- Susceptible to skin infections

DIABETES – TYPE 1 *(continued from previous page)*

NOTES:

Type 1 diabetes cannot be prevented. Fluctuations in blood glucose are frequent in children and adolescents due to many controllable and uncontrollable factors. Nutrition, exercise, insulin dosing are controllable factors. Illness, stress, hormones, and developmental factors are uncontrollable. Every child is unique in how their body responds to different insulin doses, foods, activities and this changes over time. Many factors must be considered when setting goals and planning for the care of the child with Type 1 Diabetes.

References

American Diabetes Association. (2013). *Diabetes care in the school and day care setting, 36* (Supplement 1), S75-S79. doi: 10.2337/dc13-S075. Retrieved from http://care.diabetesjournals.org/content/36/Supplement_1/S75.full

American Diabetes Association. (2015). Standards of medical care in diabetes – 2015. *Journal of Clinical and Applied Research and Education- Diabetes Care, 38 (1), S70 – S76. Retrieved from* http://diabetes.teithe.gr/UsersFiles/entypa/STANDARDS%20OF%20MEDICAL%20CARE%20IN%20DIABETES%202015.pdf

Bobo, N. & Silverstein, J. (2010). Designing diabetes management training for school personnel using a three-level approach. *NASN School Nurse, 25*, 216-218. doi: 10.1177/1942602X10375719

Butler, S., Kaup, T., Swanson, M.A., & Hoffman. S. (2013). Diabetes management in the school setting. *In J. Selekman (Ed.), School nursing a comprehensive text* (2nd ed.) (pp. 872-895). Philadelphia, PA: F. A. Davis.

Cleveland Clinic. (2015). Diabetes Basics. Retrieved from http://my.clevelandclinic.org/health/diseases_conditions/hic_diabetes_Basics/

National Association of School Nurses. (2015). *Helping administer to the needs of students with diabetes in school (HANDS).* Silver Spring, MD: Author.

National Association of School Nurses. (2014). *Managing diabetes at school: Tools for the school nurse.* Silver Spring, MD: Author.

National Association of School Nurses. (2012). Diabetes *management in the school setting* (Position Statement). *Retrieved from* https://www.nasn.org/PolicyAdvocacy/PositionPapersandReports/NASNPositionStatementsFullView/tabid/462/ArticleId/22/Diabetes-Management-in-the-School-Setting-Adopted-January-2012

National Diabetes Education Program. (2012). *Helping the student with diabetes succeed: A guide for school personnel.* Retrieved from http://www.ndep.nih.gov/publications/PublicationDetail.aspx?PubId=97&redirect=true#main

DIABETES – TYPE 2

DEFINITION/ETIOLOGY:

Type 2 Diabetes, formerly called adult-onset or non-insulin dependent diabetes, was once an adulthood disease. With the rising incidence of obesity, there is also a rise in Type 2 diabetes in our youth, particularly those 10 years of age and older. Currently, 20-25% of new cases of diabetes in youth are children with Type 2 Diabetes. Statistics are limited due to the lack of diagnosis and proper screening. With an increased focus on this growing pediatric issue, guidelines and recommendations have been developed for screening and treatment, leading to diagnoses that are more accurate.

Type 2 diabetes is defined by impaired secretion of the hormone insulin from the beta cells of the pancreas, insulin-resistance, or a combination of both processes. This "results from a progressive insulin secretory defect on the background of insulin resistance" (ADA, 2013a). This is unlike Type 1 diabetes where there is an absolute insulin deficiency. Insulin is a hormone that is necessary to convert food into energy for normal body functioning. Without enough insulin, food is converted into high glucose levels in the blood stream, depriving the brain and muscles of glucose. The accumulation of glucose within the blood stream damages tissues and blood vessels, leading to nephropathy/kidney disease, retinopathy/eye disease, neuropathy/nervous system, gastroparesis (slowing of the digestive system), heart disease, risk of stroke, poor wound healing and amputations.

Type 2 Diabetes results from a physiological resistance to rising levels of insulin in the presence of being significantly overweight and physically inactive. The addition of high blood pressure and abnormal blood lipids, especially low HDLs and high triglycerides, to diabetes forms a triad called metabolic syndrome that poses a risk for cardiovascular disease associated with diabetes. Obesity is a common precursor. While there is a genetic predisposition for Type 2 Diabetes, it requires an "environment" to develop - usually being overweight (especially with a body type that stores excess fat around the waist more than the hips) due to high calorie diet and too little activity. Detected early, type 2 can be treated by changes in diet and daily activity but may require oral medication and, at times, insulin injections.

COMORBID CONDITIONS:
- Polycystic Ovarian Syndrome (PCOS)
- Hypertension
- Dyslipidemia
- Fatty liver

DIABETES – TYPE 2 *(continued from previous page)*

RISK FACTORS:
- Obesity- BMI 85th-94th and >95th percentile for age and gender
- Family history of Type 2 Diabetes
- Ethnicity - Hispanic, Non-Hispanic white, African American, Asian/Pacific Islander
- Sedentary lifestyle
- Low socioeconomic status
- Small-for-gestational age birth-weight
- Maternal history of gestational diabetes during pregnancy during the child's gestation

Type 2 Diabetes risk factor identification is an important aspect of prevention and control.

SIGNS AND SYMPTOMS:
Hyperglycemia:
- Increased thirst
- Increased urination
- Increased hunger
- Unexplained weight loss/no weight change
- Vaginal yeast infections
- Fatigue
- Slow healing wounds
- Vision changes
- Acanthosis Nigricans (later sign of insulin resistance) - dark, velvety textured skin primarily noted in the axillary, inner elbow, posterior neck and groin areas that signify insulin resistance that may or may not be present with Type 2 Diabetes

Hypoglycemia:
- Shakiness
- Dizziness
- Pale skin
- Weakness
- Confusion
- Behavior change/irritability/emotional
- Loss of consciousness**
- Seizure**

*Some children do not demonstrate any outward symptoms of hypoglycemia or may have hypoglycemic unawareness (inability to recognize symptoms of low blood glucose).
**Severe hypoglycemia is not as common with Type 2 Diabetes, but should be considered when on insulin management.

DIABETES – TYPE 2 *(continued from previous page)*

MANAGEMENT/TREATMENT:

1. Monitor blood glucose levels with glucometer if ordered (may also have a continuous glucose monitoring system- CGM) per healthcare provider orders. Testing recommendations are for those who are taking insulin or oral medications with a risk of hypoglycemia, who may be initiating or changing treatment regimens or have concurrent illnesses.

2. Metformin (only oral medication approved for children with Type 2 Diabetes), may be ordered. Metformin is recommended as a first-line therapy, unless initial diagnosis included DKA. If there is significant hyperglycemia, insulin may be initiated to reverse glucose toxicity. Insulin delivery systems and dosages vary. There is potential to discontinue insulin, begin oral therapy and progress to management with diet, and exercise only (unlike Type 1 Diabetes where insulin is the only option for treatment).

3. Exercise to improve blood glucose control because of decreased insulin resistance. Additionally, weight maintenance or weight loss may minimize complications of diabetes. Activity recommendations are for 60 minutes of exercise daily.

4. A healthy, well balanced diet is recommended for all children. If child or youth is being treated with insulin, dosing is usually related to total carbohydrate count of each meal along with blood glucose level.

5. Treatment of hypoglycemia follows "The Rule of 15"- 15 grams of carbohydrate and recheck in 15 minutes for mild hypoglycemia. Moderate episodes of hypoglycemia may require the use of glucose gel if alert, but unable to follow directions. Emergency glucagon administration for episodes of severe hypoglycemia and the child is unconscious or has a seizure. (See Diabetes Emergencies Guidelines). **While glucagon may not be prescribed for the child with Type 2 Diabetes, it should be considered if the child is treated with insulin.

6. Treatment of hyperglycemia per the child's emergency plan. Encourage drinking water. Urine or blood ketone testing as ordered by healthcare provider during episodes of hyperglycemia and illness. (See Diabetes Emergencies Guidelines). **Often ketone testing is NOT ordered for children with Type 2 Diabetes due to decreased risk for DKA.

** **Severe hypoglycemia is not as common with Type 2 Diabetes, but should be considered when on insulin management.**

DIABETES – TYPE 2 *(continued from previous page)*

General Management

Diabetes requires an individualized care and lifestyle plan balancing daily dietary intake, physical activity, medication (if ordered) and self-monitored blood glucose. Children can learn to use glucometers and, in time, to self-administer insulin as ordered. A lab test called Hemoglobin A1c (HbA1c) measures the past 3-4 months' fasting and post meal blood glucose levels to indicate the effectiveness of blood glucose control. While a non-diabetic HbA1c ranges from 4-6%, the goal for the child with Type 2 Diabetes is <7% (Copeland et.al, 2013).

A team approach including students, families, healthcare providers, and school staff (food services, physical education, counseling staff, teachers, bus drivers and administration) led by the school nurse, can assist with risk reduction as well as disease management. The school nurse is the coordinator of care in school, but all staff that have responsibility for the student should have basic training to understand Type 2 Diabetes and the needs of these students. Diabetes management training for school personnel is recommended to follow three levels of training. Level One training should be provided as basic information to all personnel. Level Two training is more in depth for those who have direct contact with the child during the school day. Level Three training is in-depth training for a small group of unlicensed personnel who will assist with specific diabetes management for the student, for those states that allow the registered nurse to delegate tasks (see your state Nurse Practice Act).

Healthcare provider orders provide the basis of the Diabetes Medical Management Plan (DMMP). From the DMMP, the school nurse develops an individualized healthcare plan (IHP) to guide management throughout the school day. An emergency healthcare plan (ECP) is developed to help guide the management during episodes of hypo/hyperglycemia. These documents are necessary attachments to Section 504 and IEP accommodation plans recommended for all children with Type 2 Diabetes. The individualized healthcare plan should be adapted to the student's developmental level. As appropriate, the plan includes immediate access to diabetes supplies and permission to self-manage tasks in the classroom or least restrictive setting. The plan also addresses emergency evacuation/school lock-down instructions.

DIABETES – TYPE 2 *(continued from previous page)*

FOLLOW-UP:
- Routine blood glucose monitoring, if ordered
- Monitor height, weight, and blood pressure
- Dietary goals – reinforce need for healthy eating habits
- Review carbohydrate counting/plate method for healthy nutrition
- Encourage routine exercise - at least 60 minutes of moderate to vigorous activity daily

POTENTIAL COMPLICATIONS:
Short term
- Hypoglycemia
- Hyperglycemia

Long term
- Cardiovascular disease
- Nephropathy
- Neuropathy
- Retinopathy
- Susceptible to skin infections
- Gastroparesis

DIABETES – TYPE 2 *(continued from previous page)*

References

American Diabetes Association. (2015). Standards of medical care in diabetes – 2015. *Journal of Clinical and Applied Research and Education- Diabetes Care, 38 (1), S40 – S44. Retrieved from* http://diabetes.teithe.gr/UsersFiles/entypa/ STANDARDS%20OF%20MEDICAL%20CARE%20IN%20DIABETES%202015.pdf

American Diabetes Association. (2013). *Diabetes care in the school and day care setting, 36* (Supplement 1), S75-S79. doi: 10.2337/dc13-S075. Retrieved from http://care.diabetesjournals.org/content/36/Supplement_1/S75.full

Copeland, K.C., Silverstein, J., Moore, K.R., Prazar, G.E., Raymer, T., Shiffman, R.N.,..., & Flinn, S. K. (2013). Management of newly diagnosed type 2 diabetes mellitus (T2DM) in children and adolescents. *Pediatrics, 131,*364-382. *doi: 10.1542/ peds.2012-3494*

Flint, A. & Aslanian, S. (2011). Treatment of Type 2 diabetes in youth. *Journal of Clinical and Applied Research and Education Diabetes Care, 34*(2), S177-S183. doi: 10.2337/dc11-s215. Retrieved from http://care.diabetesjournals.org/ content/34/Supplement_2/S177.full.pdf+html /

National Association of School Nurses. (2015). *Helping administer to the needs of students with diabetes in school (HANDS).* Silver Spring, MD: Author. Retrieved from http://www.nasn.org/ContinuingEducation/ LiveContinuingEducationPrograms/HANDS

National Association of School Nurses. (2014). *Managing diabetes at school: Tools for the school nurse.* Silver Spring, MD: Author.

National Diabetes Education Program. (2012). *Helping the student with diabetes succeed: A guide for school personnel.* Retrieved from http://www.ndep.nih.gov/publications/PublicationDetail.aspx?PubId=97&redirect=true#main

Today Study Group. (2010). Design of a family-based lifestyle intervention for youth with type 2 diabetes: The TODAY study. *International Journal of Obesity 2010, 34*(2), 217-26. doi: 10.1038/ijo.2009.195. Retrieved from http://www.ncbi.nlm.nih.gov/pmc/articles/PMC2822093/

DIABETES EMERGENCIES (Also see Diabetes Type I)

DEFINITION/ETIOLOGY:
A diabetic emergency is a life-threatening condition. Diabetic emergencies occur when there is a severe imbalance between insulin and blood glucose in the body. There are two types of diabetic emergencies: hypoglycemia and hyperglycemia.

HYPOGLYCEMIA

Hypoglycemia is low blood sugar and is considered a medical emergency. Causes are:
- Too much insulin
- Not enough food or student eats less than insulin dose calculated
- Delayed snack or missed meal
- Too much exercise without snack before
- Some prescribed or over-the-counter medication

SIGNS AND SYMPTOMS: HYPOGLYCEMIA
- Vary from person to person
- Symptoms develop rapidly without warning
- Children may not always demonstrate outward symptoms
- Young children especially may not recognize symptoms of hypoglycemia

Mild	Moderate	Severe
o Blurred vision o Difficulty concentrating or inattention o Headache, hungry o Irritable o Nausea and/or vomiting o Shaky, stomach ache, o Sweaty and/or pale	o Disoriented o Confusion o Poor coordination o Restlessness o Mood changes (aggression, crying, bizarre behavior) o Drowsy	o Inability to swallow o Seizures o Unconscious

DIABETES EMERGENCIES *(continued from previous page)*

MANAGEMENT/TREATMENT: HYPOGLYCEMIA

Hypoglycemia low blood sugar (<70 mg/dL or > 70 mg/dL with symptoms)

- Follow student's Emergency Care Plan (ECP). Note student specific blood glucose targets.
- If possible, check blood sugar and follow ECP, immediately give 15 gram fast-acting carbohydrate such as one of the following:
  - 3 or 4 glucose tablets
  - 4 oz. fruit juice or regular soft drink (not diet)
  - 1-2 Tablespoons of honey or sugar
  - 1 tube glucose gel
- Follow with protein snack plus if it is more than a one hour until meal time.
- Recheck blood glucose level 15 minutes after treatment.
- If blood glucose level is still below target range, repeat treatment, contact parent/ guardian.

Severe hypoglycemic reaction:

- If student becomes unconscious, has a seizure or is unable to swallow, administer glucagon IM or SQ per licensed healthcare provider's order.
- Call 911 if glucagon is administered.
- Position student on side as vomiting is a side effect of glucagon.

HYPERGLYCEMIA

Hyperglycemia is high blood sugar and is not considered a medical emergency in the acute stage. Untreated hyperglycemia can progress to ketoacidosis, which is a medical emergency.

Causes are:

- Late or missed insulin
- Illness, infection, stress, hormonal response (e.g., menses)
- Expired insulin
- Problem with insulin pump
- Excess food intake (for amount of insulin or binge eating)
- Insufficient exercise

DIABETES EMERGENCIES *(continued from previous page)*

SIGNS AND SYMPTOMS: HYPERGLYCEMIA

- Usually develops slowly

Mild	Moderate (mild symptoms plus)	Severe (DKA)
○ Increased thirst ○ Increased urination ○ Stomach ache ○ Blurred vision ○ Fatigue ○ Hunger, headache ○ Pale	○ Inability to concentrate ○ Abdominal cramps ○ Nausea ○ Dry Mouth ○ Light headed	○ Nausea and/or vomit ○ Abdominal cramps ○ Lethargic ○ Breath that smells fruity ○ Respiratory problems, Shortness of breath ○ Weakness ○ Confused ○ Moderate to Large ketones

MANAGEMENT/TREATMENT: HYPERGLYCEMIA (Blood sugar > 300)

- Follow student's ECP.
- Check urine for ketones and report findings.
- Encourage water and moderate exercise only if ketones are negative.
- Repeat ketone testing in 1-2 hours or next void.
- Supplemental insulin may be ordered by licensed healthcare provider.
- Notify parent/guardian.

ROLE OF THE SCHOOL NURSE:

- Develop and implement an Individualized Healthcare Plan (IHP) and an Emergency Plan (ECP) from student's Diabetes Medical Management Plan which includes:
  - ○ Specific detailed procedures and responsibilities performed by school staff
  - ○ Glucagon administration and storage
  - ○ Specific Section 504 Plan
  - ○ Disaster Plan
- Provide diabetes training (Level I, II or III based on need know) to teachers, cafeteria manager, bus driver and sports coaches.
- Manage and monitor trained staff.
- Distribution of the ECP to appropriate classrooms and staff.
- Students with insulin pumps require the nurse and staff (as appropriate) to be oriented to the specific unit.

DIABETES EMERGENCIES *(continued from previous page)*

FOLLOW UP:
- Monitor student for continued sign or symptoms of hypoglycemia or hyperglycemia.
- Report incidence to parents/guardians as required by ECP.
- Inventory supplies used to treat hypoglycemia or hyperglycemia.

PREVENTION:
- Obtain from history and review signs and symptoms of hypoglycemia and hyperglycemia experienced with individual student (if known).
- Consistent routine (meal times, carbohydrate intake and physical activity).
- Notify parents/guardians in advance of schedule changes and special events.
- Provide a snack if physical activity occurs just before lunch period or in the late afternoon.
- Keep a fast-acting carbohydrate accessible during exercise.
- Keep emergency glucose/sugar in key places, especially in large schools (PE, nurse's office, locker, main office).

NOTES:
- Check state laws, nurse practice act and school district policy to determine what tasks of diabetes care can be delegated to Unlicensed School Personnel.
- Glucagon usually works within 10 minutes.
- Student should wear Medic Alert identification.

ADDITIONAL RESOURCES:
- American Diabetes Association. Provides staff training tools and sample diabetes management and Section 504 plans. www.diabetes.org
- National Association of School Nurses. Helping Administer to the Needs of Students with Diabetes in School (HANDS) is a continuing education resource. http://www.nasn.org/ContinuingEducation/LiveContinuingEducationPrograms/HANDS
- National Diabetes Education Program. Diabetes Resources for Schools and Youth http://www.ndep.nih.gov/hcp-businesses-and-schools/Schools.aspx

DIABETES EMERGENCIES *(continued from previous page)*

References

American Diabetes Association. (2015). *Ketoacidosis.* Retrieved from http://www.diabetes.org/living-with-diabetes/complications/ketoacidosis-dka.html

American Diabetes Association. (2014). *Hyperglycemia.* Retrieved from http://www.diabetes.org/living-with-diabetes/treatment-and-care/blood-glucose-control/hyperglycemia.html

American Diabetes Association. (2014). *Hypoglycemia.* Retrieved from http://www.diabetes.org/living-with-diabetes/treatment-and-care/blood-glucose-control/hypoglycemia-low-blood.html

Butler, S., Kaup, T., Swanson, M., & Hoffmann, S. (2013). Diabetes management in the school setting. In J. Selekman (Ed.), *School nursing: A comprehensive text* (2nd ed.) (pp. 888-892). Philadelphia, PA: F.A. Davis

Mayo Clinic. (2015). *Diabetic coma.* Retrieved from http://www.mayoclinic.com/print/diabeticcoma/DS00656/METHOD=print&DSECTION=all

National Association of School Nurses. (2015). *Helping administer to the needs of students with diabetes in school (HANDS).* Retrieved from http://www.nasn.org/ContinuingEducation/LiveContinuingEducationPrograms/HANDS

National Association of School Nurses. (2014). Managing *diabetes at school: Tools for the school nurse.* Silver Spring, MD: Author.

National Diabetes Education Program. (2012). *Helping the student with diabetes succeed: A guide for school personnel.* Retrieved from http://ndep.nih.gov/publications/PublicationDetail.aspx?PubId=97

DIARRHEA

DEFINITION/ETIOLOGY:
Diarrhea is an increase in the number of stools (3 or more per day) and a loosening/softening in consistency in relation to the patient's normal stooling pattern. Severe diarrheal stools are watery, may be green and/or contain mucous or blood. Diarrhea can be acute or chronic. Acute diarrhea is typically caused by parasites, bacterial or viral infections. Diarrhea is considered chronic if it lasts longer than two weeks. There are many causes of diarrhea. The most common causes of diarrhea are viruses, bacteria, parasites, and medications.

Below is a partial list of common causes leading to diarrhea.

Infections
- Acute gastroenteritis (viral) – norovirus, viral hepatitis, rotavirus
- Bacterial diarrhea – salmonella, shigella, E. Coli, campylobacter
- Parasites (Giardia, cryptosporidium)

Diseases of the colon
- Celiac disease
- Crohn's disease
- Ulcerative colitis
- Irritable Bowel Syndrome (IBS)

Psychogenic diarrhea
- Fear/anxiety
- Encopresis

Other
- Cystic fibrosis
- Parasites (round worms, tapeworms)
- Gastrointestinal
- Food allergy/Food intolerance/Lactose intolerance
- Antibiotic diarrhea
- Laxatives
- Artificial sweeteners
- Constipation with fecal retention

DIARRHEA *(continued from previous page)*

SIGNS AND SYMPTOMS:
- Abdominal pain, abdominal cramps, or bloating
- Viral gastroenteritis – vomiting and frequent watery diarrhea stools
- Bacterial enteritis often causes a rapid onset of diarrhea without vomiting and greater than four diarrhea stools per day with blood or mucous
- May have signs of dehydration (decreased urine output, thickening of saliva, thirst, feeling dizzy when standing up, etc.)
- Vital signs—may have increased pulse and lower blood pressure if dehydrated
- Fever is sometimes present, but usually not high
- Weight loss

MANAGEMENT/TREATMENT:
1. Treatment is dependent on etiology. Treat underlying cause.
2. Monitor for signs and symptoms of dehydration (tachycardia, hypotension, lethargy).
3. If signs of dehydration are present, refer immediately.
4. If well hydrated but acutely ill, notify parent/guardian.
5. If all symptoms are mild, observe in clinic and offer preferably oral rehydrating solution or clear liquids. Notify parent/guardian.
6. Although many cases of diarrhea are not caused by an infectious disease, public health guidelines may call for the exclusion of the child from school or childcare if the feces are not able to be contained in a diaper or in a toilet.
7. Very young children who attend school, significantly developmentally delayed children of any age, or children whose physical disabilities include lack of bowel control, are the children who may need to be excluded for diarrhea, even if the cause is known to be non-infectious.
8. **Diarrhea from suspected or known food borne-illnesses is reportable to the health department, in most states.**
9. Instruct parent/guardian to notify healthcare provider immediately if no urine output for 12 hours, temperature 102°F or greater, blood or mucous noted in stool, severe abdominal pain, no tears when crying , irritability or lethargy.

FOLLOW UP:
- Obtain diagnosis and assess the risk to fellow students.
- Examine child on re-entry to school (temperature and hydration status).
- Give medication as prescribed.
- Report any relapse.

DIARRHEA *(continued from previous page)*

POTENTIAL COMPLICATIONS:
Dehydration is a complication of intense diarrhea due to the loss of excess fluids and electrolytes. Dehydration limits the body's ability to carry out normal functions due to the lack of water/fluid intake. **Serious consequences can result if lost fluids are not replenished. Note:** Immunocompromised individuals are increased risk of dehydration.

NOTES:
Prevention

- Proper handwashing prevents the spread of viral diarrhea.
- Guard against contaminated food.
- Watch what you eat and drink if traveling to developing countries.
- Educate parent/guardian(s) on vaccine preventable diarrhea (rotavirus).

References

American Academy of Pediatrics. (2013). *Diarrhea*. Retrieved from http://kidshealth.org/parent/infections/common/diarrhea.html#

Centers for Disease Control and Prevention (CDC). (2013).*Norovirus*. Retrieved from http://www.cdc.gov/norovirus/about/overview.html

Mayo Clinic. (2013). *Diarrhea*. Retrieved from http://www.mayoclinic.org/diseases-conditions/diarrhea/basics/definition/con-20014025

Merck Manual. (2013). *Diarrhea in children*. Retrieved from http://www.merckmanuals.com/professional/pediatrics/approach_to_the_care_of_normal_infants_and_children/diarrhea_in_children.html?qt=diarrhea&alt=sh

National Digestive Diseases Information Clearinghouse (NDDIC). (2013). *Diarrhea*. Retrieved from http://www.niddk.nih.gov/health-information/health-topics/digestive-diseases/diarrhea/Pages/facts.aspx

WebMD. (2015). *Diarrhea: Why it happens and how to treat it*. Retrieved from http://www.webmd.com/digestive-disorders/digestive-diseases-diarrhea?page=2

DIPHTHERIA

DEFINITION/ETIOLOGY:

Diphtheria is an acute, highly contagious, potentially life-threatening infection caused by *Corynebacterium diphtheriae* that can either invade the pharyngeal site or present as a cutaneous infection. In the respiratory system the bacteria produces a toxin. It is transmitted from person-to-person through respiratory droplets (coughing or sneezing). Persons can also become infected by coming in contact fomites, an object (telephone, keyboard, doorknobs, toys, and dish) that has been contaminated by an infected person. Contact with infected skin lesions can also spread the infection. Humans are the only known reservoir for *C. diphtheria*. Today, diphtheria is rare in the United States and other developed countries due to widespread vaccination programs.

SIGNS AND SYMPTOMS:
Pharyngeal/Respiratory Diphtheria

- Weakness
- Sore throat
- Fever and chills
- Swollen glands (neck)
- Difficulty swallowing
- Loss of appetite
- Within 2-3 days, a thick coating (pseudomembrane) can build up in the throat or nose; may cause difficulty breathing
- The toxin may be absorbed into the heart, kidneys, and nerves

The normal incubation period is 2 to 5 days, although it could range 1 to 10 days from the time of exposure to onset of symptoms. Diagnosis is determined by symptoms (gray colored pseudomembrane covering nose/throat). Definite diagnosis is made by laboratory results of throat or lesion swabs – confirming the presence of toxin in the body. Treatment begins when a diagnosis of Diphtheria is suspected.

DIPHTHERIA *(continued from previous page)*

MANAGEMENT/TREATMENT:
- Hospitalization.
- Diphtheria Antitoxin (DAT) to counteract toxin.
- Antibiotics (penicillin or erythromycin) to kill and eliminate bacteria.
- If experiencing respiratory difficulties – healthcare provider may remove pseudomembrane covering nose and/or throat.
- Isolation until no longer able to infect others, usually after completing a 48 hour antibiotic regime.
- Untreated person who is infected may be contagious for up to 4 weeks. If the person is treated appropriately, the contagious period can be limited to less than 4 days.
- Diphtheria is a reportable disease (local health department).
- Follow local and state health department guidelines regarding potential outbreak control and management.

FOLLOW-UP:
- Recovery from diphtheria is not always followed by life-time immunity- post recovery vaccination is needed.

POTENTIAL COMPLICATIONS:
- Obstructed airway
- Myocarditis, endocarditis
- Polyneuropathy
- Paralysis
- Pneumonia
- Respiratory failure
- Septic arthritis
- Mortality rate with treatment is 1 in 10
- Mortality rate without treatment is 1 in 2

NOTES:
Cutaneous Diphtheria
- Rare in the U.S. Persons with poor hygiene or living in crowded conditions are those most often seen with diphtheria.
- Cutaneous diphtheria presents as a scaling rash, lesions, of blisters that can occur anywhere on the body. Lesions may be painful and swollen. The infection is treated by thoroughly cleaning the skin with soap and water and with antibiotics.

DIPHTHERIA *(continued from previous page)*

Prevention
- Vaccine (primary and post-exposure).
- Post exposure antibiotics.
- Diphtheria is a vaccine preventable disease (VPD) when diphtheria vaccine is appropriately given to infants and children, to pre-teens and teens, and to adults.
- Adults should receive Td vaccine every 10 years.
- Childhood vaccination should be routine.
- Follow CDC, AAP, and /or State Departments of Health recommendations for immunization schedules.

References

Centers for Disease Control and Prevention. (2013). *Diphtheria.* Retrieved from http://www.cdc.gov/diphtheria/index.html

Center for Disease Control and Prevention (CDC). (2015). Diphtheria. In J. Hamborsky, A. Kroger, & S. Wolfe (Eds.), *Epidemiology and prevention of vaccine-preventable diseases, the pink book: Course textbook (13th ed.).* Washington D.C. Public Health Foundation. Retrieved from http://www.cdc.gov/vaccines/pubs/pinkbook/dip.html

Mayo Clinic. (2014). *Diphtheria.* Retrieved from http://www.mayoclinic.com/diphtheria/DS00495

Medline Plus. U.S. National Library of Medicine. (2015). *Diphtheria.* Retrieved from https://www.nlm.nih.gov/medlineplus/diphtheria.html

Merck Manual. (2013). *Diphtheria).* Retrieved from http://www.merckmanuals.com/professional/infectious_diseases/gram-positive_bacilli/diphtheria.html?qt=diphtheria&alt=sh

Selekman, J., & Coates, J. (2013). Disease prevention. In J. Selekman (Ed.), *School nursing: A comprehensive text (2nd ed.)* (p. 503). Philadelphia, PA: F.A. Davis.

EAR PAIN

DEFINITION/ETIOLOGY:

Otalgia or earache/pain can be caused by external or middle ear conditions or by referred pain from other sources. Infections of the ear are one of the most common diseases of childhood. The incidence of middle ear infection increases in winter and spring. Conditions of the ear can be responsible for transient hearing loss in students and therefore can have a great impact in the educational setting.

External ear including external auditory canal
- Infection/inflammation (otitis externa, cellulitis, furuncle or abscess, perichondritis of the pinna)
- Cerumen (wax) impaction
- Trauma
- Foreign object
- Tumor or growth

Middle ear - Eustachian tube and Mastoid
- Infection/inflammation (otitis media, middle ear effusion, mastoiditis)
- Trauma
- Tumor or growth
- Allergies

Referred ear pain
- Pharyngeal lesions (peritonsillar abscess, retropharyngeal abscess, nasopharyngeal fibroma)
- Mouth lesions (acute stomatitis or glossitis, dental problem)
- Laryngeal and esophageal sources, e.g., laryngeal ulceration, esophageal foreign body, esophageal reflux (acid reflux)

Other
- Temporomandibular joint (TMJ) dysfunction

EAR PAIN (*continued from previous page*)

SIGNS AND SYMPTOMS:

- **Otitis externa**, or inflammation of the external ear canal, is also called "swimmer's ear." It is commonly seen after frequent exposure to moisture or swimming. *Pseudomonas aeruginosa* is the most common pathogen responsible for otitis externa and *staphylococcus aureus* is also common. The student has pain which may begin gradually or suddenly, and is increased with pressure on the tragus or when the pinna is moved. Otorrhea (discharge coming from the external canal) is common. Erythema (redness) of the ear canal, itching and irritation, pressure and fullness in the ear may be reported. There may be hearing loss if there is enough swelling to occlude the canal.

- **Otitis Media (OM)** is an acute inflammation of the middle ear. It is the most common cause of ear pain, and may accompany a simple "cold". The tympanic membrane is dull, often bulging and sometimes erythematous (red). It often resolves spontaneously. Ear pain, fever, inability to sleep, lethargy, diarrhea and vomiting may be present. Sudden hearing loss may occur. Otitis media may also be classified as Acute Otitis Media (AOM) referring to a sudden onset and the presence of a middle ear effusion.

- **Middle Ear Effusion (**MEE) may complicate an upper respiratory infection. A collection of watery fluid fills the middle ear canal and can interfere with hearing. In most cases, the fluid is absorbed spontaneously within 3 months, but if it persists, it can lead to a hearing loss. The child is often asymptomatic and afebrile but may have mild or intermittent ear pain, fullness, or "popping" in the ear, dizziness, or loss of balance.

- **Otitis Media with Effusion (OME)** is an accumulation of serous fluid in the middle ear without signs and symptoms of acute infection. Between 50 and 79% of children may develop OME after a course of antibiotics for AOM. Bubbles or fluid levels may be seen behind the tympanic membrane.

- **Impacted Cerumen** may cause ear pain if the cerumen hardens and touches the tympanic membrane. Although cerumen is a naturally forming lubricant and protector of the ear canal, excessive production may block the ear canal causing hearing loss until removed.

EAR PAIN (*continued from previous page*)

- **Foreign Objects** may be placed in the ear canal by small children. If present for more than a few days it is likely there will be foul smelling discharge or pain from abrasions to the auditory canal.

Mastoiditis is a severe condition caused by extension of a middle ear infection into the periosteum of the skull. Symptoms would include displacement of the pinna away from the skull, erythema, edema and tenderness on palpation. This would require prompt evaluation from a healthcare provider.

Severe ear pain may be a sign of a ruptured eardrum or foreign body, especially if the onset is sudden.

MANAGEMENT/TREATMENT:

1. The student with severe pain should be evaluated promptly. If a live insect is the cause of pain, inspection by otoscope may be difficult because the light may aggravate an insect and cause additional pain. Notify parents/guardians and advise taking the child to his/her healthcare provider.

2. For otitis externa, the parents/guardians should be advised to take the student to the healthcare provider. Clean any drainage gently from pinna of the ear using clean technique/standard precautions and apply a warm dry compress to the affected ear to relieve pain. Topical antibiotic treatment (eardrops) may be prescribed, but only after confirming that the eardrum is intact. In the eardrum has been perforated a nontoxic topical medication will be ordered. Swimming should be discouraged for 7-10 days and moisture in the ear should be avoided for 4-6 weeks. The parent/guardian should be advised to have the child use ear plugs when swimming. Prevent recurrence (which is common) by instilling 2-3 drops of isopropyl alcohol in the ear canals after swimming, showering or during hot humid weather. Otitis externa should resolve in 7 days.

3. For healthy school-aged children with OM, guidelines recommend observation and pain management for 48 to 72 hours as the majority of OM will resolve spontaneously.

4. Removal of cerumen should be done in the office of the healthcare provider and may be done using a curette or irrigation.

EAR PAIN (*continued from previous page*)

FOLLOW UP:

Screening hearing acuity and comparing the result with a previous screen can be helpful after the student recovers from an acute ear infection. If mild hearing loss is found on screening in the absence of any other signs or discomfort, re-check after about 3 weeks. Most OME will resolve without treatment, but if OME persists for 3 months or at any time, there is a language delay, learning problem, or a significant hearing loss is suspected, a medical referral is indicated.

References

Bowden, V. R. & Greenberg, C. S. (Eds.). (2014). The child with altered sensory status. In *Children and their families: The continuum of care (2nd edition) (pp. 1462-1516). Philadelphia PA: Lippincott Williams and Wilkins.*

Medline Plus, U.S. National Library of Medicine. (2014). *Earache.* Retrieved from http://www.nlm.nih.gov/medlineplus/ency/article/003046.htm

Yellon, R. & Chi, D. (2012). Otolaryngology. In B. J. Zitelli, S. McIntire, & A. J. Nowalk (Eds.), *Atlas of pediatric physical diagnosis* (6th ed.) (p.918). Philadelphia, PA: Elsevier Saunders.

EATING DISORDERS

An eating disorder is marked by severe disturbances in eating behavior, such as extreme reduction of food intake or extreme overeating, along with feelings of significant concern about body weight or shape. Eating disorders have complicated genetic, biological, behavioral, and social causes. According to the National Institute of Mental Health, eating disorders primarily affect females. However, males can also be vulnerable to eating disorders. Two main types are anorexia nervosa and bulimia nervosa. A third category is eating disorders not otherwise specified or EDNOS. These are similar to anorexia or bulimia with slightly different characteristics, such as binge-eating disorder. Eating disorders will often surface during adolescence but can occur at any age. People with eating disorders frequently have other psychiatric disorders including depression, substance abuse, or anxiety. They also can develop serious physical complications such as heart or kidney disorders that can be fatal.

ANOREXIA NERVOSA

DEFINITION/ETIOLOGY:
Anorexia is characterized by induced and sustained weight loss. Speculation on traits that may lead to this disorder are low self-esteem, rigid self-control, fear of maturation, obsession with appearance, and perfectionism.

SIGNS AND SYMPTOMS:
The term anorexia is a misnomer since loss of appetite is rare.
- Refusal to maintain body weight at minimal normal weight for age and height, e.g., weight loss leading to body weight at least 15% below that expected; or failure to make expected weight gain during period of growth.
- Obsessed with their weight. Intense fear of gaining weight or becoming fat, even though underweight.
- Disturbance in the way in which one's body weight, size, or shape is experienced, e.g., the person claims to "feel fat" even if emaciated, believes that one area of the body is "too fat" even when obviously underweight.
- Weight loss accomplished by reduction in total food intake, often with extensive exercising.
- Frequently there is self-induced vomiting, use of laxatives, enemas or diuretics (in such cases Bulimia Nervosa may also be present).
- Often undiagnosed until weight loss is marked. By the time the person is profoundly underweight, there are other signs, such as hypothermia, bradycardia, hypotension, edema, lanugo (fine hair), and a variety of metabolic changes.

EATING DISORDERS *(continued from previous page)*

- Other symptoms may include abnormal laboratory tests (CBC, electrolytes, liver, kidney, etc.), fatigue, insomnia, thinning of hair, dizziness, and/or constipation.
- Amenorrhea - in most cases, amenorrhea follows weight loss, but may appear before noticeable weight loss has occurred.

MANAGEMENT/TREATMENT:
1. **Initial diagnosis** is most important.
   a. Often not suspected at home because child is not seen unclothed.
   b. Alert the PE teacher to monitor.
2. Refer for psychiatric evaluation and counseling as appropriate.
3. Effective treatment is long term.
4. Establish liaison with parents/guardians, healthcare provider, and therapists – develop multidisciplinary approach in health plan in consultation with healthcare provider and therapist along with school mental health staff.

FOLLOW UP:
- Provide safe haven in school health office where the student can freely discuss problems.
- Monitor for secondary physical effects of under-nutrition.
- Relapse is common.
- **Significant mortality if not treated:** involuntary commitment may be considered if refusal to seek psychiatric care.

COMPLICATIONS:
Under-nutrition can become severe enough to affect secondary endocrine, metabolic, and electrolyte disturbances of bodily functions, including osteoporosis. Prolonged anorexia may lead to alcohol and substance addiction, fertility problems and death due to cardiac arrhythmia, congestive heart failure, or suicide.

BULIMIA NERVOSA

DIAGNOSIS/ETIOLOGY:
No single etiological factor; may be combined neurochemical, developmental, cultural, psychological, family, and environment. Dieting is often precursor to disordered eating. A higher rate of reported sexual abuse is seen in females. In order to qualify for this diagnosis, person must have had a minimum of one binge eating episode per week for at least three months.

EATING DISORDERS *(continued from previous page)*

SIGNS AND SYMPTOMS:
- Recurrent episodes of binge eating
- Rapid consumption of a large amount of food in a discrete period of time, usually done in secrecy
- A feeling of lack of control over eating behavior during the eating binges
- Self-induced vomiting, use of laxatives or diuretics, strict dieting or fasting
- Vigorous exercise in order to prevent weight gain
- Persistent over concern with body shape and weight
- Chapped, cracked, irritated, or sore fingers from self-induced vomiting
- If person purges by vomiting, may have tooth enamel damage and sore throats
- Frequent trips to bathroom following meal
- Although most people with Bulimia Nervosa are within a normal weight range, some may be slightly underweight and others may be overweight. Extreme thinness (25% below normal weight) may result
- A depressed mood that may be part of a depressive disorder is commonly observed

MANAGEMENT/TREATMENT:
1. Refer for nutritional counseling, family therapy and/or psychotherapy as appropriate.
2. Cognitive Behavioral Therapy (CBT) may benefit to help focus on and solve problems related to bulimia. CBT may be individual or group-based and is effective in changing binge-eating /purging behaviors and attitudes towards eating.
3. Develop multidisciplinary approach (described in an individualized healthcare plan).
4. Psychotherapeutic drugs may be prescribed if depression is present.

FOLLOW UP:
- Monitor behavior and compliance to mental health and eating plan.
  Note: Eating binges may be planned. The food consumed during a binge often has a high caloric content, a sweet taste, and a texture that facilitates rapid eating. The food is usually eaten in secrecy. The food is usually gobbled rapidly with little chewing. Once eating has begun, additional food may be sought to continue the binge. A binge is usually terminated by the physical pain of abdominal distention allowing either continued eating or termination of the binge and often reduces post-binge anguish. In some cases, vomiting may itself be desired so that the person will binge in order to vomit or will vomit after eating a small amount of food. Although eating binges may be pleasurable, disparaging self-criticism and a depressed mood often follow.
- Frequent weight fluctuations due to alternating binges and fasts are common. Often persons with bulimia feel that their life is dominated by conflicts about eating.

EATING DISORDERS *(continued from previous page)*

COMPLICATIONS:

- Some people with this disorder are subject to psychoactive substance abuse or dependence, most frequently involving sedatives, amphetamines, cocaine, or alcohol.
- Dehydration may lead to kidney failure.
- Repeated vomiting can cause inflammation or tears in the lining of the esophagus and erosion of tooth enamel.
- Electrolyte imbalance may lead to cardiac arrhythmia.
- Under-nutrition can become severe enough to affect secondary endocrine, metabolic, and electrolyte disturbances of bodily functions, including osteoporosis.
- Prolonged bulimia may lead to alcohol and substance addiction, mental health issues, fertility problems and death due to cardiac arrhythmia, congestive heart failure, or suicide.

> **NOTE: Anorexia and bulimia are two serious life-threatening conditions that are curable if identified early, treated by trained therapists, and supplemented by support groups.**

Resources

- National Eating Disorders Association (NEDA) - http://www.nationaleatingdisorders.org/who-we-are
- National Association of Anorexia Nervosa and Associated Disorders - http://www.anad.org/

References

American Psychological Association. (2011). *Eating disorders*. Retrieved from http://www.apa.org/helpcenter/eating.aspx

Mayo Clinic. (2015). *Bulimia nervosa*. Retrieved from http://www.mayoclinic.org/diseases-conditions/bulimia/basics/definition/con-20033050

Mayo Clinic. (2015). *Eating disorders*. Retrieved from http://www.mayoclinic.org/diseases-conditions/eating-disorders/basics/definition/con-20033575

Medline Plus. (2015). *Eating disorders*. Retrieved from https://www.nlm.nih.gov/medlineplus/eatingdisorders.html#summary

Merck Manual. (2014). *Anorexia nervosa*. Retrieved from http://www.mayoclinic.org/diseases-conditions/eating-disorders/basics/definition/con-20033575

National Eating Disorders Association. (n.d.). Get the facts on eating disorders. Retrieved from https://www.nationaleatingdisorders.org/get-facts-eating-disorders

National Institute of Mental Health. (2014). *Eating disorders*. Retrieved from http://www.nimh.nih.gov/health/publications/eating-disorders/complete-index.shtml

Selekman, J., Diefenbeck, & Guthrie, S. (2013.). Mental health concerns. In J. Selekman (Ed.), *School nursing: A comprehensive text* (2nd ed.) (pp. 956-959). Philadelphia, PA: F.A. Davis.

ECZEMA (Atopic Dermatitis)

DEFINITION/ETIOLOGY:
Eczema is a form of noncontagious dermatitis or inflamed skin. Atopic (allergic nature) dermatitis is a common type of eczema characterized by acute or chronic skin eruptions. Eczema affects about 1 in 10 children. Symptoms almost always develop before age 5. More than half of these children will outgrow it before they are teenagers. Most states require the exclusion of children from school if they have signs or symptoms of communicable diseases. Eczema may be difficult to distinguish from other rashes. An unidentified rash is a classic symptom of some communicable diseases. Therefore, children should be excluded unless the rash is identified as non-communicable.

SIGNS AND SYMPTOMS:
- **Acute:** Skin is intensely itchy, moist, weepy, red, with generalized rash, usually in the antecubital and popliteal area, face and neck. Usually seen in children under age two years.
- **Chronic or atopic:** Areas of involvement are wrist, neck, ankles (feet), antecubital and popliteal area, face and neck. Usually dry, scaly, easily irritated. May be red or depigmented. Usually seen in school age children. Crusting may be present. Atopic eczema is chronic and characterized by remissions and exacerbations. Be aware of the Allergy Triad: Allergies-Eczema-Asthma either with the child or with positive family history.
- **"Itch-scratch cycle":** Scratching or rubbing itchy skin causes further irritation and traumatizes sensitive tissue that increases the risk of secondary infection. Itching can also cause skin damage that eventually leads to thickened brownish areas on the skin (lichenification).
- Symptoms range from a small patch to a painful rash affecting large areas of the body.

DIFFERENTIAL DIAGNOSES:
- Seborrheic dermatitis (severe dandruff)
- Fungal infections
- Contact dermatitis, e.g. poison ivy
- Irritant dermatitis, e.g. friction from tight clothing
- Psoriasis

ECZEMA (Atopic Dermatitis) *(continued from previous page)*

MANAGEMENT/TREATMENT:
Eczema tends to come and go; periods of mild or no symptoms and then times of severe symptoms or "flare ups".

1. Keep skin hydrated:
   - Keep baths brief. Pat dry.
   - Avoid excessive soap exposure; use mild soap or lipid-free cleanser (e.g. Cetaphil®, Aquaphil®).
   - Apply an emollient (moisturizer) or a cool washcloth to itchy areas.
2. Antibiotic ointment for secondary infection may be prescribed.
3. Oral antihistamine to relieve itching, used at bedtime, watch for drowsiness.
4. Keep fingernails short to minimize skin damage when scratching.
5. Use soft cotton clothing and bedding. Avoid wool or rough fabrics. Do not rub skin with washcloth.
6. Control temperature and humidity extremes (high or low); gently pat sweaty skin dry.
7. Treatment is aimed at avoiding triggers that may cause flare-ups and breaking the "itch-scratch cycle".
8. Flare-ups may be seasonal, due to factors like irritants, allergens, or stress or you may not be able to identify cause.

FOLLOW UP:
- Secondary infection is common, especially due to scratching. Resembles impetigo at the edges of eczematous skin; may show as isolated circular crusts with moist or dry pus underneath.
- Observe for cellulitis or lymphangitis.
- Study flare-ups for possible allergies to chemicals, foods, or environmental factors, e.g., dust mites.
- Medical evaluation is necessary for any severe diet restrictions.
- Advise others that eczema is not contagious (unless a secondary infection is present).
- Children are subject to teasing and social distancing which exacerbates stress and low self-esteem.
- Emotions do not cause atopic dermatitis but can trigger the "itch-scratch cycle".
- Anger and frustration can lead to flushing and itchiness.

ECZEMA (Atopic Dermatitis) *(continued from previous page)*

- Sleep disturbances are common, particularly during flare-ups. If the child is tired or irritable, ask the parent/guardian about night symptoms and management.
- Encourage patience. Some parents/guardians try different products without allowing enough time for anyone to show effectiveness.
- Involve children in their care by asking about their experiences and giving them choices and some control over treatment, such as who applies the topical product, and privacy.

References

American Academy of Pediatrics. (2015). *Eczema*. Retrieved from http://kidshealth.org/parent/infections/skin/eczema_atopic_dermatitis.html

Mayo Clinic. (2014). *Atopic dermatitis (eczema)*. Retrieved from http://www.mayoclinic.org/diseases-conditions/eczema/basics/definition/con-20032073

Morelli, J. G. & Prok, L.D. (2014). Skin. In W.W. Hay, R.R. Deterding, M.J. Levin, & M. Abzug. (Eds.), *Current diagnosis and treatment pediatrics* (22nd ed.) (pp.426-445). New York, NY: McGraw Hill Education, Inc.

National Eczema Association. (n.d.). *Eczema tools for school: An educator's guide*. Retrieved from https://nationaleczema.org/living-with-eczema/tools-for-school/

Zheng, T., Yu, J., Oh, M. H., & Zhu, Z. (2011). The atopic march: Progression from atopic dermatitis to allergic rhinitis and asthma. *Allergy Asthma Immunology Research, 3*(2), 67-73. doi: 10.4168/aair.2011.3.2.67

ENCOPRESIS

DEFINITION/ETIOLOGY:

Encopresis is defined as stool incontinence by a child of an age that should be able to control bowel movements, usually over 4 years old. Most cases are due to chronic constipation that results in the large intestine stretching and filling with stool. This leads to involuntary soiling or leakage of liquid stool around the larger stool mass. This is considered functional encopresis and 90% of cases fall into this category. Organic causes, or constipation due to a medical origin, are less common. The incontinence occurs as stool leaks around the impaction and it cannot be controlled by the child.

The cause for encopresis is unclear but may be due to physiologic and/or psychological factors. Physiologic factors may include inadequate fluid intake, change in diet, lack of exercise, stress, and inappropriate use of laxatives. It may be seen with a change in routine such as the start of a school year, when access to the bathroom is more controlled, or the child is too busy playing to use the bathroom. It also may be secondary to an anal fissure causing painful bowel movement.

Nonfunctional encopresis is less common and may be due to congenital anal strictures or bands, or Hirschprung's Disease (congenital megacolon) or other organic anomalies (rare). Psychological factors may include "withholding" stool due to excessively stringent and/or too early toilet training (less common) or other emotional problems. The child may be too young to be toilet trained; children between 3 and 5 often are not yet fully trained. Research supports that children with psychological disorders have a higher incidence of encopresis, such as oppositional defiant disorder. Additionally, major life or family adjustment may be a factor as well as possible physical or sexual abuse.

Prevalence: Constipation is seen in 16-37% of school-aged children. Encopresis occurs in 4% of pre-school aged children, and 1-2% of school-aged children. In autistic children, the rate climbs to 10-20%.

SIGNS AND SYMPTOMS:
- Fecal impaction with leaking of liquefied stool around impaction (most common)
- Large stools that block up the toilet
- Fecal soiling of clothes
- Needing to have a bowel movement with little or no warning or involuntary bowel movement
- Fecal odor

ENCOPRESIS *(continued from previous page)*

SIGNS AND SYMPTOMS: *(continued)*
- Loss of appetite
- Abdominal pain
- Urinary symptoms: urinary tract infections, urine incontinence, bedwetting
- Sometimes anemia and/or under nutrition
- Hypo active or absent bowel sounds may indicate bowel obstruction or acute constipation

EMOTIONAL/BEHAVIORAL FINDINGS:
- Student may be aggressive/disruptive or passive/withdrawn, depending on personality.
- Poor peer acceptance, scape-goating.
- Emotional problems including obsessive/compulsive and oppositional defiant behaviors
- Feelings of shame, embarrassment and low self-esteem.
- Often behaviors are secondary to the encopresis, and dissipate once the encopresis is resolved.

MANAGEMENT/TREATMENT:
1. Be aware of the medical treatment plan to develop a school plan (IHP) that will meet the student's needs during the school day.
2. Always consult with a healthcare provider before starting any treatment e.g., laxatives.
3. Differentiate between staining of underpants with small amounts of stool and pants that contain a full-size bowel movement. Children with impaction show lesser amounts of stool.
4. Make change of clothing plus wash-up facilities available. Protect child's problem from other children as much as possible.
5. Disimpaction: Healthcare provider may prescribe a "clean out" that may include mineral oil, enemas, laxatives, suppositories or a combination of things.
6. Disimpaction is followed by mild laxatives (bulking agents as first choice, then osmotic laxatives such as Miralax®, then stimulants), bowel training, and increased fiber and fluids in diet. The school nurse should work with the parents/guardians, if possible, so that the enemas and laxatives do not "work" during school or school bus times.

ENCOPRESIS *(continued from previous page)*

MANAGEMENT/TREATMENT: *(continued)*

7. Bowel training includes a toileting schedule encouraging the child to sit on the toilet for 10-15 minutes after each meal in a private, non-stressful environment. Have child put feet on a small foot stool when sitting on the toilet to have a bowel movement. This puts pressure on the abdomen, making a bowel movement easier.
8. Start school counseling and/or professional mental health counseling for help with associated emotional/behavioral problems.
9. Liaison with healthcare provider/medical facility to ensure that a digital rectal exam has been done (it is surprising how often this is overlooked, especially at mental health clinics).
10. Enlist parent or other person in home to assist with diet, prescribed laxatives, and regular bowel training. The home and school plan for times, rewards or behavioral techniques, appropriate foods, etc., should be jointly developed so that the school staff and family are consistent in their management.

COMPLICATIONS

- Child may experience ridicule, shame and social outcast from friends and family.
- Teachers may be disgusted or frustrated.
- Parents/guardians may experience guilt, anger, or frustration.
- Low self-esteem.

FOLLOW UP:

- The goal is to prevent constipation and maintain good bowel habits.
- Long term success depends on how well the plan of care is followed.
- Maintain liaison with classroom and PE teacher, parents and healthcare provider.
- Maintain toilet schedule at school that matches child's usual BM habits.

Resources

University of Virginia School of Medicine has a wealth of information on their website, including an extensive reference list.
http://www.medicine.virginia.edu/clinical/departments/pediatrics/clinical-services/tutorials/constipation/encopresis

Printable informational flyer for parents/guardians: http://www.gikids.org/files/documents/digestive%20topics/english/Constipation%20and%20fecal%20soiling.pdf

ENCOPRESIS *(continued from previous page)*

Books for children:
- <u>Clouds and Clocks: A Story for Children Who Soil,</u> by Matthew Galvin
- <u>Everyone Poops,</u> by T. Gomi

Websites for Children:
- Are Your Bowels Moving? http://kidshealth.org/kid/stay_healthy/body/bowel.html
- The Real Deal on the Digestive System http://kidshealth.org/kid/htbw/digestive_system.html

References

Boston Children's Hospital. (n.d). *Encopresis*. Retrieved from http://www.childrenshospital.org/conditions-and-treatments/conditions/e/encopresis/overview

Cincinnati Children's. (2013). *Encopresis in Children*. Retrieved from http://www.cincinnatichildrens.org/health/e/encopresis/

Garman, K., & Ficca, M. (2012). Managing encopresis in the elementary school setting: The school nurse's role. *The Journal of School Nursing, 28*(3), 175-180. doi: 10.177/1059840511429685

Goldson, E., & Reynolds, A. (2014). Child development and behavior. In W. Hay, M. Levin, R. Deterding, & M. Abzug (Eds.), *Current diagnosis and treatment pediatrics* (22nd edition) (pp. 95-96). McGraw Hill Education, Inc.

John, R. & Chewey. L. (2013). Common complaints. In J. Selekman (Ed.), *School nursing: A comprehensive text* (2nd ed.) (pp. 615-616). Philadelphia, PA: F.A. Davis.

Kids Health. (2015). *Encopresis (Soiling)*. Retrieved from http://kidshealth.org/parent/general/sick/encopresis.html?tracking=P_RelatedArticle#

Mayo Clinic. (2014). *Encopresis*. Retrieved from http://www.mayoclinic.org/diseases-conditions/encopresis/basics/lifestyle-home-remedies/con-20029758

Mosca, N., & Schatz, M., (2013) Encopresis: Not just an accident. *NASN School Nurse, 28*(5), 218 - 221. doi: 10.1177/1942602X13500994

University of Virginia, School of Medicine. (2011). *About encopresis*. Retrieved from http://www.medicine.virginia.edu/clinical/departments/pediatrics/clinical-services/tutorials/constipation/encopresis

ENURESIS

DEFINITION/ETIOLOGY:

Enuresis (involuntary urination) is repeated, spontaneous urinary voiding in clothes or in bed after the age when toilet training should be complete (usually age 5 years or under). Enuresis is typically diagnosed after the age of five. It does not usually indicate a physical or emotional problem. It is twice as common in boys. Enuresis usually takes the form of bed wetting.

CAUSES:
- Idiopathic hereditary type (primary nocturnal enuresis) is the most common
- If both parents had a history of enuresis, the rate of nocturnal enuresis found in children is approximately 80%
- Sleep apnea
- Chronic constipation
- Some children have unusually deep sleep patterns
- Child is too young to be toilet trained; children 3-5 need a bathroom in or near classroom
- Meatal stenosis in boys
- Boys with excessively long foreskin with poor hygiene
- Chronic urinary tract infection
- Small bladder capacity, irritable bladder, poor sphincter control, or other organic conditions
- Various emotional/psychological problems, including sexual abuse
- Stress

SIGNS AND SYMPTOMS:
- Urine-stained and wet clothes
- Odor
- Urgency to void
- Bed wetting
- Emotional/behavioral problems, but not as pervasive or common as in children with encopresis
- Symptoms of chronic infection: poor nutritional status plus anemia, itching, foul odor, low-grade fever, stained underpants from constant dribbling, redness and/or impetigo in genital area
- Small caliber of urinary stream in boys with meatal stenosis
- Infection under an excessively long foreskin

154

ENURESIS (continued from previous page)

MANAGEMENT/TREATMENT:
1. Bed wetting
   - Children may outgrow bed wetting without any intervention.
   - Behavior modification with rewards may help.
   - Bladder control training.
   - Limiting fluids at bedtime alone does not appear to be effective.
   - Alarm devices which wake child when the bed is wet – most effective long-term strategy.
   - Healthcare provider may prescribe medication – drugs can decrease bed wetting; results are often not sustained after treatment is stopped.
   - Oral desmopressin (DDAVP) along with limiting fluids reduces urine production in children with normal bladder capacity.
      - ✓ Side effect – DDAVP increases the potential for seizures.
   - Anticholinergic agents such as oxybutynin chloride and tolterodine; the combination of desmopressin acetate and oxybutynin chloride may be efficacious in children with overactive bladder or dysfunctional voiding who show daytime response to anticholinergic therapy but continue to wet at night.

2. At school:
   - Protect privacy of child's problem from other children.
   - Eliminate shame, guilt or punishment.
   - Make toilet, washing, and change of clothing facilities available.
   - Keep extra clothing at school.
   - Help child make pre-need trips to bathroom.
   - Use clock to help remind child of the need to use the bathroom.
   - Liaison with parent/guardian(s) and healthcare provider as necessary.
   - The healthcare provider may request a diary to understand the pattern of daytime urination and bowel movements, diet, etc.
   - Educate the child that, during sleep, his/her brain may not "hear" his/her full bladder's signal to help him/her understand the condition and how medication or other interventions (alarm) may help.

ENURESIS (continued from previous page)

FOLLOW-UP:
- If prescribed, monitor for side effects of medication.
- Monitor for medical conditions – enuresis may be a symptom of a physical condition (diabetes mellitus, diabetes insipidus, sickle cell anemia, urethral obstruction, renal failure etc.). There may be a correlation between pinworms and nocturnal enuresis.
- If indicated, refer to healthcare provider for further diagnostic workup
- **RED FLAG** – enuresis could be a sign of sexual abuse; monitor; if indicated, report to child protective services per school and state guidelines.

Possible Complications
- Contributes to poor self-esteem
- Disrupts family interactions
- May disrupt peer/social interactions
- Genital rash

NOTES:
- Children with significant ADHD are more likely to experience nocturnal enuresis.

References

American Psychiatric Association. (2013). *Diagnostic and statistical manual of mental disorders* (5th ed.). Washington, DC: Author.

John, R. & Chewey, L. (2013). Common complaints. In J. Selekman (Ed.), *School nursing: A comprehensive text* (2nd ed.) (pp. 578-640). Philadelphia: F. A. Davis.

Ju, H. T., Kang, J. H., Lee, S. D., Oh, M. M., Moon, D. G., Kim, S. O., ... & Woo, S. H. (2013). Parent and physician perspectives on the treatment of primary nocturnal enuresis in Korea. *Korean Journal of Urology*, 54(2), 127-134. doi: 10.4111/kju.2013.54.2.127.

Mayo Clinic. (2014). *Bed-wetting*. Retrieved from http://www.mayoclinic.org/diseases-conditions/bed-wetting/basics/definition/con-20015089

Merck Manual. (2014). *Urinary incontinence in children*. Retrieved from http://www.merckmanuals.com/professional/pediatrics/incontinence_in_children/urinary_incontinence_in_children.html?qt=enuresis&alt=sh

Perrin, N., Sayer, L., & While, A. (2013). The efficacy of alarm therapy versus desmopressin therapy in the treatment of primary mono-symptomatic nocturnal enuresis: A systematic review. *Primary Health Care Research & Development*, 16(1), 21-31. 1-11. doi: 10.1017/S146342361300042X

Robson, Lane. (2015). *Enuresis treatment & management*. Retrieved from http://emedicine.medscape.com/article/1014762-treatment

EYE TRAUMA

DEFINITION/ETIOLOGY:

Ocular injuries can involve the eyelids, the eyeball and the bones surrounding the eye. Eye injuries in children commonly result from blunt trauma, sharp objects, sport injuries or projectiles. Baseball is the leading cause of sports-related injuries. Facial injuries often accompany eye trauma.

Chemical burns to the eye are ophthalmologic emergencies and must be referred for immediate emergency care.

Corneal abrasion may result from a direct contact injury, contact lens, or a foreign body with or without penetration.

Foreign Body injuries to the eye may present as either non-penetrating or penetrating. Penetrating injuries are ophthalmologic emergencies and must be referred for immediate emergency care.

SIGNS AND SYMPTOMS (general):

- Pain
- Difficulty with vision
- Redness in the sclera
- Blood in or around the eye
- Hematoma
- Tearing
- Photosensitivity
- Foreign body in eye or under eyelid
- Sensation of foreign body
- Irregular size or shape of the pupil

ASSESSMENT

- Obtain history and nature of physical injury or chemical exposure.
- Assess visual acuity first by using Snellen Chart or "E" test (preschool children). Each eye should be checked individually. The only exception is an acute chemical exposure/injury that requires immediate irrigation (flush with water).
- If student is unable to open eye, do not force.
- Check for visible contusion/lacerations on lids or eye ball.
- Check for blood in anterior chamber (between iris and cornea), called "hyphema".

EYE TRAUMA *(continued from previous page)*

ASSESSMENT *(continued)*
- Check extra-ocular movements.
- Check for double vision (diplopia).
- Check for unequal or irregular pupils.
- Check pupil responses.

MANAGEMENT/TREATMENT (for all eye injuries)
- Instruct - do not rub eye.
- Do not attempt to remove penetrating objects.

Emergency referral to healthcare provider:
- All cases with chemical burn after irrigation with copious amount of water or saline.
- Impaired vision in any way.
- Painful eye or feels like a foreign object.
- Contusion or laceration on eyelid or eyeball.
- Red eye persists for more than one hour (suggests corneal abrasion or foreign object).

Eye trauma without above symptoms:
- Small abrasion or laceration of skin around the eye- without other symptoms- can be washed and left uncovered.
- Red spot limited to the sclera (white of the eye) is typically related to coughing or vomiting (subconjunctival hemorrhage will resolve spontaneously).
- Cold pack may be useful for minor trauma if healthcare provider referral is not necessary.
- Avoid using any eye drops or ointments. Ophthalmic corticosteroids are contraindicated, as they tend to promote growth of fungi and reactivate herpes simplex virus.

Chemical Burn
Ophthalmic burns to the cornea and conjunctiva are an **ophthalmic emergency** and treatment should begin immediately. The eye will be painful, sensitive to light (photophobic) and exhibit excessive tearing (lacrimation).
1. Determine chemical if possible. Alkali burns are generally worse than acid burns. If chemical is known, contact poison control (1-800-222-1222) for further information regarding specific emergency treatment. Send available chemical (name of chemical and ph) information with student to emergency treatment center.

EYE TRAUMA *(continued from previous page)*

2. *Immediately,* flush/irrigate eye with copious amounts of water or saline solution while both eyelids are held open. If only one eye has been exposed to the chemical, attempt to irrigate the eye with the person lying on his/her side. If possible, pour water from the inner corner flowing toward the outer corner.
3. Notify parent/guardian.
4. Refer for emergency medical treatment. Eye should be examined by an ophthalmologist as soon as possible, no longer than 24 hours after exposure.
5. Cool compress to the surrounding area may provide comfort.

Corneal Abrasion

The eye will be painful, sensitive to light (photophobic) and exhibit excessive tearing (lacrimation).

1. Remove contact lens, if present.
2. Examine the eye for the presence of a foreign body. The absence of a *visible* foreign body does not negate the presence of or irritation from a foreign body.
3. Notify parent/guardian.
4. Refer to ophthalmologist for evaluation and necessary treatment.
5. To minimize eye movement, patch <u>both</u> eyes with gauze pads prior to travel to healthcare provider or ophthalmologist.

Foreign Body (non-penetrating)

The eye will be painful, sensitive to light (photophobic), exhibit excessive tearing (lacrimation), and have the sensation of a foreign body presence in the eye.

1. Remove contact lens, if present.
2. Examine the eye for the presence of a foreign body. To visualize foreign object, have student look up and down and from side to side. It may be necessary to invert the upper lid to see the presence of a foreign body.
3. If foreign body (speck of dirt, sand, eyelash, etc.) is obvious, try to remove it by gently flushing with warm water from inner to outer area of eye. If foreign object is visualized in corner of eye or in the lower lid, attempt to remove object by touching object with clean moistened cotton swab.
4. If these attempts and maneuvers fail, notify parents/guardians and refer to the healthcare provider.
5. To minimize eye movement, patch <u>both</u> eyes with gauze pads prior to travel to healthcare provider or ophthalmologist.

EYE TRAUMA *(continued from previous page)*

Foreign Body (penetrating)

The patient will experience intense pain, sensitivity to light (photophobic), exhibit excessive tearing (lacrimation) and redness. You may be able to visualize the penetrating object.

Penetrating injuries are ophthalmologic emergencies. Do not attempt to remove the object or flush the eye.

- Cover the injured eye with an eye shield or small paper cup. Anchor in place. Patch other eye to minimize eye movement.
- Notify parent/guardian.
- Refer to emergency medical center or ophthalmologist for *immediate* care.

FOLLOW UP:

- If student returned to class, re-examine eye later that day and on the following day. Continue to monitor for pain and infection.
- For eye trauma without emergency symptoms, re-check visual acuity the 3-4 days after treatment and refer to healthcare provider if there is difference from prior screening.
- If seen by the healthcare provider, implement healthcare provider's instructions for care after initial evaluation and treatment.
- Healthcare provider may recommend not wearing contact lens for a few days following eye trauma requiring emergency care. This may have implications for reading and classroom work.

NOTES:

Prevention

Stress the importance of wearing protective eyewear when participating in contact and ball sports, working with metal and glass projects, hammering metal on metal, and handling chemicals.

EYE TRAUMA *(continued from previous page)*

References

American Academy of Ophthalmology. (2015). *Recognizing and treating eye injuries.* Retrieved from http://www.geteyesmart.org/eyesmart/living/eye-injuries/index.cfm

American Academy of Ophthalmology. (2013). *Clinical statement: Protective eyewear for young athletes.* Retrieved from http://one.aao.org/CE/PracticeGuidelines/ClinicalStatements_Content.aspx?cid=1fda605b-97b9-47e3-90d1-11b7a9607797

MedlinePlus. (2015). *Eye emergencies.* Retrieved from http://www.nlm.nih.gov/medlineplus/ency/article/000054.html

Merck Manual. (2014). *Corneal abrasions & foreign bodies.* Retrieved from http://www.merckmanuals.com/professional/injuries_poisoning/eye_trauma/corneal_abrasions_and_foreign_bodies.html?qt=corneal%20abrasions&alt=sh

Merck Manual. (2014). *Eye contusions and lacerations.* Retrieved from http://www.merckmanuals.com/professional/injuries_poisoning/eye_trauma/ocular_burns.html

Merck Manual. (2014). *Subconjunctival hemorrhages.* Retrieved from http://www.merckmanuals.com/professional/eye-disorders/conjunctival-and-scleral-disorders/subconjunctival-hemorrhages

FAINTING (Syncope)

DEFINITION/ETIOLOGY:
Syncope is a brief, partial or complete loss of consciousness due to diminished oxygen supply to the brain. It may be caused by low blood sugar, standing in place for a long time, headache, seizure, drugs, depression or panic attack or may be as a result of more serious situation such as head injury, neurological disorders or an underlying condition such as heart disease/complications.

In children and adolescents most episodes of syncope are benign and most commonly result from vaso-vagal episodes. These are commonly precipitated by trigger events such as unpleasant sights or smells, anxiety, emotional stress, anticipated pain or fear.

Orthostatic hypotension is also a common cause of syncope. This occurs when the child stands and there is a transient increase in the heart rate and inadequate cerebral perfusion resulting in low blood pressure. Dehydration may also be a contributing cause.

Although rare, syncope may be due to cardiac disease such as dysrhythmias or valvular disease. Syncope due to cardiac disease often occurs suddenly and may present on exertion and with generalized weakness and pallor. If an arrhythmia occurs the child often presents with a brief loss of consciousness, palpitations and no warning.

SIGNS AND SYMPTOMS:
- Loss of consciousness may be preceded by pale, cool, diaphoretic skin, lightheadedness, tunnel vision, nausea, frequent yawn, and/or restless feeling.
- Loss of consciousness (usually brief).
- As person begins to lose consciousness, they may have a brief eye roll and/or body twitching.
- Fainting related to hyperventilation is often accompanied by numbness around the mouth and fingers.
- How fainting may be different from a seizure:
    - Fainters usually know when it is going to happen.
    - Seizures occur with no warning except occasional aura.
    - Seizure twitching is more severe and lasts longer.
    - Post seizure sleep is longer and deeper.
    - Fainters usually remember what happened after they wake up.

FAINTING (Syncope) *(continued from previous page)*

MANAGEMENT/TREATMENT:
1. If observe person about to faint, instruct them to lie down to prevent falling.
2. Help ease person to floor or reclining position.
3. Place person on back with no pillow and elevate feet about 12 inches to encourage blood flow to head.
4. Roll person to side if they vomit.
5. As person awakens, do not allow them to stand immediately (be prepared to have person resume reclining position if dizzy).
6. If person does not awaken within 1 minute, <u>call 911</u>. Prepare for possibility of CPR.
7. If fainting is as a result of head injury, <u>seek immediate medical care</u>.
8. If person is known to have diabetes, proceed with diabetes emergency action plan.
9. Refer to the healthcare provider to rule out serious cause of syncope.
10. If student sustained injury from fainting episode – administer first aid.
11. Syncope with chest pain needs immediate medical evaluation.

FOLLOW UP:
- Determine history of fainting and if applicable, results of past medical evaluation for fainting.
- If prior evaluation determined no cause or need for medical intervention, educate frequent fainters about safety; when experiencing warning symptoms, sit down in a chair, position head between knees close to floor. If they are embarrassed to do this in public, they can pretend to remove something from their shoe. Educate students with postural hypotension about getting up slowly.

NOTE:
It is important to note that after medical workup the etiology of some cases of syncope remain unknown. Inhaling ammonia or amyl nitrite is **not** recommended.

References

John, R. & Chewey. L. (2013). Common complaints. In J. Selekman (Ed.), *School nursing: A comprehensive text* (2nd ed.) (pp. 587-590). Philadelphia, PA: F.A. Davis.

Mayo Clinic. (2014). *Fainting: First aid*. Retrieved from http://www.mayoclinic.org/first-aid/first-aid-fainting/basics/art-20056606

Mayo Clinic. (2013). *Vasovagal syncope*. Retrieved from http://www.mayoclinic.com/health/vasovagal-syncope/DS00806/DSECTION=symptoms

Merck Manual. (2015). *Syncope*. Retrieved from http://www.merckmanuals.com/professional/SearchResults?query=syncope

FEVER

DEFINITION/ETIOLOGY:

Fever is a physiological response to inflammation or an infection which probably helps the body's defense mechanism. Fever is one of the body's responses to illness or injury, but it can also be a result from heat exposure. Fever is not always cause for alarm, but sometimes it is a sign of a serious problem.

Fever can improve the immune response at lower temperatures and impair some microorganisms and viruses. However, fever can be uncomfortable, dehydrate, and stress the cardio-respiratory system. An oral temperature of over 100.4° Fahrenheit is considered a fever.

SIGNS AND SYMPTOMS:
- May feel cold or shiver with an elevated temperature.
- May have signs and symptoms of infectious disease such as cough, diarrhea, vomiting, general weakness and muscle ache.
- Skin may feel sensitive to touch; described as "prickly".
- Eyes may appear glassy.
- Face may be flushed.
- Skin will be warm to touch.
- Dehydration with extended increased temperature.
- There is generally an increase of 10 pulse beats for every degree of fever and respirations increase 4 breaths per minute per degree.

MANAGEMENT/TREATMENT:
1. Assess vital signs.
2. Ensure accurate temperature reading; wait several minutes to take temperature if student has been out in cold or if has just consumed hot or cold liquid.
3. Provide comfort measures and cool compress on the forehead.
4. Remove extra outer clothing (but not to point to create shivering which will increase temperature).
5. Give fluids to drink.
6. Assess for signs of infectious disease and use social distancing.
7. Follow school exclusion policies for elevated temperature.
8. Fever that causes enough discomfort to need medication probably indicates that the student should not be in school.

FEVER *(continued from previous page)*

9. Follow school policy regarding over-the-counter (OTC) medications. Since a low grade fever may be beneficial, withhold acetaminophen unless healthcare provider orders it.
10. Recheck the student's temperature 30-60 minutes after giving medication and note if medication was effective.

NOTES:

- Children with fever, headache, neck stiffness, petechiae or purpura may have significant illness and should be evaluated by a healthcare provider.
- A healthcare provider should evaluate children with fever and who are lethargic, unusually drowsy, altered level of consciousness, or extremely pale or cyanotic.
- Never give aspirin to a child or teen under 19 during episodes of fever-causing illnesses as aspirin has been linked to the life-threatening disorder Reye's syndrome.
- Some children are prone to seizures from a high fever.
- Children can return to school when the temperature has been normal for 24 hours without medication.

References

John, R. & Chewey, L. (2013). Common complaints. In J. Selekman (Ed.), *School nursing: A comprehensive text (2nd ed.)* (pp. 580-582). Philadelphia, PA: F. A. Davis.

Mayo Clinic. (2014). *Fever.* Retrieved from http://www.mayoclinic.org/diseases-conditions/fever/basics/definition/con-20019229

Merck Manual. (2013). *Fever.* Retrieved from http://www.merckmanuals.com/professional/pediatrics/symptoms-in-infants-and-children/fever-in-infants-and-children

Sullivan, J.E., Farrar, H.C., and the American Academy of Pediatrics' Section on Clinical Pharmacology and Therapeutics, Committee on Drugs. (2011). *Fever and antipyretic use in children.* Retrieved from http://pediatrics.aappublications.org/content/127/3/580.full

The Nemours Foundation. (2013). *Fever and taking your child's temperature.* Retrieved from http://Kidshealth.org/parent/general/body/fever.html#

FIFTH DISEASE (Erythema Infectiosum)

DEFINITION/ETIOLOGY:

"Fifth Disease" is named that because it was identified after rubeola, rubella, scarlet fever, and roseola. It is caused by Human Parvovirus (*parvovirus B19*)—related to, but not the same as dog parvovirus. It is a common viral infection and occurs in preschool and school aged children. Transmission or spread is by droplets from respiratory secretions or secondarily by hands before the rash appears. About 50% of adults have had the disease as children and thus are immune. The incubation period is 4-14 days but can be as long as 21 days. Rash symptoms occur 1-3 weeks after infection.

SIGNS AND SYMPTOMS:

- About a week after exposure, the patient may develop a low grade fever, headache, cold symptoms and or muscle aches which may last 5-7 days, after which the child recovers with no other symptoms.
- About 1-3 weeks after the fever goes away, a distinctive rash may appear. The rash has a slapped cheek appearance and a faint, lacy rash on the trunk, arms and legs may develop about 1 day later.
- Adults, especially women, may have joint pain and swelling at this stage. The rash fades in 1-2 weeks but may recur for several weeks brought on by exposure to sunlight, heat, exercise, or stress.
- Often there is neither fever nor rash with this disease (sub-clinical form).

MANAGEMENT/TREATMENT:

1. The most contagious period is just before onset of fever, gradually declining during the next week and low to absent by the time the rash appears. An outbreak of this disease often occurs in late winter and spring. Therefore, Fifth Disease may be suspected in the pre-rash, infective stage, if it has occurred in other family members. Transmission of Fifth Disease is enhanced by household contact. A susceptible parent/guardian has a 50% chance of catching the disease from their child. In contrast, during an extensive school outbreak, about 20% of susceptible teachers may develop the infection.
2. Children with the rash of Fifth Disease do not need to be isolated because they are *no longer contagious by the time the rash appears.*
3. Pregnant women who become infected in the *first 4-5 months are at a risk of spontaneous abortion.*

FIFTH DISEASE (Erythema Infectiosum) *(continued from previous page)*

4. Available data suggest that a susceptible woman exposed to her own infected child during the first 20 weeks of pregnancy runs an increased risk (about 1-2%) of having a spontaneous abortion.
5. If the exposure is at school or another job site, the risk is lower because of less intimate contact.
6. Hand washing and proper tissue disposal should be scrupulously practiced.
7. Encourage pregnant family members and staff that expect to have contact with children in school to consult with their healthcare provider about their risk for infection. A blood test to determine if they are already immune may help to alleviate their concern.
8. No treatment is usually required.

POTENTIAL COMPLICATIONS:
- Children with unusual long-term blood disease such as sickle cell anemia, immunodeficiency, etc. need special consideration.
- *Exposed pregnant women need advice from their healthcare provider or an infectious disease specialist.*
- Testing for susceptibility may be available.
- Teachers and day care workers are at increased risk of exposure, but a routine policy of exclusion of pregnant women from these work places is not recommended.

FIFTH DISEASE (Erythema Infectiosum) *(continued from previous page)*

References

American Academy of Pediatrics. (2015). Parvovirus B19. In L. K. Pickering, C. J. Baker, D. W. Kimberlin, & S. S. Long (Eds.), *Red Book: 2015 report of the committee on infectious diseases, (30th ed.)* (pp. 593-596). American Academy of Pediatrics: Elk Grove Village, IL.

American Academy of Pediatrics. (2013). Fifth disease (human parvovirus B19). In S. Aronson, & T. Shope (Eds.), *Managing infectious diseases in child care and schools (2nd ed.)* (pp. 93-94). Elk Grove Village, IL: American Academy of Pediatrics.

Brice, S. L. (2013). Viral diseases of the skin. In E. T. Bope & R. D. Kellerman (Eds.), *Conn's current therapy 2013* (pp. 288-289). Philadelphia: Saunders Elsevier.

Garcia, L. T. (2013). Parvovirus B19 infection. In F. J. Domino (Ed.), *The 5-minute clinical consult 2013 (21st ed.)* (pp. 952-953). Philadelphia: Wolters Kluwer Health/Lippincott Williams & Wilkins.

Hahn, W., & Tammaro, D. (2014). Fifth disease (parvovirus infection). In F. F. Ferri (Ed.), *2014 Ferri's clinical advisor: 5 books in 1* (p. 427). Philadelphia: Mosby Elsevier.

March of Dimes. (2012, March). *Fifth disease and pregnancy. Pregnancy complications.* Retrieved February 4, 2014, from http://www.marchofdimes.com/pregnancy/complications_fifthdisease.html

Medline Plus, U.S. National Library of Medicine. (2013a). *Fifth disease.* Retrieved from http://www.nlm.nih.gov/medlineplus/ency/article/000977.htm

Medline Plus, U.S National Library of Medicine. (2013b). *Fifth disease.* Retrieved from http://www.nlm.nih.gov/medlineplus/fifthdisease.html#cat59

National Center for Immunization and Respiratory Disease, CDC. (2012). *Parvovirus B19 (fifth disease) fact sheet.* Retrieved from http://www.cdc.gov/ncidod/dvrd/revb/respiratory/parvo_b19.htm

FOOD ALLERGY (Also see Allergies and Anaphylaxis)

DEFINITION/ETIOLOGY:

A food allergy is an exaggerated immune system response to a particular protein found in that food (most commonly milk, eggs, peanuts, tree nuts, soy, wheat, fish, and shellfish, or some other specific food). Food intolerance is an adverse reaction to certain foods but which does not involve the immune system. In a true food allergy, the immune system reacts to exposure to a certain food. The body produces an abnormally large amount of an antibody called Immunoglobulin E (IgE) during an exposure. These antibodies go to work destroying these food allergens by releasing histamines which then trigger the symptoms of an allergic reaction, Food allergies may develop at any time, even after eating the food repeatedly in the past without having problems. Symptoms may occur after that allergic individual consumes or is exposed to even a small amount of the food.

MILD SIGNS AND SYMPTOMS:
- Hives on any part of the body
- Rash or eczema
- Diarrhea and mild abdominal cramping
- Nausea and/or vomiting
- Nasal congestion or sneezing
- Itchy mouth

SEVERE/ANAPHYLAXIS SIGNS AND SYMPTOMS:
- Uneasiness and agitation
- Sense of impending doom
- Rapid pulse, palpitations, thready or unobtainable pulse
- Swelling of face, lips, tongue, and/or eyelids
- Blue or gray color around the lips or nail beds
- Dizziness
- Difficulty breathing, coughing and/or wheezing
- Trouble swallowing
- vomiting
- Fall in blood pressure
- Fainting, unresponsiveness

Not __ALL__ signs and symptoms need be present in anaphylaxis.

> **Please note:** Symptoms of anaphylaxis may appear within 1 to 15 minutes and progress rapidly. In some cases, the severe reaction may be delayed. Although most serious reactions occur within the first hour of contact with the allergen, anaphylaxis has been known to occur up to several hours later. Severe allergic reactions may be a precursor to anaphylaxis.

FOOD ALLERGY *(continued from previous page)*

MANAGEMENT/TREATMENT:

An Individualized Healthcare Plan (IHP) and an emergency plan should be developed for any student with food allergies. Many allergic reactions are not severe enough to cause anaphylaxis. Intervention may not be necessary unless the student develops one of the following. <u>Follow local school policy and procedures.</u>

1. SKIN: Rash or hives. May be alleviated with an oral or topical antihistamine or steroid.
2. GASTROINTESTINAL: Nausea or mild diarrhea. Offer small sips of water, avoid dehydration. If vomiting, severe diarrhea or abdominal cramping may indicate anaphylaxis.
3. RESPIRATORY: Wheezing, repetitive coughing or throat clearing, shortness of breath, change in voice, difficulty swallowing, or chest tightness Treat as anaphylaxis. Bronchodilators should not be given in place of epinephrine for anaphylactic reactions but may be beneficial for asthma symptoms after epinephrine has been given.
4. CARDIOVASCULAR: Fainting, shock. Treat as anaphylaxis.
5. ANAPHYLAXIS: inject adrenalin (epinephrine) medication as quickly as possible, followed by **immediate call to 911** and transport to a hospital emergency department. (Despite initial improvement after first injectable epinephrine (adrenalin), symptoms often recur).
6. A copy of the students record should be sent with the emergency medical services (EMS) and should include:
   - Allergen to which student is reacting, if known
   - Signs and symptoms of distress
   - Emergency measures instituted
   - Student's response to emergency measures
   - Time of all activities, including giving injectable epinephrine (adrenalin)
   - Signature of nurse and phone number
   - Give used epinephrine auto injector to EMS
7. **If student's anaphylaxis symptoms have not improved or have relapsed within 15 minutes after first dose of epinephrine, a repeat dose may be needed.** (Plans need to be made in advance with parents/guardians for 2 doses of injectable epinephrine (adrenalin) to be in place if school does not stock injectable epinephrine [adrenalin])
8. Monitor blood pressure. Lay student down and elevate legs if blood pressure is low.
9. Cover with blankets if necessary to keep warm; don't allow blankets to interfere with handling or observation.
10. Notify parents/guardians and healthcare provider.

FOOD ALLERGY (*continued from previous page*)

FOLLOW UP:
- Avoid contact and exposure to foods which trigger allergic reactions. May need access to food labels for food served at school.
- Develop an **Individualized Healthcare Plan** with input from the healthcare provider and family that includes specific actions to prevent exposure, staff training, and the emergency action plan with individualized orders.
- Assess the student's classroom and school for possible environmental triggers that may cause allergic reactions.
- Environmental controls to avoid the symptoms that cause allergic reactions.
- Suggest to parent/guardian that child wear a Medic Alert bracelet or tag.
- If injectable epinephrine (adrenalin) is ordered, suggest student keep the product/device at hand at all times (depending on age and maturity level) and replace if expired or used.

NOTES:
Controlling Food Allergies
Food allergy reactions and life-threatening anaphylaxis may occur at school or during school-sponsored activities. The risk of accidental exposure to trigger foods can be reduced in the school setting if schools communicate with students, parents, and healthcare providers to minimize risks and provide a safe educational environment for food-allergic students. Schools need to ensure that:
1. Staff (i.e., teachers, cafeteria personnel, lunch, playground and bus monitors) and parent/guardian are educated about food allergies and preventive measures, e.g., checking food and container labels;
2. Individual healthcare plans are developed for students known to have a food allergy; and
3. There is immediate access to emergency medications, including epinephrine, and local emergency medical services.

Children that have asthma in addition to their food allergy have a greater risk of anaphylaxis after exposure.

FOOD ALLERGY (*continued from previous page*)

Resources

- Center for Disease Control and Prevention - Voluntary Guidelines for Managing Food Allergies In Schools and Early Care and Education Programs. http://www.cdc.gov/healthyyouth/foodallergies/pdf/13_243135_A_Food_Allergy_Web_508.pdf
- Food Allergy Research & Education (FARE) - extensive website with tools and resources for schools including sample action plans http://www.foodallergy.org
- Food Allergy Anaphylaxis In School: What School Staff Need to Know – online training module. http://www.allergyhome.org/schools/management-of-food-allergies-in-school-what-school-staff-need-to-know/
- NASN Food Allergy and Anaphylaxis Toolkit – retrieve from http://www.nasn.org/ToolsResources/FoodAllergyandAnaphylaxis

References

American Academy of Allergy, Asthma & Immunology. (2015). *Food Allergy Overview.* Retrieved from http://www.aaaai.org/conditions-and-treatments/allergies/food-allergies.aspx

American Academy of Allergy, Asthma & Immunology. (2013). *What you should know about anaphylaxis.* Retrieved from http://www.aaaai.org/Aaaai/media/MediaLibrary/PDF%20Documents/Libraries/What-you-Should-Know-about-Anaphylaxis.pdf

American Academy of Pediatrics. (2010). *Clinical report - Management of allergy in the school setting.* http://www.aaaai.org/Aaaai/media/MediaLibrary/PDF%20Documents/Practice%20and%20Parameters/AAP-managing-food-allergy-in-schools-2010.pdf

Centers for Disease Control and Prevention. (2013). *Voluntary guidelines for managing food allergies in schools and early care and education programs.* Washington, DC: US Department of Health and Human Services.

Food Allergy Research & Education (FARE). (n.d.). *Food allergy action plan.* Retrieved from http://www.foodallergy.org/faap

Food Allergy Research & Education (FARE). (n.d.).*Managing students with food allergy during a shelter in place emergency.* Retrieved from http://www.foodallergy.org/managing-food-allergies/at-school/shelter-in-place

Food Allergy Research & Education (FARE). (2015). *About food allergies.* Retrieved from http://www.foodallergy.org/about-food-allergies

Hogate, S., Giel, J. & Selekman, J. (2013). Allergy. In J. Selekman (Ed.), *School nursing: A comprehensive text* (2*nd* ed.) (pp. 784-838). Philadelphia, PA: F.A. Davis.

National Association of School Nurses. (2012*). Allergy/anaphylaxis management in the school setting* (Position statement). Retrieved from http://www.nasn.org/PolicyAdvocacy/PositionPapersandReports/NASNPositionStatementsFullView/tabid/462/ArticleId/9/Allergy-Anaphylaxis-Management-in-the-School-Setting-Revised-June-2012

FOODBORNE ILLNESS

DEFINITION/ETIOLOGY:

Foodborne Illness (food poisoning) is an illness that results from consuming or handling contaminated food or beverages. Foodborne illnesses are associated with the lack of adequate knowledge regarding food preparation, storage, hygiene and increasing amounts, and types of imported foods.

NOTIFICATION

It is important to have established criteria with the local or state health department about when and how they are to be involved if a foodborne illness is known or suspected. Many such illnesses are reportable not only to the local or state department of health but also to the Centers for Disease Control and Prevention (CDC). It is important to involve the health department almost immediately because of the actions they can take to identify whether or not the illness is indeed foodborne and to prevent further spread of the outbreak.

CAUSE

Foodborne illness arises from the ingestion of food that is contaminated with bacteria, viruses, parasites, or chemicals both natural and manufactured. An outbreak is generally defined by the CDC as "an incident in which two or more persons experience a similar illness after ingesting a common food, which epidemiologic analysis implicates as the source of the illness".

Outbreaks have been associated with consumption of cold foods, including salads, sandwiches and bakery products. Liquid items (e.g., salad dressings or cake icing) that allow a virus to mix evenly have also been implicated in outbreaks. Food can be contaminated at its source (e.g., oysters harvested from contaminated waters have been associated with widespread outbreaks). Rough, wet, uncooked foods (such as salads) and contaminated produce are at highest risk of transmission of norovirus. Most foodborne outbreaks of norovirus illness arise from direct contamination of food by a food handler immediately before the food is eaten.

FOODBORNE ILLNESS *(continued from previous page)*

Top Five Pathogens Causing Foodborne Illness	Top Five Pathogens Causing Hospitalization	Top Five Pathogens Causing Death
Norovirus	Salmonella nontyphoidal	Salmonella, non typhoidal
Salmonella	Norovirus	Toxoplasma gondii
Clostridium perfringens	Campylobacter	Listeria monocytogenes
Campylobacter	Toxoplasma gondii	Norovirus
Staphylococcus	E.coli	Campylobacter

(CDC 2014)

SIGNS AND SYMPTOMS:
- History of exposure to suspect food
- Frequent vomiting
- Often abdominal pain
- Hyperactive bowel sounds
- Diarrhea may be present after the onset of vomiting
- Little or no fever
- Chills
- Dehydration
- Depend on the type and amount of the source
- Last for a few hours to several days
- Range from mild to severe and death

MANAGEMENT/TREATMENT:
1. Report cluster of cases to health department; they will usually:
   a. Investigate food source (possible cultures)
   b. Interview individuals (possible stool cultures)
   c. Inspect food preparation area and handlers
2. Refer individuals to healthcare provider or emergency room (some students may require hospitalization; others merely antibiotics for treatment).
3. Replace fluids and electrolytes.

FOODBORNE ILLNESS *(continued from previous page)*

FOLLOW UP:
- Obtain results of any cultures taken and determine from treating healthcare provider if any student returning to school might pose a threat to others (e.g., carrier state of Salmonella).
- Monitor student's state of hydration, temperature and general status.
- Report relapses and new cases to health department.
- Additional information for student/family education can be found at CDC (www.cdc.gov), National Food Safety Program (www.foodsafety.gov) which hosts National Food Safety Education Month (September) and the Food and Drug Administration (http://www.fightbac.org/).

POTENTIAL COMPLICATIONS:
- Dehydration (In severe cases, dehydration can be deadly)
- Hemolytic uremic syndrome (rare - affects children under 10 years old)
- Thrombotic purpura

NOTES:
- Children are at greatest risk for diarrhea and dehydration when exposed to foodborne illness.
- The food handler is the most common source of food contamination (this includes volunteers who conduct food events at school).

PREVENTION:
- Hand washing by food handlers is the single most effective means of minimizing foodborne illness transmission.
- Follow recommended or required techniques for food storage, preparation, and holding (hot or cold, covered, etc.).
- Sanitize food preparation and serving areas and of items used to prepare and serve food.
- Most food if properly cooked/heated is rendered harmless (temperature depends on the type of food).
- Avoid cross contamination by separating foods.
- Refrigerate food promptly.
- Uncooked foods such as salads require the greatest care with preparation because *E. coli*, norovirus and hepatitis A can be transmitted.
- Sometimes food suppliers are the source of contamination (eggs, poultry, ground meat, instant mashed potatoes).

FOODBORNE ILLNESS *(continued from previous page)*

References

Ball, J., Binder, R., & Cowen, K. (Eds.). (2012). Child and adolescent nutrition. *Principles of Pediatric Nursing: Caring for Children (5th ed.)* (pp. 349, 353). Upper Saddle River, NJ: Pearson Education, Inc.

Centers for Disease Control and Prevention. (2015). *Foodborne germs and illness.* Retrieved from http://www.cdc.gov/foodsafety/foodborne-germs.html

Centers for Disease Control and Prevention. (2014). *CDC Estimates of foodborne illness in the United States.* Retrieved from http://www.cdc.gov/foodborneburden/

Mayo Clinic. (2014). *Food poisoning.* Retrieved from http://www.mayoclinic.org/diseases-conditions/food-poisoning/basics/definition/con-20031705

Medline Plus, U.S. National Library of Medicine. (2015). *Foodborne illness.* Retrieved from http://www.nlm.nih.gov/medlineplus/foodborneillness.html

National Digestive Diseases Information Clearinghouse. (2014). *Foodborne illness.* Retrieved from http://digestive.niddk.nih.gov/ddiseases/pubs/bacteria/#1

National Institute of Allergy and Infectious Disease. (2015). *Foodborne diseases.* Retrieved from http://www.niaid.nih.gov/topics/foodborne/Pages/Default.aspx

U.S. Department of health and Human Services. (2015). *Food poisoning.* Retrieved from http://www.foodsafety.gov/poisoning/index.html

U.S. Food and Drug Administration. (2015). *What you should know about government response to foodborne illness outbreaks.* Retrieved from http://www.fda.gov/Food/ResourcesForYou/Consumers/ucm180323.htm

FOREIGN BODIES: Eye, Ear (including earwax), Nose

DEFINITION/ETIOLOGY:
It is not uncommon for children to present with a foreign body in the eye, ear, or nose. A variety of inanimate objects and vegetable materials can get in the ear and nose. Environmental materials such as dust, dirt, sand, and insects can also get in the eyes, ears, and nose. Children may put foreign objects such as beads, small stones, beans, sponges, food, etc. into their nose and ears.

SIGNS AND SYMPTOMS:
- *Eye:* pain, tearing, irritation, inflammation.
- *Ear:* initially usually no discomfort. Later may complain of pain, itching in ear canal or purulent drainage from affected ear.
    - o   Child may report something in ear.
    - o   Object may be visible in ear canal.
- *Nose:* usually no symptoms at first. After few days, a unilateral sero-purulent foul-smelling or bloody discharge may be present.
    - o   Child may report putting something in nose.
    - o   May have difficulty breathing through obstructed nostril.
    - o   Object may be visible in nose.

MANAGEMENT/TREATMENT:

EYE (see also Eye Trauma)
1. Never remove an intraocular foreign body or if history indicates there was a projectile object involved. Refer immediately to ophthalmologist.
2. Pull down lower lid with tip of index finger. If foreign body can be seen in the sac of the lower lid, remove with a moistened cotton-tipped applicator.
3. If not successful after 1-2 attempts or if foreign body is in any other location, refer to healthcare provider.
4. To minimize eye movement, patch <u>both</u> eyes with 4x4 gauze pads prior to travel to healthcare provider or ophthalmologist.

Minor irritation from foreign object, e.g., glitter, sand in eye:
1. Fill paper cup to brim with tap water.
2. Have student position irritated eye in water, look into cup, and blink eye, much like opening eyes in swimming pool. *Or*
3. Flush eye at eyewash station or with hand held eyewash bottle.

177

FOREIGN BODIES: Eye, Ear (including earwax), Nose *(continued from previous page)*

MANAGEMENT/TREATMENT (continued):

EAR
1. ***Do not*** *try to remove unless foreign body can be easily seen and grasped with forceps, tweezers or fingers and can be removed safely. Frequently swabs, forceps, tweezers and fingers push the object farther into the ear canal.*
2. If the object is an insect, do not attempt to examine with an otoscope as the light may irritate the insect causing it to move and creating discomfort for the student. Take the student into a dark room and shine a flashlight into the ear and the insect may crawl toward the light and out of the ear canal. The insect may have caused inflammation in the ear canal. Even if successful in removing insect, refer child to healthcare provider for follow-up care.
3. If policy/protocol permits and with parent/guardian's permission, ear wax may be treated by instilling mineral oil into ear and after 10 minutes turn onto affected side and allow draining.
4. If these attempts are not successful, refer to healthcare provider.

NOSE
1. Try having child blow nose forcibly while holding the unaffected nostril shut.
2. ***Do not*** *attempt to remove object unless object can be seen and can be grasped with forceps or fingers and can be removed safely.*
3. While removing visible object, press the nose above the object so you cannot push it farther in. If foreign object is visualized in both nares – refer to healthcare provider. Do not attempt to remove objects.
4. Seek immediate medical care if child is having difficulty breathing.
5. Refer to healthcare provider if foreign object removal is unsuccessful.

FOLLOW UP:
1. *Eye:* Ask teacher to report any further symptoms. Recheck visual acuity 3-4 days after treatment.
2. *Ear:* No, follow up if object has been removed.
3. *Nose:* None if object removed. Check for cessation of nasal discharge.

Also, see School Nurse Guideline – Eye Trauma.

FOREIGN BODIES: Eye, Ear (including earwax), Nose *(continued from previous page)*

References

Eyes:

Medline Plus, U.S. National Library of Medicine. (2013). *Eye pain*. Retrieved from http://www.nlm.nih.gov/medlineplus/ency/article/003032.htm

Medline Plus, U.S. National Library of Medicine. (2015*). Eye emergencies*. Retrieved from http://www.nlm.nih.gov/medlineplus/ency/article/000054.htm

Ears:

Mayo Clinic. (2014). *Foreign object in the ear: First aid*. Retrieved from http://www.mayoclinic.com/print/fiRST-aid/HQ00061

Mayo Clinic. (2015). *Earwax blockage*. Retrieved from http://www.mayoclinic.com/health/earwax-blockage/DS00052

Medline Plus, U.S. National Library of Medicine. (2014). *Ear emergencies*. Retrieved from http://www.nlm.nih.gov/medlineplus/ency/article/000052.htm

Merck Manual. (2014). *External ear obstructions, foreign bodies*. Retrieved from http://www.merckmanuals.com/professional/ear_nose_and_throat_disorders/external_ear_disorders/external_ear_obstructions.html

Foreign Objects:

John, R., & Chewey, L. (2013). *Common complaints*. In J. Selekman (Ed.), *School nursing: A comprehensive text* (2nd ed.) (pp. 578-640). Philadelphia: F. A. Davis.

Nose:

Medline Plus, U.S. National Library of Medicine. (2013). *Foreign body in the nose*. Retrieved from http://www.nlm.nih.gov/medlineplus/ency/article/000037.htm

Merck Manual. (2013). *Nasal foreign bodies*. Retrieved from http://www.merckmanuals.com/professional/ear_nose_and_throat_disorders/nose_and_paranasal_sinus_disorders/nasal_foreign_bodies.html

FRACTURE
(see also Sprains of Ankle or Knee)

DEFINITIONS/ETIOLOGY:
A fracture is a broken bone most frequently associated with an injury to surrounding tissue caused from direct trauma. Fractures may also be caused from diseases that weaken the bone such as osteogenesis.
- Simple fracture – the bone is lined up and does not need to be set, just immobilized
- Hairline fracture – a fine crack; this may not show immediately on x-ray
- Greenstick fracture – split on one side but not the other
- Displaced fracture – end of bones are not lined up and may actually overlap
- Impacted fracture – two broken ends are jammed together
- Compound fracture – both ends are apart and one or both protrudes through broken skin

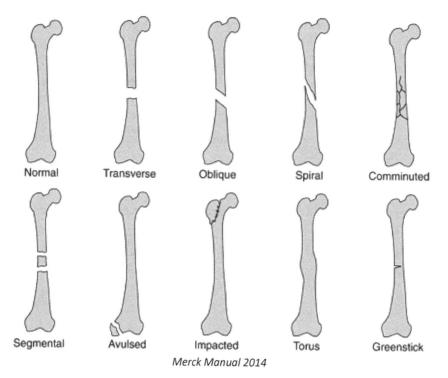

Merck Manual 2014

FRACTURE *(continued from previous page)*

SIGNS AND SYMPTOMS:
- Asymmetry compared to opposite side, but not always present.
- Deformity is associated with severe pain.
- Swelling and discoloration are not always present, but the likelihood of a fracture is greater if discoloration appears within 30 minutes.
- Suspect "stress" fracture if painful from excess exercise, jogging, gymnastics, ballet training, etc. Produces pain without swelling at site of fracture, especially on movement.
- Most frequently missed fractures: ribs, fingers/toes (chipped), elbow, knee, and end of the radius in the forearm.
- Other signs of a fracture:
  - Pain and swelling
  - Difficulty moving an affected extremity
  - Tenderness
  - Bruising
  - Numbness
  - Stiffness

MANAGEMENT/TREATMENT:
1. Treatment depends on the type and severity of the injury and may include pain relievers, *PRICE* - protection, rest, ice, compression, and elevation. If using ice, wrap in a towel before applying to the area.

2. Do not move the student until an assessment is complete.

3. Do not move the student if a fracture of the leg bones, pelvis or head, neck or spine is suspected unless the student is in grave danger by being left where he is. If a student must be moved under these circumstances, utilize multiple people and devices such as backboards or other large flat items in order to keep the student immobilized.

4. Inspect for deformity, pain, bleeding, protruding bone and edema.

5. Stop bleeding if present.

6. Calm student. Watch for signs of shock and treat symptoms.

FRACTURE *(continued from previous page)*

MANAGEMENT/TREATMENT: *(continued)*

7. Check for pulses near injury; if skin color is white/pale or pulse is absent, gently reposition only until circulation improves. If limb resists movement, stop.

8. Immobilize beyond joints above and below ends of suspected fracture, leaving the limb in position.

9. Treatment depends on the type and severity of the injury and may include pain relievers, *PRICE* - protection, rest, ice, compression, and elevation. If using ice, wrap in a towel before applying to the area.

10. Do not move the student until an assessment is complete.

11. Do not move the student if a fracture of the leg bones, pelvis or head, neck or spine is suspected unless the student is in grave danger by being left where he is. If a student must be moved under these circumstances, utilize multiple people and devices such as backboards or other large flat items in order to keep the student immobilized.

12. Inspect for deformity, pain, bleeding, protruding bone and edema.

13. Stop bleeding if present.

14. Calm student. Watch for signs of shock and treat symptoms.

15. Check for pulses near injury; if skin color is white/pale or pulse is absent, gently reposition only until circulation improves. If limb resists movement, stop.

16. Immobilize beyond joints above and below ends of suspected fracture, leaving the limb in position.

17. Splint only with a pillow if calling for emergency services. Raise body part above the heart if possible.

18. Cover exposed bone with sterile/clean bandage. DO NOT wash or probe.

FRACTURE *(continued from previous page)*

19. Summon emergency services and/or parent/guardian, depending on:
    - Severity and need for special transportation
    - Discolored or numb
    - Limb or joint is deformed
    - Bone is piercing the skin
    - Heavy bleeding

20. Monitor pulse(s) and breathing rate, checking for shock, every five minutes until emergency services arrive.

21. Fingers/Toes:
    - If suspect fracture, tape to adjacent finger/toe ("buddy" splint). Refer to be seen within the day, sooner if deformity is present.
    - Jammed finger: buddy tape to adjacent digit. Check onset of discoloration; usually within 12-15 hours if fractured and more than 15 hours if only "jammed."

22. Splint only with a pillow if calling for emergency services. Raise body part above the heart if possible.

23. Cover exposed bone with sterile/clean bandage. DO NOT wash or probe.

24. Summon emergency services and/or parent/guardian, depending on:
    - Severity and need for special transportation
    - Discolored or numb
    - Limb or joint is deformed
    - Bone is piercing the skin
    - Heavy bleeding

25. Monitor pulse(s) and breathing rate, checking for shock, every five minutes until emergency services arrive.

26. Fingers/Toes:
    - If suspect fracture, tape to adjacent finger/toe ("buddy" splint). Refer to be seen within the day, sooner if deformity is present.
    - Jammed finger: buddy tape to adjacent digit. Check onset of discoloration; usually within 12-15 hours if fractured and more than 15 hours if only "jammed."

FRACTURE *(continued from previous page)*

FOLLOW-UP:
- Splint/cast care as directed.
- Check fingers/toes for adequate circulation and sensation.
- Assist with modifications for classes, writing, keeping cast dry, etc.
- Assess proper crutch use.
- Promote mobility.

POTENTIAL COMPLICATIONS:
- Damage to blood vessels
- Fat embolism
- Nerve damage
- Osteomyelitis
- Compartment Syndrome

OTHER MUSCULOSKELETAL CONCERNS
- Dislocation – injury to a joint in which the ends of your bones are forced from their normal positions. Can occur in major joints such as the shoulder, hip, knee, elbow and ankle or in the smaller joints (fingers, thumbs and toes)
- Subluxation – partial dislocation
- Sprain – tearing or stretching of ligament (caused by injury)
- Strain - tearing or stretching of muscle or tendon (caused by overuse)

SIGNS AND SYMPTOMS:
- Joint looks visibly deformed or out of place
- Area swollen
- Immovable
- Area intensely painful

Complications
- Failure to reduce subluxation/dislocation
- Nerve damage
- Blood vessel damage

FRACTURE *(continued from previous page)*

MANAGEMENT/TREATMENT: depends on the severity of the injury
- The healthcare provider may try to gently maneuver the dislocated bone back into place (this is called reduction).
- If dislocation is severe – may need local or general anesthesia.
- May need to immobilize joint with a sling or splint.
- May need RICE (rest, ice, compression, elevation).

NOTES:
- Encourage children to wear protective gear such as helmets, elbow pads, kneepads and shin pads while biking, roller blading, and participating in contact sports.
- Repeated fractures can be an indication of other health conditions.
- Child abuse should be considered if there are reoccurring fractures without a medical indication or if the type of fracture is uncommon for a particular age group.
- Compartment Syndrome (mostly in lower limbs) is rare but can occur when there is swelling in a muscle group that has a fibrous covering. The lining does not allow for swelling from the injury and excessive pressure is place on the muscle that decreases blood flow to the muscle and can cause damage. Compartment Syndrome can also be caused from a splint or cast.
- The most common fractures in children are the clavicle, distal forearm, ulna, tibia and femur.

Resources

Medline Plus. (2012). Creating a Sling. http://www.nlm.nih.gov/medlineplus/ency/presentations/100137_1.htm

References

American Academy of Pediatrics. (2013). Alterations in musculoskeletal function. In S. Aronson, & T. Shope (Eds.), *Managing infectious diseases in child care and schools* (2nded.) (p.p.979-979). Elk Grove Village, IL: American Academy of Pediatrics.

Cleveland Clinic. (2013). *Fractures.* Retrieved from http://my.clevelandclinic.org/services/orthopaedics-rheumatology/diseases-conditions/hic-fractures

Mayo Clinic. (2015). *Fractures (broken bones): First aid.* Retrieved from http://www.mayoclinic.com/health/first-aid-fractures/FA00058

The Merck Manual. (2014). *Overview of fractures.* Retrieved http://www.merckmanuals.com/professional/injuries-poisoning/fractures-dislocations-and-sprains/overview-of-fractures-dislocations-and-sprains

HEADACHE(S)

DEFINITION/ETIOLOGY:

Headaches are common in children and have a wide range of causes with many levels of severity. Headaches are thought to be caused by changes in chemicals, nerves, or blood vessels in the area which send pain messages to the brain and bring on a headache. Children get the same types of headaches as adults and headaches are often hereditary. Headaches can be caused by a variety of triggers or certain infections.

Headaches can be considered <u>primary</u> meaning that they are not due to any underlying condition or <u>secondary or organic</u> meaning it is secondary to another disease or disorder.

Primary Headaches: (Generally recurrent, episodic and sporadic in presentation)
- Migraine
- Cluster
- Tension type

Secondary Headaches:
- Tumors
- High blood pressure
- Head injuries
- Sinusitis
- Other disease processes

Other Important Causes to Consider:
- Fatigue (probe reason if inadequate sleep), skipped breakfast, not wearing vision correction
- Sinusitis
- Central nervous system bleeding
- Increased intracranial pressure (chronic progressive headache)
- Tension
- Exertion
- Hormonal (associated with menstrual cycles)

HEADACHE(S) *(continued from previous page)*

SIGNS AND SYMPTOMS:
Findings with principal causes:

- **Tension-type headache**: the most common type in adolescence, "dull/achy," diffuse, bilateral, radiates to cervical neck, nausea may accompany but rarely vomiting. It is described as a general pain around the head. Precipitating factors include emotional stress and fatigue.

- **Vascular headaches:**
  - **Migraine:** "throbbing/pounding," usually unilateral. Generalized headaches are more common than unilateral headaches in children. It is common to experience nausea, vomiting, and sensitivity to light which makes it difficult to carry out activities of daily living. About 1/3 of migraine sufferers also experience an "aura" prior to the headache which may be described as a visual disturbance such as blinking lights or loss of vision. The presence of auras is less common in children than adults. Hunger may precede a childhood migraine. Dizziness, light-headedness, pallor, or purple bags around the eyes may also occur. Headaches last between 4 and 72 hours and are often hereditary.
  - **Cluster:** Often described as "burning/stabbing," often felt most around one eye. These headaches generally start suddenly and are of short duration but may reoccur for several months at a time. They are most common in spring and autumn.

- **Exertion** (exercise-related): Straining (Valsalva maneuver) triggers severe throbbing, **usually at the base of the head**; felt as a dull ache for 4-6 hours and may recur in later weeks or months upon exertion.

- **Secondary to other conditions**, e.g., sinusitis, dental problem, eye strain. May be associated with other symptoms such as cough, fever or blurred vision. A headache associated with sinusitis may present as a sense of fullness or throbbing in the frontal or temporal areas.

HEADACHE(S) *(continued from previous page)*

- **Pathological conditions**:
  - ○ **Traction headaches:** brain tumor, intracranial hemorrhage or disorder of cerebrospinal fluid pressure.
  - ○ **Infection/inflammation:** meningitis, encephalitis and brain abscess. The nature of headache is sudden onset, increasingly severe within days, may be persistently one sided or localized. Headaches are followed in time by abnormal neurological signs, such as vomiting without nausea, headaches that awaken the person, staggering gait and/or confusion.

ASSESSMENT:

- History: Ask about occurrences, such as surrounding events (injury, stressor such as lack of food or sleep), frequency, duration, cyclic nature, location, and severity of headache (e.g., stops playing, causes school absenteeism). Determine associated symptoms and use of any medications or other care.
- **The most important part of the evaluation is to ascertain if this is a benign condition or a pathological condition**. If exam is abnormal, especially neurological exam and history (e.g., irritability, mental confusion, fatigue or blurred/altered vision), then there is heightened concern for a more serious pathological condition causing the headache.

MANAGEMENT/TREATMENT:

1. If student has a suspected pathological condition underlying the headache, notify the parent/guardian immediately and refer to the student's healthcare provider.

2. For benign conditions, headache diaries are useful for evaluation. The school nurse, working with the student's healthcare provider, can suggest a long-term plan.

3. Intervention is based on the cause.
   Non-medication measures
   - Rest in quiet, darkened room
   - Cool or warm cloth on forehead
   - Stress management/relaxation techniques
   - Eliminate precipitating factors
   - Biofeedback, good posture and daily exercise

HEADACHE(S) *(continued from previous page)*

Medications
- **Tension headache**: Non-prescription analgesics. No food or caffeine restrictions unless the food is a confirmed trigger.
- **Migraine type**: Treat the headache as soon as it starts; do not wait for nausea or other symptoms. Prompt treatment turns off the mediators of inflammation and should be available at school. Over-the-counter analgesics, including acetaminophen, nonsteroidal anti-inflammatory drugs (NSAID) such as ibuprofen and naproxen may be effective if given at the onset of the headache. Triptans and serotonin antagonists are commonly prescribed but should not be used more than 4-6 times per month. School absences or inability to perform at school due to migraine suggests that prophylactic agents are indicated. Prophylactic agents (such as tricyclic antidepressants (amitriptyline), propranolol, and calcium channel blockers) are used when auras present or in severe cases.
- **Cluster headache**: Children are usually referred to pediatric neurologists.

FOLLOW UP:
- Gauge continuing symptoms with a headache diary.
- Reevaluation is warranted any time initial impressions do not fit, when symptoms persist or worsen with time, or when new symptoms emerge.
- Monitor complications such as side effects of medications and disruption of activities (e.g. school absences, poor academic performance).
- Assist those with migraine or tension headache to follow their medical and non-medical regimens.
- Healthy lifestyle strategies such as adequate sleep, good diet and relaxation techniques can be helpful.

POTENTIAL COMPLICATIONS:
Headaches can be painful and debilitating but are generally not due to dangerous conditions. However, occasionally headaches can be a sign of something more serious including very severe high blood pressure greater than 180/110 mm Hg, stroke, brain tumor, or meningitis.

HEADACHE(S) *(continued from previous page)*

It is critical to seek emergency medical care if a headache
- **gets worse over days or weeks**
- **is accompanied by impaired neurological function**
- **is accompanied by persistent nausea and vomiting**
- **is accompanied by fever or stiff neck**
- **is accompanied by seizure, mental disturbance, or loss of consciousness**
- **is different than usual headaches, strikes suddenly with great intensity, or**
- **wakes the patient from sleep and is worse when laying down**

NOTES: (PREVENTION)

Migraine-specific preventive interventions:
- Meals should not be skipped; a morning snack can help if hunger is a trigger. The role of specific food triggers is controversial, but parents/guardians may want child to avoid one food at a time to see if there is a benefit.
- Stay well hydrated; dehydration is a trigger for some migraines.
- Regular sleep routines and stress management.
- Daily exercise (20-30 minutes).

References

Anatomical Chart Company. (2014). Pathology- Understanding headaches and migraines. *Classic Anthology of Anatomical Charts 7th ed. Volume 2*, p. 6. Philadelphia, PA: Lippincott Williams and Wilkins.

Buck M.L. (2013). Use of topiramate in preventing pediatric migraine. Retrieved from http://www.medicine.virginia.edu/clinical/departments/pediatrics/education/pharm-news/current/201307.pdf

Hershey, A.D., Kabbouche, M.A., & O' Brien, H.O. (2016). Headache. In R.M. Kliegman, B.S. Stanton, J. St. Geme, & N.F. Schor (eds.), *Textbook of pediatrics: Expert consult (20th ed.)* (p. p. 2863-2872). Philadelphia, PA: Elsevier.

Kids Health from Nemours. (n.d.). *Headaches.* Retrieved from http://kidshealth.org/parent/general/aches/headache.html

MediResource Inc. (n.d.). *Headaches.* Retrieved from http://bodyandhealth.canada.com/channel_condition_info_details.asp?channel_id=42&relation_id=10900&disease_id=67&page_no=2#Treatment

HEART MURMURS

DEFINITION/ETIOLOGY:
A murmur is defined as an extra or unusual sound heard during a heartbeat. Murmurs can be functional (innocent) or pathologic (abnormal) indicating possible cardiac disease or a malfunction in the cardiac system.

A heart murmur is a common finding among children. Up to 50-75% of children will have an innocent murmur at some point in their childhood. Innocent murmurs are often heard in the newborn period, especially in the first few days of life.

Murmurs should be described based on the following characteristics:
- Location and radiation (where the murmur is heard best)
- Relation to the cardiac cycle and duration (whether heard following S1 or throughout the cycle)
- Intensity
  - Grade 1 barely audible
  - Grade 2 soft but easily audible
  - Grade 3 moderately load with no palpable thrill (a vibratory feeling over the sternum)
  - Grade 4 loud with a thrill
  - Grade 5 audible with the stethoscope barely touching the chest
  - Grade 6 audible with no stethoscope
- Quality (harsh, musical or high, medium or low in pitch)
- Variation with position (audible changes when the student is supine, sitting standing or squatting

SIGNS AND SYMPTOMS:
The following should also be assessed in the presence of a murmur
- Arterial rate and rhythm
  - Tachycardia may be indicative of cardiovascular or respiratory compromise.
- Arterial pulse quality and amplitude
  - A bounding pulse can be indicative of a cardiac abnormality
  - A weak or thread pulse can be indicative of poor cardiac output
- Blood pressure in all 4 extremities
  - A decreased blood pressure in the lower extremities can be indicative of a coarctation of the aorta
- Color of skin, nail beds, lips
- Respiratory rate and rhythm

191

HEART MURMURS *(continued from previous page)*

Symptoms suggestive of cardiac pathology
- Chest pain associated with shortness of breath or murmur
- Family history of Marfan Syndrome or sudden death of young family members
- Increased precordial activity
- Decreased femoral pulses
- Abnormal second heart sound
- Increased intensity of a murmur when the student stands
- A murmur of grade 4 or higher
- Palpitations
- Lightheadedness or syncope

MANAGEMENT/TREATMENT:
Any previously undiagnosed murmur heard in the school aged child should be evaluated by the healthcare provider. A murmur in the absence of any other abnormal finding is not a medical emergency but evaluation is warranted.

Children with a newly diagnosed murmur will often be referred to a pediatric cardiologist and will be evaluated with a cardiac ultrasound for diagnosis.

FOLLOW-UP:
When innocent murmurs are found in a child the parent should be assured of that these are normal heart sounds of the developing child.

References

American Heart Association. (2013). *Heart murmurs*. Retrieved from http://www.heart.org/HEARTORG/Conditions/More/CardiovascularConditionsofChildhood/Heart-Murmurs_UCM_314208_Article.jsp#.VijfCCsjlgQ

Bernstein, D. (2016). In R.M. Kliegman, B.S. Stanton, J. St. Geme, & N.F. Schor (eds.), *Textbook of pediatrics: Expert consult* (20th ed.) (p.p. 2163-2167). Philadelphia, PA: Elsevier.

Cleveland Clinic. (2015). *Heart murmur*. Retrieved from http://my.clevelandclinic.org/services/heart/disorders/heart-valve-disease/heart-murmur

Mayo Clinic. (2015). *Heart murmurs*. Retrieved from *http://www.mayoclinic.org/diseases-conditions/heart-murmurs/basics/definition/con-2002870*

Menashe, V. (2007). Heart murmurs. *Pediatrics in Review, 28*(4), e19 -e22. doi: 10.1542/pir.28-4-e19

National Heart, Lung and Blood Institute, U.S. Department of Health and Human Services. (2012). *Explore heart murmurs*. Retrieved from http://www.nhlbi.nih.gov/health/health-topics/topics/heartmurmur

HEAT-RELATED ILLNESS

DEFINITION/ETIOLOGY:

Heat-related illness occurs when the body's temperature-regulating mechanisms are over-whelmed. Core body temperature may rise above a safe level. Initially, the loss of salt and potassium from heavy perspiring may lead to **muscle cramps,** referred to as **heat cramps.** If the person is not cooled, this may lead to **heat exhaustion** due to dehydration. The most serious form of heat illness is **heatstroke** which can lead to shock, brain damage, and death.

- Hot environments such as outdoors on a hot and humid day or indoors in a hot, poorly ventilated area are the most common causes of heat-related illness.
- Certain medications (beta-blockers, diuretics, some medications used to treat depression, psychosis, or ADHD) can alter the body's response to heat and sun.
- Heat-related illness is also associated with alcohol, inappropriate use of drugs, prolonged exertion, dehydration, heart disease, not drinking enough fluids during activity and wearing too much clothing.

SIGNS AND SYMPTOMS:

HEAT CRAMPS
- Muscle cramps often in the abdomen or legs
- Excess perspiration
- Weakness (fatigue), lightheadedness
- Thirst

HEAT EXHAUSTION
- Cool, pale and clammy skin
- Heavy sweating
- Weakness or tiredness
- Dizziness, lightheadedness, or fainting
- Headache
- Nausea/vomiting
- Muscle cramping
- Rapid heart rate
- Dark Urine

HEAT-RELATED ILLNESS *(continued from previous page)*

HEAT STROKE
- Hot, red, dry skin
- Absence of sweating
- Temperature above 104°F
- Rapid, weak pulse
- Extremely high body temperature (above 103°F, orally and may be up to 106°F)
- Rapid, shallow breathing
- Nausea
- Confusion/lack of coordination
- Unconsciousness/seizures
- Throbbing headache
- Dizziness

MANAGEMENT/TREATMENT:
HEAT CRAMPS
1. Move person to cool place and instruct person to rest.
2. If person is alert, give sips of fluids (water, sports drink, or make salted drink of one teaspoon of salt per quart of water) 4 oz. every 15 minutes.
3. Do not give liquids with caffeine.
4. Do not give salt tablets.
5. If person does not improve or if worsens call EMS.

HEAT EXHAUSTION
1. Move person to cool place.
2. Stop activity and instruct person to lie down and elevate feet 8-12 inches.
3. Loosen clothing.
4. Apply cool, wet cloths to neck, armpits, and groin.
5. Use fan to cool (evaporation) and/or move to air-conditioned area.
6. If conscious, administer sips of fluids (may use sports drink with carbohydrate content under 6 percent).
7. If nausea or vomiting occurs, discontinue fluids.
8. Seek immediate medical attention if symptoms are severe, worsen, or last over an hour.
9. Seek medical attention immediately, if person has high blood pressure or heart problems.

HEAT-RELATED ILLNESS *(continued from previous page)*

HEAT STROKE
1. Call 911.
2. Move the victim to a cooler environment.
3. Reduce body temperature with cold bath or sponging, wet sheets, or towels.
4. Monitor body temperature and continue cooling efforts until body temperature reaches 101°F.
5. Remove clothing, use fans, air-conditioners.
6. Do not give fluids to drink.
7. Be alert for vomiting and prevent aspiration.
8. Monitor consciousness and prepare to administer CPR, if necessary.

NOTE: Untreated heat cramps and exhaustion may lead to Heat Stroke.

HEAT STROKE IS A SEVERE MEDICAL EMERGENCY. SUMMON EMERGENCY MEDICAL ASSISTANCE OR GET THE VICTIM TO A HOSPITAL IMMEDIATELY. DELAY CAN BE FATAL.

PREVENTION:
1. Provide information about temperature and heat index during extreme heat conditions.
2. Follow local news and weather channels or contact the local health department for health and safety updates.
3. Provide education:
   a. Drink plenty of fluids.
   b. Do not wait until thirsty to drink fluids.
   c. During heavy exercise in a hot environment, drink two to four glasses (16-32 ounces) of cool fluids every hour.
   d. Encourage limiting activities to morning and evening (avoid mid-day sun) and providing opportunities for frequent rest in shady areas.
   e. Wear loose-fitting, lightweight and light colored clothing.

HEAT-RELATED ILLNESS *(continued from previous page)*

PREVENTION *(continued)*

4. Initiate efforts to promote "Sun Safety" for students, faculty and staff, and parents.
   - Sunburn causes the loss of body fluids and effects the body's ability to cool itself.
   - Promote an awareness campaign to SLIP, SLOP, SLAP, SEEK, SLIDE on days with high temperatures, high heat index, and outdoor activities in bright sunlight.
     - SLIP on a long sleeve shirt.
     - SLOP on sunscreen of SPF 15 or higher (the most effective products marked "broad spectrum" or "UAV/UVB protection" on the labels). Sunscreen must be applied liberally and frequently.
     - SLAP on a hat. (A broad brimmed hat gives the most protection.)
     - SEEK shade.
     - SLIDE on sunglasses.

5. Recommend programs and efforts to prevent heat related health emergencies:
   - Hydration and extended "rest/time out" during athletic and sport events/ practices.
   - Indoor (air conditioning) classes for physical education on high heat index days.
   - Contribute to playground planning efforts to include areas of shade for respite from heat and sun.

References

American Cancer Society. (2013) *American Cancer Society: Skin cancer prevention activities.* Retrieved from http://www.cancer.org/healthy/morewaysacshelps you stay well/acs-skin-cancer-prevention-activities

Cancer Council Australia. (2015) *Slip Slop Slap Seek Slide. Retrieved from http://www.cancer.org.au/preventing-cancer/sun-protection/campaigns-and-events/slip-slop-slap-seek-slide.html*

Center for Disease Control and Prevention. (2015). *Extreme heat prevention guide.* Retrieved from http://www.bt.cdc.gov/disasters/extremeheat/heat_guide.asp

Hockenberry, M., Baker, R., & Mondozzi, M. (2013). The Child with integumentary dysfunction. In M. Hokenberry, E. In Chg) & D. Wilson (Eds), *Wong's Essentials of Pediatric Nursing.* (9th ed.) (p.p. 1047-1048) St. Louis, MO: Elsevier/Mosby.

Mattey, E. (2013). Growth and development: Preschool through adolescence. In J. Selekman (Ed.), *School nursing: A comprehensive text* (2nd ed.) (p. 346). Philadelphia, PA: F.A. Davis.

Medline Plus, U.S. National Library of Medicine. (2014). *Heat emergencies.* Retrieved from http://www.nlm.nih.gov/medlineplus/ency/article/000056.htm

Schraga, E.D. (2013). *Cooling techniques for hyperthermia.* Retrieved from http://emedicine.medscape.com/article/149546-overview

HEMOPHILIA

DEFINITION/ETIOLOGY:
Hemophilia is a common hereditary blood clotting disorder, primarily affecting males. The severity of hemophilia depends on the amount of clotting factor in the blood (ranging from mild to severe). Clotting factor is a protein in the blood that is needed for normal clotting. There is no cure for hemophilia. Hemophilia is a life-long disease.

TYPES:
- *Hemophilia A*: classic hemophilia (80% of cases), usually severe
- *Hemophilia B*: "Christmas disease"—first diagnosed in child whose last name was Christmas (15% *of cases),* severity varies
- *Hemophilia C*: usually mild with bleeding problems only after surgery or major injury

SIGNS AND SYMPTOMS:
- External bleed: excessive bleeding from mild cuts or abrasions, bruises easily, frequent nose bleeds that are difficult to stop. External bleeds are typically not a problem; hemophiliacs bleed longer, not faster.
- Internal bleeding may occur anywhere in body. **This is a serious problem**. Symptoms of internal bleeding depend on the location of the bleeding, the amount of bleeding, and structures/functions of the body affected. **If you suspect an internal bleed, seek medical treatment immediately!** Below are examples of internal bleeds:

Location of Bleed	Potential symptom(s)
Kidneys	• Blood in urine • Flank pain
Joint bleed (frequently affects elbows, knees and ankles)	• Can occur without obvious injury • Feeling of tightness in joint • Swelling around joint • Warm to touch • Pain around joint
Intracranial bleed	• Headache (painful) • May have neck pain/stiffness • Altered mental function • Recurrent vomiting • Double vision • Seizures

HEMOPHILIA *(continued from previous page)*

Location of Bleed	Potential symptom(s)
Intra-abdominal bleeding	• Lightheaded • Short of breath • Shock • Decreased blood pressure • Gastrointestinal bleed – may vomit bright red blood or have black tarry stools, bruising around umbilical area

MANAGEMENT/TREATMENT:
Specific orders should be obtained for all students with a diagnosis of hemophilia. Students must have an Individualized Healthcare Plan and Emergency Plans. They may be eligible for Section 504 or special education services.

Student may be receiving frequent transfusions with special blood products. Open communication between parent/guardian(s) and school staff, including the school nurse, is important in providing safe and effective care in the school setting for students with hemophilia.

School policies and procedures can provide guidance in caring for hemophilia in the school setting. A school nurse may be needed to be available for continuity of care and success in school for students with hemophilia.
1. **If you suspect an internal bleed; seek medical treatment immediately.**
2. Apply firm pressure for 10 minutes over skin lacerations or abrasions.
3. Apply ice pack to small bleeds under the skin.
4. Carefully observe student following minor trauma for possible internal bleeding.
5. Notify parent/guardian after all accidents (even if there is no visible sign of injury).
6. NO ASPIRIN or IBUPROFEN (prolongs bleeding time) nor other medications without healthcare provider's orders.
7. No injections at school unless under a healthcare provider's order because of possible hemorrhage into muscle.
8. Follow healthcare provider's orders for PE participation. Contact and hard ball sports are contraindicated.
9. Establish liaison with playground supervisors, PE teacher, parent/guardian(s), and healthcare provider.
10. Educate student about play and sport safety. Restrict activity as little as possible within medical limits.

HEMOPHILIA *(continued from previous page)*

11. May receive transfusions; increased risk of infection through blood products.
    a. Educate parent/guardian regarding the importance of being up-to-date on Hepatitis A and B vaccination.

FOLLOW UP:

- Provide accommodations for frequent doctors' appointments.
- Observe for early bleeding episodes. Many children do not report early bleeding even if they know it is beginning. Children with hemophilia can learn about the signs and symptoms of internal bleeding and are encouraged to notify an adult when he or she senses bleeding to prevent long-term damage.
- Encourage non-contact sports: golf, swimming.
- Resume activity gradually after external bleeding episode.
- Follow healthcare provider's activity orders following an internal bleeding episode.
- Help student feel at ease if returns to school in a wheelchair or with a sling to relieve pressure.
- Educate child/parent/guardian regarding injury prevention when riding bicycle; wear kneepads, elbow pads, helmets, etc.
- If indicated, (with parent permission) provide hemophilia education to classmates.
- Promote good oral hygiene to prevent dental extractions.

POTENTIAL COMPLICATIONS:

- Internal bleeding
- Joint damage
- Infections

NOTES:

People with hemophilia can live relatively normal lives with proper treatment. However, prognosis is guarded without adequate treatment.

References

Centers for Disease Control and Prevention. (2014). *Hemophilia*. Retrieved from http://www.cdc.gov/ncbddd/hemophilia/facts.html

Mayo Clinic. (2014). *Hemophilia*. Retrieved from http://www.mayoclinic.com/health/hemophilia/DS00218

Merck Manual. (2015). *Hemophilia*. Retrieved from http://www.cdc.gov/ncbddd/hemophilia/facts.html

National Heart, Lung, and Blood Institute. (2011). *Signs and symptoms of hemophilia*. Retrieved from http://www.nhlbi.nih.gov/health/health-topics/topics/hemophilia/signs.html

Selekman, J., Bochenek, J. & Lukens, M. (2013). Children with chronic conditions. In J. Selekman (Ed.), *School nursing: A comprehensive text* (2nd ed.) (pp. 700-783). Philadelphia, PA: F. A. Davis.

HEPATITIS (VIRAL, TYPES A, B, AND C)

DEFINITION/ETIOLOGY:

The term hepatitis describes inflammation of the liver. Hepatitis may be caused by alcohol, drugs, autoimmune diseases, metabolic diseases, and viruses. Acute viral hepatitis is the most common cause of jaundice (conjugated hyperbilirubinemia) in childhood and adolescence. Three types of hepatitis (A, B, C) are reportable illnesses in most states. These viruses affect the liver and produce similar symptoms. The incubation period, the mode of transmission, and results of serologic tests help to distinguish the different types of viral hepatitis.

The five types of viral hepatitis are Hepatitis A (HAV), Hepatitis B (HBV), Hepatitis C (HCV), Hepatitis D (HDV), and Hepatitis E (HEV). In the United States, HAV is the most common cause of acute hepatitis and HCV is the most common cause of chronic hepatitis. The information provided in this guideline will focus on HAV, HBV, and HCV infections in the pediatric population.

CAUSE

Hepatitis: Characteristics of Virus Types			
	Hepatitis A	**Hepatitis B**	**Hepatitis C**
Transmission	Transmission is almost always person to person via fecal-oral route, contaminated water/food	High concentrations parenteral, blood, blood products Moderate concentrations saliva, vaginal fluids and semen Sexual contact, drug use	Parenteral, blood , blood product, sexual contact, drug use In children perinatal transmission is the most prevalent mode of transmission
Incubation period	2-6 weeks (average 4 weeks)	1-6 months (average 3 mos.)	2 weeks – 6 months (average 6-7 weeks)
May be a carrier	Not long-term	Yes	Yes

HEPATITIS (VIRAL, TYPES A, B, AND C) *(continued from previous page)*

	Hepatitis A	Hepatitis B	Hepatitis C
Treatment (acute)	Immune globulin within 2 weeks of exposure	Hepatitis B immunoglobulin after exposure	None
Treatment (chronic)	Supportive	Supportive	Supportive –interferon see below
Vaccine	Available (recommended 2 doses, the second dose 6 to 12 months after the first dose, for all children 12 months and older)	Available (recommended shortly after birth with 2 additional doses)	Not available

SIGNS AND SYMPTOMS:
- Fever, malaise, fatigue, headache, joint pain
- Dark urine and lighter-color stools
- Loss of appetite, nausea, vomiting, stomachache
- Jaundice (yellow eyes and skin)
- Enlargement and/or tenderness of the liver on palpation
- Most cases in young children are mild

HEPATITIS A (HAV)
- **HAV infection occurs throughout the world but is most common in developing countries.**
- Symptomatic hepatitis A infection occurs in approximately 30% of infected children younger than six years of age; most infected children have no jaundice. Among older children and adults, infection usually is symptomatic and typically lasts several weeks, with jaundice occurring in approximately 70% of cases.
- The highest titer of HAV in stool occurs during one to two weeks before the onset of illness. HAV is transmitted from person-to-person or by contamination by food and water. The risk of transmission subsequently diminishes by one week after onset of jaundice. However, HAV can be detected in stool for long periods, especially in young children.

HEPATITIS (VIRAL, TYPES A, B, AND C) *(continued from previous page)*

- Post-exposure prophylaxis: Immune globulin (IG) is recommended for un-immunized close personal contacts within two weeks after exposure, e.g., member of household, day care center for un-immunized employees and all younger children not yet toilet trained. In a center in which all children are toilet trained, IG is recommend for only the children in the same rooms as the index case. Exposure at **regular school** is _not_ considered a close contact and IG is not recommended except under unusual circumstances.
- Children with hepatitis A should be referred to the healthcare provider and excluded for 1 week after onset of illness.
- Adults with acute HAV infection who work as food handlers or in child care settings should be excluded until one week after onset of the illness, until the IG prophylaxis program has been completed, or as directed by the health department.
- Active immunization (HAV vaccine) is effective for children and adults.

HEPATITIS B (HBV)
- HBV has two phases, acute and chronic. Acute HBV is new and is short-term, occurring shortly after exposure to the virus. Chronic HBV is ongoing and long-term lasting longer than six months. Chronic HBV may not go away completely.
- Young children usually do not have jaundice or other symptoms. Sometimes, HBV affects other parts of the body resulting in arthritis, rash or thrombocytopenia. More than 90% of infants who are infected perinatally will develop chronic infection, whereas 25%-50% of children infected between one and five years of age and 10% of infected older children and adults develop a chronic case.
- HBV virus is transmitted through blood and body fluids, including exudates, semen, cervical secretions and uncommonly with saliva. Person-to-person contact can occur in any setting involving interpersonal contact over an extended period. HBV virus can survive in the environment for one week, so transmission from shared objects, such as razor blades or toothbrushes also may occur but is uncommon. Among adolescents and adults, those at highest risk include users of injection drugs and those with multiple sexual patters.
- HBV is almost always preventable. Pre-exposure HBV immunization is the universally recommended preventive measure for infants, un-immunized children and adolescents.
- School nurses, athletic trainers, and teachers of students who are severely developmentally delayed and positive for Hepatitis B surface antigens (HBsAg) are candidates for immunization.

HEPATITIS (VIRAL, TYPES A, B, AND C) *(continued from previous page)*

- Most children with hepatitis B should be admitted to school without restrictions. If the student has weeping sores, or behaviors that would lead to bleeding exclusion may be necessary.
- Post-exposure prophylaxis: Hepatitis B Immune Globulin (HBIG) is indicated for people at risk of developing HBV due to recent exposure of body fluids of someone infected with HBV. This includes babies of mothers infected with HBV, healthcare workers, emergency first responders, and morticians. HBIG is effective because it provides temporary induced immunity by the transfer of immunoglobulin.

HEPATITIS C (HCV)
- Acute disease tends to be mild and insidious in onset and most infections are asymptomatic. Persistent infection with HCV occurs in 50% to 60% of infected children but without significant liver damage.
- Risk factors are blood transfusions, kidney dialysis, and injected illicit drug use.
- Treatment is with interferon-alfa alone or in combination with ribavirin in chronic hepatitis C in adults. Combination therapy results in higher sustained response rates in 40% of cases but has not received FDA approval for those less than 18 years of age.
- Direct acting antivirals have shown good results in the treatment of HCV but studies are pending in children.
- Children with chronic infection should be screened periodically for chronic hepatitis because of potential risk of chronic liver disease. Viral titers should be checked yearly.

MANAGEMENT/TREATMENT:
1. Notify the parent/guardian of symptoms of concern and refer to healthcare provider.
2. Follow state regulations and school policy on reporting to health department.
3. Recommendations for immune globulin are only for those with close contact, not general classroom contact. Immune globulin recommendation depends on type of hepatitis and indications. HAV: serologic testing of contacts is not recommended, because testing may delay administration of IG. HBV: serologic test for anti-HBs is recommended in exposed person with previous immunization but unknown response. Work with Public Health authorities.
4. Use good hand washing techniques at all times and instruct children as necessary.

HEPATITIS (VIRAL, TYPES A, B, AND C) *(continued from previous page)*

FOLLOW UP:

- Educate campus personnel and students on Universal/Standard Precautions.
- Teach about specific routes of transmission, incubation periods, and signs of infection.
- Athletes should cover existing cuts, abrasions, wounds, or other areas of broken skin with a dressing.
- Inquire about other cases in family and after-school care, group or club.
- Inform about requirements and availability of Hepatitis A and Hepatitis B vaccines.

References

American Academy of Pediatrics. (2015). Hepatitis A, B, C. In L. K. Pickering, C. J. Baker, D. W. Kimberlin, & S. S. Long (Eds.), *Red Book: 2015 report of the committee on infectious diseases, (30th ed.)* (pp. 391-430). American Academy of Pediatrics: Elk Grove Village, IL.

American Academy of Pediatrics. (2013). Hepatitis A infection; Hepatitis B infection. In S. Aronson, & T. Shope (Eds.), *Managing infectious diseases in child care and schools (2nd ed.)* (pp. 101-104). Elk Grove Village, IL: American Academy of Pediatrics.

Buggs, A. M. (2014). *Hepatitis: Viral.* Retrieved from http://emedicine.medscape.com/article/185463-overview

Centers for Disease Control and Prevention (CDC). (2015a). Hepatitis A. In W. Atkinson, C. Wolfe, & J., Hamborsky (Eds.), *Epidemiology and prevention of vaccine-preventable diseases* (13th ed.). Washington DC: Public Health Foundation. Retrieved from http://www.cdc.gov/vaccines/pubs/pinkbook/hepa.html

Centers for Disease Control and Prevention (CDC) (2015b). Hepatitis B. In W. Atkinson, C. Wolfe, & J., Hamborsky (Eds.), *Epidemiology and prevention of vaccine-preventable diseases* (13th ed.). Washington DC: Public Health Foundation. Retrieved from http://www.cdc.gov/vaccines/pubs/pinkbook/hepb.html

Centers for Disease Control and Prevention. (2015c). *Viral hepatitis.* Retrieved from http://www.cdc.gov/HEPATITIS/

Jensen, K. & Balistreri, W. (2016). The digestive system. In R.M. Kliegman, B.F. Stanton, J.W. St. Geme, & N.F. Schor (Eds.), *Nelson Textbook of Pediatrics (20*th *ed.) (p.38).* Philadelphia, PA: Elsevier Saunders

HERPES SIMPLEX - ORAL (cold sore, fever blister)

DEFINITION/ETIOLOGY:

An acute, viral infection with a local primary lesion (cold sore or fever blister occurring on the lips, mouth or face), which is frequently latent and has a tendency to recur. Most persons are initially infected by school age. During the first infection people may shed the virus for at least a week and possibly several weeks after signs and symptoms appear. The virus remains dormant in the body and may recur when triggered by local skin trauma, sun exposure, or systemic changes such as fatigue, menstruation, fever or stress. Recurrent episodes are due to reactivation of latent herpes simplex virus (HSV). People with recurrent sores shed the virus for 3-4 days after symptoms appear. Two to five percent of healthy persons with no visible lesions carry herpes simplex virus in their saliva. The virus is often spread by people with no signs or symptoms, often adults and is spread by direct contact through kissing or contact with open sores.

Etiology: *Herpes simplex virus*, type 1 is the usual cause of mouth sores and herpes simplex virus, type 2 is the usual causative for most genital herpes lesions. At times, type 1 may cause infection in the genital area and type 2 can cause infection in the mouth.

SIGNS AND SYMPTOMS:

- Painful superficial, fluid filled blisters on an erythematous base, usually on the mouth, lips, and face, and are slow to crust over.
- May have an itchy or tingling sensation before blister appears.
- May have tender lymph nodes.
- During an episode the typical duration is 7-10 days.
- Contagious until the lesion is completely crusted over.

In the initial infection of herpes simplex virus, the symptoms are more generalized and more severe than in recurrent infections. Children may develop 10 or more small ulcers on the buccal mucosa, tonsils, inner lips tongue and gingiva. This is associated with fever and tender cervical adenopathy.

HERPES SIMPLEX - ORAL (Cold sore, fever blister) *(continued from previous page)*

MANAGEMENT/TREATMENT:
1. No exclusion from school.
2. Use good hand-washing techniques at all times.
3. There is no cure for herpes simplex.
4. Glyoxide, campho-phenique, and aloe vera relieve burning and itching briefly.
5. Blisters should be kept clean to prevent bacterial infection.
6. Lesions are contagious (spread by skin to skin contact), so hands should be washed after touching lesions.
7. Refrain from kissing when blisters are present.
8. Refer to healthcare provider if severe, frequently recurring or long lasting.
9. Some healthcare providers prescribe oral acyclovir for early use in frequently recurring or severe cases.
10. A child with type 2 lesions should be evaluated for possible sexual abuse.

FOLLOW UP:
Sunscreen on lips reduces risk of recurrence.

POTENTIAL COMPLICATIONS:
- Avoid cross-contamination. Keep hands away from eyes. Herpes simplex infections of the eye can cause scarring of the cornea which can potentially lead to blindness.
- Can cause meningitis or encephalitis if the herpes simplex virus spreads to the brain.
- Can result in dehydration due to dysphagia especially in young children.

NOTES:
The herpes simplex virus can be life-threatening to a person with a compromised immune system.

SPECIAL INFORMATION on HERPES SIMPLEX, type 2
1. Genital herpes simplex (type 2) does not require exclusion from school.
2. Oral acyclovir is prescribed to suppress painful lesions.
3. Educate staff and pregnant students about dangers to fetus if herpes simplex is acquired during pregnancy.
4. Newborn baby may acquire the infection during vaginal delivery if mother has active type 2 lesions.

HERPES SIMPLEX - ORAL (Cold sore, fever blister) *(continued from previous page)*

Reference

American Academy of Pediatrics. (2013). Herpes simplex virus. In S. Aronson, & T. Shope (Eds.), *Managing infectious diseases in child care and schools (2nd ed.)* (pp. 105-106). Elk Grove Village, IL: American Academy of Pediatrics.

American Academy of Pediatrics, Committee on Infectious Diseases. (2015). Herpes simplex. In D.W. Kimberlin, M. T. Brady, M.A. Jackson, & S.S. Long (Eds.), *Red Book: 2015 report of the committee on infectious diseases* (30th ed.) (pp.432-445). Elk Grove Village, IL: American Academy of Pediatrics.

Aronson S. & Shope T. (Eds.). (2013). Herpes simplex virus. *Managing infectious diseases in childcare and schools*, (p.105-106). Elk Grove Village, IL: American Academy of Pediatrics.

Levin, M.J., & Weinberg, A. (2014). Infections: Viral and rickettsial. In W. Hay, M. Levin, R. Deterding, & M. Abzug (Eds.), *Current diagnosis and treatment pediatrics* (22nd edition) (pp. 522, 1244-1245). McGraw Hill Education, Inc.

Smith, S. (2014). *Herpes labialis.* Retrieved from http://www.nlm.nih.gov/medlineplus/ency/article/000606.htm

HIV

DEFINITION/ETIOLOGY:

HIV stands for Human Immunodeficiency Virus. The virus spreads through body fluids that affect specific cells of the immune system called CD4 cells, or T cells. Over time, HIV destroys so many of these cells that the body cannot fight off infections and disease. When this happens, HIV infection leads to Acquired Immunodeficiency Syndrome (AIDS). Currently, there are no safe or effective cures but the disease can be controlled with proper medical care and antiretroviral therapy (ART). Before the introduction of ART in the mid-1990s, people could progress to AIDS within a few years. Presently, someone diagnosed with HIV can have a near normal life expectancy.

In 2010, the estimated number of new HIV infections was highest among individuals aged 25-34 (31%), followed by individuals aged 13-24 (26%). There were 40,500 new HIV infections in the United States in 2010. About 1.2 million people in the United States were living with HIV at the end of 2012. Blacks/African Americans continue to be disproportionately affected by HIV infection. The estimated rate of new HIV infections among blacks/African Americans (68.9 per 100,000) was 7.9 times as high as the rate in whites (8.7). Hispanic/Latinos are also disproportionately affected by HIV infection. In 2010, Hispanics/Latinos comprised 21% of the new HIV infections. The rate of new HIV infections for Hispanics/Latinos (27.5) was three times the rate for whites (8.7). HIV is largely an urban disease, with most cases occurring in metropolitan areas with 500,000 or more people.

In the United States, HIV is spread mainly by having sex with someone who has HIV (anal sex is the highest risk behavior), sharing needles, syringes, rinse water, or other equipment (works) used to prepare injection drugs with someone who has HIV. Other less common forms of transmission include:

- Being stuck with an HIV contaminated needle.
- Receiving blood transfusions, blood products, or organ/tissue transplants.
- Eating food that has been pre-chewed by an HIV-infected person.
- Being bitten by a person with HIV.
- Oral sex.
- Contact between broken skin, wounds, or mucous membranes and HIV-infected blood or blood-contaminated body fluids.
- Deep, open-mouth kissing if the person with HIV has sores or bleeding gums and blood is exchanged. HIV is not spread through saliva.
- Being born to an infected mother. HIV can be passed from mother to child during pregnancy, birth, or breastfeeding.

HIV *(continued from previous page)*

CAUSES OF HIV:
Scientists identified a specific type of chimpanzees and monkeys in West Africa as the original source of HIV infection in humans. The scientists believe simian immunodeficiency virus (SIV) was most likely transmitted to humans via contact with an infected monkey's blood during butchering or cooking allowing the virus to cross into humans and become HIV.

HIV is one of several bloodborne pathogens. Only certain body fluids from an HIV-infected person that come in contact with mucus membranes, damaged tissue, or injected directly into the bloodstream (from a needle or syringe) can transmit HIV. Mucous membranes can be found inside the rectum, the vagina, the opening of the penis, and the mouth. These fluids include:
- Blood
- Semen
- Pre-seminal fluid
- Rectal fluids
- Vaginal fluids
- Breast milk

Note: HIV is not spread by casual contact.

TESTING:
The CDC recommends that everyone between the ages of 13 and 64 is tested at least once and that high-risk groups are tested more often.

PRE-EXPOSURE PROPHYLAXSIS:
Pre-exposure prophylaxis, or PrEP, is a prevention option for people who are at high risk of getting HIV.

SYMPTOMS:
The symptoms of HIV and AIDS may vary depending on the phase of the infection. The phases of infection include primary infection, clinical latency and progression to AIDS. Table 1 provides a summary of symptoms noted in each phase of HIV infection.

HIV *(continued from previous page)*

Table 1 - Symptoms of HIV Infection

Acute or Primary Infection	Clinical Latency (inactivity or dormancy)	AIDS (Acquired Immunodeficiency Syndrome)
Flu-like illness develops within 2 – 4 weeks after the virus enters the body. **Symptoms:** • Fever • Enlarged lymph nodes • Rash • Sore throat	Sometimes called asymptomatic HIV infection or chronic HIV infection. During this phase, HIV is still active, but reproduces at very low levels. People who are on antiretroviral therapy (ART) may live with clinical latency for several decades. For people who are not on ART, this period can last up to a decade, but some may progress through this phase faster. **Symptoms:** May or may not have symptoms.	The number of CD4 cells falls below 200 cells per cubic millimeter of blood (200 cells/mm3 (Normal CD4 counts are between 500 and 1,600 cells/mm3). **Symptoms:** • Susceptible to opportunistic infections • Profuse night sweats • Fever >100°F • Chronic diarrhea • Persistent lesions on the tongue or in the mouth • Headaches • Persistent fatigue • Blurred and distorted vision • Weight loss • Skin rashes or bumps
Note: These symptoms can last anywhere from a few days to several weeks. During this time, HIV infection may not show up on an HIV test, but people who have it are highly infectious and can spread the infection to others.	**Note**: HIV remains in the body as free virus and in the infected white blood cells	

HIV *(continued from previous page)*

POTENTIAL RISKS and COMPLICATIONS:
- Infections - Tuberculosis, Salmonellosis, Cytomegalovirus, Candidiasis, Cryptococcal meningitis, Toxoplasmosis, Cryptosporidiosis
- Cancers - Kaposi's sarcoma, Lymphomas
- Other complications - Wasting Syndrome, neurological, kidney disease

MANAGEMENT/TREATMENT in the school setting:

Standard/Universal Precautions
The implementation of standard/universal precautions is advised for all school personnel to promote infection control and prevent the spread of bloodborne pathogens such as HIV/AIDS. Standard/universal precautions include the use of gloves and other protective equipment when there is a risk of exposure to human blood and body fluids known to transmit HIV. Annual training for standard/universal precautions should be provided to all school staff at the beginning of the school year. The training should include the mode of transmission for HIV and proper use of personal protective equipment.

Confidentiality
All health records, including notes and other documents referencing a student's HIV status, should be kept in a secure location. Access to confidential student records is only shared with school officials with a legitimate need to know the information. Parents/guardians and students are not required to disclose a student's HIV infection status in order for the student to enroll in and attend school. However, if the parents/guardians or student choose to disclose the HIV status to school staff, the confidentiality of this information should be emphasized.

School Attendance and School Placement
Students with HIV infections have the same right to attend school and receive educational services as any other student. The student's HIV status should not the deciding factor in determining educational services and participation in school sponsored activities. Thus, decisions regarding school attendance, school placement, or special healthcare needs should be considered on a case-by-case basis including maintaining respect for the rights to privacy of the student and family. If a parent or school official believes that a child with AIDS needs related services or placement outside the regular classroom, Section 504 requires an evaluation and placement process to determine the appropriate educational setting for a child with AIDS.

211

HIV *(continued from previous page)*

Protection

An important aspect of the school nurse's role is protecting the student with HIV/AIDS. If the school nurse, is a staff member who is aware of the student's HIV status, h/she should inform the student and/or family members whenever there are communicable diseases in the school setting that could pose a threat to the immune compromised student (such as chicken pox, strep, pertussis, etc.). This is especially important if the student has the opportunity to be exposed to the ill students.

References

American Academy of Pediatrics, Committee on Pediatric AIDS. (2000). Education of children with human immunodeficiency virus infection. *PEDIATRICS, 105*(6), 1358 – 1360. Doi: 10 1542/peds 10561358

Centers for Disease Control and Prevention. (2015). *HIV basics*. Retrieved from http://www.cdc.gov/hiv/basics/index.html

Centers for Disease Control and Prevention. (2015). *HIV transmission*. Retrieved from http://www.cdc.gov/hiv/basics/transmission.html

Mayo Clinic. (2015). *HIV/AIDS*. Retrieved from http://www.mayoclinic.com/health/hiv-aids/DS00005

National Institute of Allergy and Infectious Diseases. (2009). *HIV/AIDS symptoms*. Retrieved from http://www.niaid.nih.gov/topics/HIVAIDS/Understanding/Pages/symptoms.aspx.

United States Department of Education (2015). *Placement of schoolchildren with Acquired Immunodeficiency Syndrome.* Retrieved from http://www2.ed.gov/about/offices/list/ocr/docs/hq53e9.html

United States Department of Labor, Occupational Safety and Health Administration. (2013). *Universal precautions*. Retrieved from https://www.osha.gov/SLTC/etools/hospital/hazards/univprec/univ.html

HUMAN PAPILLOMAVIRUS (HPV)

DEFINITION/ETIOLOGY:

The Human Papillomavirus (HPV) is the most common sexually transmitted infection in the United States. HPVs are small, double-stranded DNA viruses that infect the epithelium. While there are more than 40 different strains of HPV that specifically infect the mucosal epithelium affecting the genital area, most of the HPV infections do not lead to cancer. However, some types of genital HPV can cause cancer of the cervix. HPV vaccines can help protect against strains of genital HPV which are most likely to cause genital warts or cervical cancer.

HPV is primarily transferred by skin-to-skin contact. The infection occurs when the virus enters the body through:
- A cut in the skin
- An abrasion
- A small tear in the outer layer of skin

SIGNS AND SYMPTOMS:

Most often, the immune system defeats HPV infection before warts are created. However, when warts do appear as a result of HPV infection, the appearance may vary depending on the type of HPV involved. Below are descriptions of the various types of warts resulting from HPV infection:
- **Genital warts** – flat lesions, small cauliflower-like bumps, or tiny stem-like protrusions. In women, genital warts appear on the vulva and may occur on the cervix or in the vagina. In men, genital warts appear on the penis and scrotum or around the anus. Rarely cause discomfort or pain.
- **Common warts** – rough, raise bumps occurring on hands, fingers, and around fingernails. May be painful and susceptible to bleeding/injury.
- **Plantar warts** – hard and grainy growths, commonly appear on heels or balls of feet; may cause discomfort.
- **Flat warts** – flat topped appearance, slightly raised lesions, may appear darker that regular skin color on face, neck, hands, wrists, elbows, or knees. Usually affect children, adolescents, and young adults.
- **Cervical cancer** – caused by two specific types of genital HPV; do not cause warts and no signs or symptoms in the early stages of cervical cancer. Annual Pap tests are important to detect precancerous changes in the cervix.
- **Recurrent respiratory papillomatosis (RRP)** – very rare, warts grow on the throat. May occur as in children (juvenile onset) or in adults (adult onset). Growths can block the airway causing hoarse voice and difficulty breathing.

HUMAN PAPILLOMAVIRUS (HPV) *(continued from previous page)*

Risk factors for HPV infection include:
- Number of sexual partners.
- Genital warts occur most often in adolescents and young adults.
- Weakened immune system increases the risk of HPV infections. (Note: immune systems may be weakened by HIV/AIDS or by drugs which may suppress the immune system.)
- Damaged skin.
- Personal contact.

MANAGEMENT/TREATMENT:

HPV can be managed and prevented in several ways:
- HPV vaccines are administered as a series of three shots over 6 months to protect against HPV infection and the health problems that HPV infection can cause. There are three HPV vaccines (Cervarix®, Gardasil®, and Gardasil 9®). It is recommended that girls and young women receive any of these HPV vaccines.
- It is recommended that boys receive either Gardasil® or Gardasil® of these HPV vaccines.

Vaccine	Prevents in Girls/Young Women	Prevents in Boys
Cervix®	• Cervical cancer	
Gardasil®	• Cervical vulvar, vaginal and anal cancer • Genital warts	• Anal cancer • Genital warts
Gardasil 9®	• Cervical, vulvar, vaginal and anal cancer • Genital warts	• Anal cancer • Genital warts

- HPV vaccines offer the best protection to girls and boys who receive all three-vaccine doses and have time to develop an immune response before being sexually active with another person. HPV vaccination is recommended for preteen girls and boys at age 11 or 12 years.
- Protection for sexually active individuals include the use of condoms, which may lower the risk of HPV infection, and HPV related diseases.
- Limiting the number of sex partners can lower chances of getting HPV.

HUMAN PAPILLOMAVIRUS (HPV) *(continued from previous page)*

- Coordinate with school-based health centers (when available in the school setting) to increase awareness about prevention education and immunizations available for HPV. (Note: School-based health centers provide an ideal setting for prevention education for sexually transmitted infections such as HPV.)

FOLLOW-UP:

The school nurse can assist in the management and prevention of HPV infection among children and adolescents in the following ways:

- Conduct health promotion education sessions in the school setting to increase awareness among youth and parents about HPV prevention and available vaccines.

POTENTIAL COMPLICATIONS:

1. Oral and upper respiratory lesions
2. Cancer, e.g. cancers of the genitals, anus, mouth, and upper respiratory tract.

NOTES: Genital HPV infections are transmitted through sexual intercourse, anal sex, and other skin-to-skin contact in the genital area. HPV infection is very rarely transmitted from mother to infant during delivery. However, if exposure occurs during delivery, it may cause HPV infection in the baby's genitals and upper respiratory system.

References

Atkinson, W., Wolfe, S., Hamborsky J., & McIntyre, L. (Eds.). (2015). *Epidemiology and prevention of vaccine-preventable diseases- The pink book: course textbook (13th ed.).* Washington DC: Public Health Foundation. Retrieved from http://www.cdc.gov/vaccines/pubs/pinkbook/index.html

Bellia-Weiss, T., Parsons, M., Sebach, A.M., & Rockelli, L.A. (2013).Promoting HPV prevention in the school setting. *NASN School Nurse, 28*(2), 86-93. doi: 10.1177/1942602X12463249

Centers for Disease Control and Prevention (CDC). (2015). *Human papillomavirus.* Retrieved from http://www.cdc.gov/hpv/vaccine.html

Mayo Clinic. (2015). *HPV infection.* Retrieved from http://www.mayoclinic.org/diseases-conditions/hpv-infection/basics/definition/con-20030343

HYPOTHERMIA

DEFINITION/ETIOLOGY:

Hypothermia is a medical emergency and can occur when the body loses heat faster than it can produce heat. This causes a dangerously low body temperature. The normal body temperature is 98.6°F (37°C) and hypothermia occurs as the body temperature decreases below 95°F (35°C). Hypothermia is most likely to occur at cold temperatures, but it can occur at cool temperatures (above 40°F) if a person becomes chilled from rain, sweat, or submersion in cold water. Once the body temperature decreases, the heart, nervous system, and other vital organ cannot function properly. If hypothermia is left untreated, complete failure of the heart and respiratory system can occur and lead to death.

CAUSES OF HYPOTHERMIA:
- Exposure to cold weather conditions
- Accidental exposure to or immersion in a cold body of water
- Staying out in the cold too long
- Being cold and wet
- Wearing inappropriate clothing for cold weather conditions
- Inadequate heating in the home or air conditioning is too cold

Note: The body may lose heat through various mechanisms including:
- Radiation, heat loss is due to heat radiated from unprotected body surfaces
- Conduction, movement of heat from the body to cooler objects such as the ground, a tree or water
- Convection, wind wicking away heat from exposed skin
- Insensible water loss, release of heat through the evaporation of body fluids that occurs during perspiration and breathing

SIGNS AND SYMPTOMS:

The human body automatically responds to cold weather by shivering in an attempt to create heat and warm up. Hypothermia may range from moderate to severe. The signs and symptoms include:
- Shivering (as hypothermia worsens, shivering stops)
- Lack of coordination, clumsiness, stumbling
- Slurred speech, mumbling
- Confusion, difficulty thinking
- Poor decision making
- Low energy or drowsiness

HYPOTHERMIA *(continued from previous page)*

- Lack of concern, apathy
- Progressive loss of consciousness
- Weak pulse
- Slow and shallow breathing
- Pale and cold to touch

MANAGEMENT/TREATMENT:
- **Call 911** – monitor breathing and provide cardiopulmonary resuscitation (CPR) immediately if breathing stops or seems slow and shallow.
- Move the person out of the cold (handle gently because sudden movement can trigger arrhythmia) or protect from wind/cold weather and insulate from the cold area.
- Rewarming is a top priority. Remove wet clothing and replace with warm, dry covering such as blankets, foil emergency blankets, coats or sleeping bags to trap the heat.
- Do not apply direct heat; use warm compresses and apply to the center of the body, e.g. head, neck, chest, and groin. Heat applied to the extremities (i.e. arms and legs) can force a cold block toward the central organs (i.e. heart, lungs, and brain) and can result in a decrease in the core body temperature, which can be fatal.
- Avoid massaging frostbitten skin as rubbing can cause severe damage to the tissues.

Note: Emergency medical care for hypothermia will be guided by the severity of hypothermia. Various interventions can be used to increase the body temperature back to normal including blood rewarming, warm intravenous fluids, airway rewarming, and cavity lavage.

POTENTIAL RISKS and COMPLICATIONS:
An increased risk of hypothermia may occur with various factors:
- **Age** can be a risk factor for hypothermia
  - Older age: The body's ability to regulate temperature may decrease with age. Older adults have a reduced shivering response. Decreased ability to communicate and mobility are contributing factors for the elderly.
  - Younger age: Children can lose heat faster than adults due to the larger head to body ratio in children. Inappropriate dressing in the colder weather may increase the risk of hypothermia in children.

HYPOTHERMIA *(continued from previous page)*

- **Mental illness** may interfere with judgment and can affect appropriate dressing for the weather.
- **Alcohol** can make the body feel warm inside resulting in rapid heat loss from the skin surface. Additionally, the use of alcohol and drugs may affect judgment regarding weather conditions. Medical conditions can affect the body's ability to regulate heat, i.e. underactive thyroid gland, poor nutrition, stroke, severe arthritis, chronic conditions affecting sensation, hypoglycemia, trauma, psoriasis and conditions that limit the normal circulation/blood flow.
- **Medications** can alter the body's ability to regulate temperature. Benzodiazepines, tricyclic antidepressants, opioids, barbiturates and phenothiazine's can reduce core temperature.

Complications of hypothermia may lead to the following:
- Frostbite – freezing of body tissues
- Gangrene – decay and death of tissue due to interrupted blood flow
- Chilblains – damage to the nerves and small blood vessels in the hands or feet due to prolonged exposure to cold temperatures
- Trench foot – damage to nerves and small blood vessels because of prolonged immersion in cold water
- Aspiration pneumonia
- Clotting disorders

FOLLOW-UP AND PREVENTION EFFORTS:
School nurses can play a valuable role in educating children and families about outdoor activities during the cold weather to prevent hypothermia. Prevention for keeping children warm in cold weather includes the following:
- Cover up with appropriate clothing for cold weather, e.g. hats, mittens, to prevent body heat from escaping.
- Avoid overexertion to prevent sweating and quick loss of body heat.
- Encourage children to wear layers of clothing – loose fitting and lightweight.
- Encourage children to stay as dry as possible and to change wet clothing as soon as possible.
- Limit amount of time spent outside during cold weather.
- Educate youth and adolescents about risky behaviors and the importance to abstain from alcohol and drug use, especially during periods of prolonged cold weather exposure.

HYPOTHERMIA *(continued from previous page)*

References

Auxier, G. (2015). Wilderness medicine: Your guide to treating illness or injury in the great outdoors. *Contemporary Pediatrics 32*(5), 22-26. Retrieved from http://web.a.ebscohost.com.proxy2.cl.msu.edu/ehost/pdfviewer/pdfviewer?sid=cdf6db05-41ce-4eee-be64-246764422a3f%40sessionmgr4004&vid=3&hid=4109

Centers for Disease Control and Prevention. (2012). *Emergency preparedness and response, winter weather: Hypothermia.* Retrieved from http://emergency.cdc.gov/disasters/winter/staysafe/hypothermia.asp

Davis, R.A. (2012). The big chill: Accidental hypothermia. *American Journal of Nursing, 112*(1), 38-46. doi: 10.1097/01.NAJ.0000410362.66308.17

Mayo Clinic. (2013). *Hypothermia*. Retrieved from http://www.mayoclinic.com/health/hypothermia/DS00333

U.S. National Library of Medicine, National Institutes of Health. (2013). *Hypothermia*. Retrieved from http://www.nlm.nih.gov/medlineplus/hypothermia.html

ILLNESS FALSIFICATION (Factitious Disorder)

DEFINITION/ETIOLOGY:
Illness falsification is considered a factitious disorder.

1. **Factitious disorders** are conditions in which a person acts as if he or she has an illness by deliberately producing, feigning, or exaggerating symptoms. People with factitious disorders seek painful or risky tests and operations in order to obtain attention. While the cause of factitious disorders is unknown, some theories believe there is both a biological and psychological cause. Numerous people with Factitious Disorder also experience mental health disorders especially personality disorders.

2. **Pediatric Condition Falsification (PCF)** (formerly referred to as Munchausen by Proxy) is a form of child abuse in which a parent/guardian/caregiver (most often the mother) deliberately produces false physical or psychological symptoms in a child under their care causing the victim to be regarded as ill or impaired by others. The child is presented for medical treatment and the parent or caregiver fails to acknowledge the deception. PCF often involves physical abuse, neglect, and emotional abuse. **A child who is subjected to this behavior is a victim of child abuse by PCF.**

Factitious disorders must be distinguished from **malingering** (faking illness to avoid other responsibilities). In malingering, the individual also produces the symptoms intentionally, but has a *goal that is recognizable* when the circumstances are known. For example, the falsification of symptoms to avoid a math test would be called malingering.

Medical conditions fabricated by children may go undetected or be diagnosed as somatization (see Note). Further study of children who falsify symptoms may in some cases help identify earlier experiences of PCF abuse (parent/guardian involvement) or covert parental coaching of illness falsification, and provide more effective interventions. Better understanding and identification of these children is likely to help prevent the development of more chronic adult factitious disorders.

NOTES:
Somatization refers to the occurrence of physical complaints for which medical evaluation reveals no physical pathology, or when pathology is present, the complaints are grossly in excess of what would be expected from the physical findings. Pain and somatic symptoms

ILLNESS FALSIFICATION (Factitious Disorder) *(continued from previous page)*

are problematic when, regardless of cause, they become a dominant force in the child's life and impair functioning. Somatic complaints often have associated psychiatric symptoms, particularly anxiety or depression, although the cause of the condition remains unclear.

SIGNS AND SYMPTOMS:
Factitious Disorder
- Child may present with an inconsistent medical history
- Child may seek treatment from the school nurse/health office personnel frequently
- May present with reports of symptoms that are not observable
- May demonstrate an extensive knowledge of medical terminology and descriptions of illness
- Presence of bruises or infection
- Causing self-harm
- Evidence of self-bruising or ingestion of substances to cause illness
- Presence of symptoms only when the child is alone or not being observed
- Willingness or eagerness to have medical tests, operations, or other procedures
- Reluctance by the child to have the school nurse speak with their parent/guardian(s) or healthcare providers
- Seeking treatment from multiple healthcare provider's, clinic, hospitals, etc.
- New symptoms after obtaining negative results

Pediatric Condition Falsification
- Seizures, fever, diarrhea, apnea, nervous system dysfunction, signs of bleeding (urine and stool) and rashes
- History of frequent hospitalizations, usually for a variety of nonspecific symptoms
- Most common in children under 1 and up to age 6 years old
- A parent or caregiver fabricates symptoms of illness in a child
- The child is presented for medical assessment and care, usually persistently, often resulting in multiple medical procedures and hospitalizations
- The perpetrator denies the etiology of the child's illness
- Symptoms of illness abate upon separation of the child from the perpetrator
- Improvement of symptoms occurs when child is hospitalized but return on discharge

Possible exceptions: when the child has suffered permanent damage as a result of the abuse; child is actively colluding with the parent/guardian; child has developed a psychiatric disorder.

ILLNESS FALSIFICATION (Factitious Disorder) *(continued from previous page)*

MANAGEMENT/TREATMENT:
1. Be alert to the possibility of Pediatric Condition Falsification and Factitious Disorder.
2. If there are concerns regarding illness fabrication or discrepancies between the parent/guardian's reports of health problems in the child and the school nurse's observations of the child's health:
   - Review the child's past medical history.
   - Consult with the child's healthcare provider to review the child's diagnosis and health status. Discuss implications for school attendance and participation in school activities. Inform the provider of observations of the child in the school setting.
   - Maintain a trusting relationship with the perpetrator.
   - Document child/parent/guardian interactions.
3. Information about the child's attendance, school health records, parental reports of medical/health problems, educational testing, and staff observations of health and behavioral issues are relevant and may be requested by the healthcare provider or legal authorities.
4. Be prepared to provide information should the family be referred to Child Protective Services. Follow district policy.
5. Factitious disorders are usually treated with psychotherapy and/or family therapy. Behavior modification is the first goal.
6. Medication may be prescribed to treat related disorders such as depression or anxiety.

POTENTIAL COMPLICATIONS:
Factitious Disorder including PCF
   - Absences from school which affect academic success
   - Side effects of use of drugs or medical tests used to explore cause of reported physical or psychological symptoms
   - Injury from self-inflicted medical conditions or harm
   - Fear
   - Pain and suffering
   - Loss of normal attachment to parent/caregiver (especially with PCF)
   - Loss of normal developmental experiences (i.e., kept out of school [PCF] or staying home from school in cases of Factitious Disorder)
   - Loss of normal social experiences
   - Alcohol or substance abuse
   - Death

ILLNESS FALSIFICATION (Factitious Disorder) *(continued from previous page)*

References

American Psychiatric Association. (2013). *Highlights of changes from DSM-IV-TR- DSM-5.* Retrieved from
http://www.dsm5.org/Documents/changes%20from%20dsm-iv-tr%20to%20dsm-5.pdf

Ball, J., Binder, R., & Cowen, K. (Eds.). (2012). Assessment and management of social and environmental influences. *Principles of Pediatric Nursing: Caring for Children (5th ed.)* (pp. 461-462). Upper Saddle River, NJ: Pearson Education, Inc.

Dimsdale, J.E. (2013). *Factitious disorder imposed on self.* Retrieved from http://www.merckmanuals.com/professional/psychiatric-disorders/somatic-symptom-and-related-disorders/factitious-disorder-imposed-on-self

Mayo Clinic. (2014). *Factious disorder.* Retrieved from http://www.mayoclinic.org/diseases-conditions/factitious-disorder/basics/definition/con-20031319

The Cleveland Clinic Foundation. (2013). *An overview of factitious disorders.* Retrieved from http://my.clevelandclinic.org/disorders/factitious_disorders/hic_an_overview_of_factitious_disorders.aspx

IMPETIGO

DEFINITION/ETIOLOGY:

Impetigo is a highly contagious skin infection characterized by eruptions caused by either *Streptococcal* or *Staphylococcal* bacteria. Minor skin injuries, insect bites, and dermatitis may be the portal for the infectious agent. The eruptions may proceed through vesicular, pustular, and encrusted stages. It usually appears as red bumps that form on the face (particularly around the nose and mouth) or extremities. The red bumps fill with pus, break open, and form a honey-colored crust. The lesions are usually itchy, but not painful. Symptoms usually begin 1-3 days after exposure for *Streptococcus,* usually 4-10 days for *Staphylococcus*. Infection is spread by direct contact with secretions from lesions. It is most common in ages 2-10.

SIGNS AND SYMPTOMS:
- Begins as a red sore, pimple or fluid-filled blister, most often found on face but may be anywhere on body.
- Blisters that rupture easily leave a red, raw looking base.
- Itchy blisters, filled with honey-colored fluid that may be oozing and crusting over.
- May have swollen lymph nodes near the infection (lymphadenopathy).

MANAGEMENT/TREATMENT:
- An untreated person can spread the bacteria for as long as drainage occurs from lesions. Infected individuals do not transmit the infection 24 hours after antibiotic treatment is underway.
- Parents/guardians should keep contagious children home until 24 hours after starting topical or oral antibiotic therapy. Contacts of cases do not need to be excluded.
- Hygienic measures: Wash the skin several times a day with an antibiotic soap to gently remove crusts and drainage.
- Antibiotic therapy: Mild cases may be treated with prescribed topical antibiotic ointment or antibacterial cream. Before applying the topical medication, gently remove scabs so the medication can penetrate the lesion. More severe cases may require oral antibiotics.
- Cover a draining lesion with a dressing.

FOLLOW UP:
- Encourage diligence in skin cleansing.
- Monitor completion of antibiotic course even though lesions are healed.
- Have family observe close contacts and family members for lesions. Watch for additional cases.

IMPETIGO *(continued from previous page)*

POTENTIAL COMPLICATIONS:
- Post streptococcal glomerulonephritis (PSGN) (rare)
- Spread of the infection to other parts of the body
- Cellulitis (see Skin Infection)
- Methicillin-resistant *Staphylococcus aureus* (see MRSA)

NOTES:
Prevention
- Infected person should:
  - Use a clean towel and wash cloth each time.
  - Not share towels, clothing, razors, and other personal care products with others.
  - Wash hands thoroughly after touching skin lesions.
- Caregiver should wear gloves when washing lesions and applying antibiotic medication. Wash hands thoroughly afterwards.

References

American Academy of Pediatrics. (2015). *Impetigo*. Retrieved from *https://healthychildren.org/English/health-issues/ conditions/skin/Pages/Impetigo.aspx*

Ball, J., Binder, R., & Cowen, K. (Eds.). (2012). Alterations in skin integrity. *Principles of pediatric nursing: Caring for children (5th ed.)* (p.p. 1038-1039). Upper Saddle River, NJ: Pearson Education, Inc.

Centers for Disease Control and Prevention. (2014). *Group A streptococcal (GAS) disease*. Retrieved from *http://www.cdc.gov/groupastrep/clinicians.html*

Mayo Clinic. (2013). *Impetigo*. Retrieved from *http://www.mayoclinic.org/diseases-conditions/impetigo/basics/definition/ con-20024185*

Medline Plus, U.S. National Library of Medicine. (2015). *Impetigo*. Retrieved from *http://www.nlm.nih.gov/medlineplus/ impetigo.html*

Merck Manual. (2013). *Impetigo and ecthyma*. Retrieved from *http://www.merckmanuals.com/professional/dermatologic_ disorders/bacterial_skin_infections/impetigo_and_ecthyma.html?qt=impetigo&alt=sh*

National Institute of Allergy and Infectious Diseases. (2013). *Impetigo*. Retrieved from *http://www.niaid.nih.gov/topics/ impetigo/Pages/Default.aspx*

INFLUENZA

DEFINITION/ETIOLOGY:

Influenza is a respiratory virus affecting the nose, throat, and lungs. There are three different influenza viruses: A, B and C. Most illnesses are caused by the type A and B influenza antigens. The symptoms are typically more severe with Influenza type A. Influenza type B is typically milder. Type B primarily affects children. The incubation period is 1 –4 days. May be contagious from 1 day before the symptoms start to more than 7 days after the onset of influenza. Symptoms typically last 3 – 5 days. The virus is spread by airborne respiratory droplets, hand-to-hand contact or by contact with contaminated objects. Influenza is prevalent in the United States from October to March.

SIGNS AND SYMPTOMS:
- Fever –typically (100-102°); abrupt onset; fever may last 3-4 days
- Chills
- Headache
- General muscle or body aches
- Fatigue
- Nasal congestion
- Sneezing
- Sore throat
- Chest discomfort
- Cough (nonproductive)
- Mild pink eye

MANAGEMENT/TREATMENT:
1. Encourage fluids and bedrest.
2. Healthcare provider may prescribe antiviral medication (Tamiflu® or Relenza®) for 5 days to shorten the duration of the symptoms and to reduce the risk of complications.
    - Benefit of taking antiviral medication is greatest if started within 48 hours of onset of illness.
    - If healthcare provider prescribes antiviral medication, monitor for side effects such as nausea and vomiting.
3. May administer acetaminophen if ordered to help alleviate flu symptoms (body aches, elevated temperature, etc.). Follow medication orders.
4. Do not administer aspirin to children under the age of 18. Aspirin can play a role in causing Reye's Syndrome (rare but potentially fatal disease).

INFLUENZA *(continued from previous page)*

MANAGEMENT/TREATMENT: *(continued)*
5. Instruct parent/guardian to call healthcare provider if symptoms worsen.
6. Instruct parent/guardian to keep child home from school until the child is fever free for 24 hours (without the use of antipyretics).
7. Educate parent/guardian(s) on potential complications of influenza.

FOLLOW UP:
- Refer to healthcare provider if symptoms reappear after illness has subsided.
- If need be, reiterate to the parent/guardian that the child should be kept home for 24 hours after the fever subsides (without antipyretic medication).

POTENTIAL COMPLICATIONS:
Students with chronic diseases such as asthma, diabetes, heart conditions, etc. may be at increased risk of complications.

Flu complications
- Pneumonia – most serious complication
- Sinus infection
- Ear infection
- Febrile seizure
- Bronchitis

NOTES:
Educate on the importance of:
- Yearly influenza vaccine, if an allergy to eggs talk to the healthcare provider before getting the vaccine.
- Controlling the spread of influenza, avoid crowds during peak influenza season.
- Do not share food or drink.
- Preventing the spread of influenza.
  - Promote good handwashing.
  - Cover mouth and nose with tissue when cough and/or sneeze; dispose of tissue properly; wash hands or use an alcohol-based hand sanitizer to remove germs.
  - If tissue is not available, cough and/or sneeze into shoulder or elbow.

INFLUENZA *(continued from previous page)*

References

American Academy of Pediatrics, Committee on Infectious Diseases. (2015). Influenza. In D.W. Kimberlin, M. T. Brady, M.A. Jackson, & S.S. Long (Eds.), *Red Book: 2015 report of the committee on infectious diseases* (30th ed.) (pp. 476-493). Elk Grove Village, IL: American Academy of Pediatrics.

American Academy of Pediatrics. (2013). Influenza. In S. Aronson, & T. Shope (Eds.), *Managing infectious diseases in child care and schools (2nd ed.)* (p.p. 111-112). Elk Grove Village, IL: American Academy of Pediatrics.

Centers for Disease Control and Prevention. (2015a). *Influenza (flu).* Retrieved from http://www.cdc.gov/flu/index.htm

Center for Disease Control and Prevention (CDC). (2015b). *Influenza.* In J. Hamborsky, A. Kroger, & S. Wolfe (Eds.), *Epidemiology and prevention of vaccine-preventable diseases, the pink book: Course textbook (13th ed.).* Washington D.C. Public Health Foundation. Retrieved from http://www.cdc.gov/vaccines/pubs/pinkbook/flu.html

Mayo Clinic. (2015). *Influenza (flu).* Retrieved from http://www.mayoclinic.org/diseases-conditions/flu/basics/definition/con-20035101

Merck Manual. (2014). *Influenza.* Retrieved from http://www.merckmanuals.com/professional/infectious_diseases/respiratory_viruses/influenza.html?qt=Influenza&alt=sh

Selekman, J., & Coates, J. (2013). Disease prevention. In J. Selekman (Ed.), *School nursing: A comprehensive text* (2nd ed.) (pp.473-515). Philadelphia, PA: F. A. Davis.

LACERATIONS

DEFINITION/ETIOLOGY:
A laceration is a tearing or jagged wound of the soft tissue. Soft tissue tears/cuts (lacerations) are common in children and are often the result of falls, blows, collisions or contact with sharp objects. Lacerations can occur anywhere on the body, but in children that most lacerations in children are on the face (60%) or upper extremities (25%).

SIGNS AND SYMPTOMS:
- Torn or jagged wound of the soft tissue
- Wound edges may be separated

MANAGEMENT/TREATMENT:
1. Educate student in the proper process to wash, apply pressure and apply bandage to their wound. Encouraging supervised self-care minimizes bloodborne pathogen exposure and encourages student to become more participatory in their own self-care.
2. Treatment for superficial lacerations include:
   - Wear gloves if assisting student to clean and cover.
   - Apply firm pressure with sterile or clean dressing until bleeding stops.
   - Clean wound and surrounding skin with tap water, sterile water or normal saline. Note: *Hydrogen peroxide is not appropriate for fresh wounds; it damages tissues and interferes with healing*
   - If debris is in wound, refer to healthcare provider for follow-up treatment.
   - If necessary, dry and bandage or apply butterfly dressing. Refer for follow-up with a healthcare provider.
3. Treatment for cuts which are contaminated, deeper, or located on the face or flexor surface (knee, elbow) include:
   - Apply firm pressure until bleeding stops.
   - Cover with sterile dressing.
   - May apply cold pack to prevent swelling.
   - Refer to healthcare provider.
   - If sutures are needed, they must be placed within 6 hours.
4. Review immunization record; check last tetanus date; provide copy to parent/guardian to accompany to healthcare provider referral.

LACERATIONS *(continued from previous page)*

FOLLOW UP:
- Change bandage as needed.
- Note signs and symptoms of infection that require a revisit to healthcare provider.
  - Early signs and symptoms of infection include: increased pain, redness around the edge of wound, swelling and tenderness.
  - Late signs and symptoms of infection include: fever, purulent drainage and lymphangitis (infection of the lymph vessel caused by a bacterial infection); look for red streak from infected area to armpit or groin.
- Observe for signs of cellulitis.
- Refer student to healthcare provider if exhibits signs of wound or systemic infection.
  - If there are sutures, watch for swelling which causes tension on sutures and tissues.
  - Observe sutures for signs of infection; infection appears first as a tiny red circle around each stitch.
- Follow healthcare provider orders or local protocol if wound irrigation and dressing change is require/needed during the school day.

POTENTIAL COMPLICATIONS:
- Wound infection
- Lymphangitis
- Cellulitis

NOTES:
Watch for pyogenic granuloma:
- Small raised red benign growth.
- Lesion is vascular; bleeds easily.
- Pyrogenic granulomas appear following an injury (typically to the hand, arm or face).
- Small pyogenic granulomas often resolve on own; larger lesions may need to be surgically removed.

LACERATIONS *(continued from previous page)*

References

Cunha, J.P. (2014). Cuts or lacerations overview. *Emedicinehealth*. Retrieved from http://www.emedicinehealth.com/cuts_or_lacerations/article_em.htm

John, R., & Chewey, L. (2013). Common complaints. In J. Selekman (Ed.), *School nursing: A comprehensive text* (2nd ed.) (pp. 578-640). Philadelphia, PA: F. A. Davis.

Medline Plus. U.S. National Library of Medicine. (2013). *Lymphangitis*. Retrieved from http://www.nlm.nih.gov/medlineplus/ency/article/007296.htm

Medline Plus. U.S. National Library of Medicine. (2013). *Wounds*. Retrieved from http://www.nlm.nih.gov/medlineplus/wounds.html

The Merck Manual, Professional Edition. (2013). *Lacerations*. Retrieved from http://www.merckmanuals.com/professional/injuries_poisoning/lacerations/lacerations.html?qt=lacerations&alt=sh

National Library of Medicine. (2012). *Pyogenic granuloma*. Retrieved from http://www.ncbi.nlm.nih.gov/pubmedhealth/PMH0002435/

Spiro, D.M., Zonfrillo, M.R. & Meckler, G.D. (2010). Wounds. *Pediatrics in Review, 31*(8), 326-334. Retrieved from http://pedsinreview.aappublications.org

WebMD. (2010*). First aid & emergencies*. Retrieved from http://firstaid.webmd.com/tc/cuts-topic-overview

LEAD POISONING (Plumbism)

DEFINITION/ETIOLOGY:

Lead is a natural metal occurring in the environment. Lead poisoning occurs when there is a build-up of lead in the body. People are exposed to lead by eating food or drinking water or inhaling air that is contaminated with lead. Old homes may have lead in the water pipes or may be painted with lead based paints. Children may be exposed to lead by playing in soil that has been contaminated with lead and/or eating lead-based paint chips. Lead poisoning most often occurs in young children under the age of six. Lead poisoning is often considered a chronic disorder.

SIGNS AND SYPMTOMS:

Symptoms are minimal at first. Symptoms are not obvious until blood levels become elevated. If not treated may have irreversible effects. Lead poisoning can affect every organ in the body.

Signs and symptoms of acute lead poisoning
- Irritable/moody
- Anorexia
- Fatigue
- Difficulty concentrating
- Gastrointestinal symptoms – abdominal pain/vomiting/constipation

Signs and symptoms of chronic lead poisoning
- Developmental delays
- Cognitive deficits (risk increases with whole blood level $\geq$ 10 µg/dL)
- Seizure disorders
- Aggressive behaviors
- Anemia (lead interferes with hemoglobin formation)
- Hearing loss
- Peripheral neuropathy
- Muscle and joint pain
- Kidney damage

LEAD POISONING *(continued from previous page)*

Blood level ≥ 50 µg/dL
- Gastrointestinal symptoms
  - Abdominal cramping (chronic)
  - Constipation
- Hand tremors
- Irritability/changes in mood

Blood level ≥ 100 µg/dL
- Encephalopathy

MANAGEMENT/TREATMENT:
- Eliminate source of lead exposure
- Children with blood lead levels of 5 µg/dL should be monitored; the child's vitamin and nutritional status should be assessed; children with diets low in fat and high in iron and calcium absorb less lead
- Chelation therapy for children diagnosed with encephalopathy or with blood lead levels greater than 45 µg/dL

FOLLOW-UP:
- Refer student to support team to evaluate if child is eligible for Special Education or Section 504 accommodations.
- Lead poisoning is preventable. Consider writing a newsletter article educating parent/guardian(s) on lead poisoning prevention and the signs and symptoms of lead poisoning.

POTENTIAL COMPLICATIONS:
- Learning disabilities
- Irreversible organ damage
- Seizures
- Encephalopathy
- Death – high lead levels cause brain damage and kidney failure which ultimately lead to death

LEAD POISONING *(continued from previous page)*

NOTES:
Cultural implications. The following products *may* contain lead:

- Some folk remedies (Greta or Azarcon – Hispanic home remedy)
- Kohl – traditional cosmetic
- Some ethnic healthcare products (Litargirio – used as deodorant)
- Imported herbal products/medicinal herbs may contain lead
- Daw tway – digestive home remedy from Thailand
- Some candies from Mexico
- Toys produced overseas may contain lead

References

Centers for Disease Control and Prevention. (2015). *Lead poisoning*. Retrieved from http://www.cdc.gov/nceh/lead/

Mayo Clinic. (2014). *Lead poisoning*. Retrieved from http://www.mayoclinic.com/health/lead-poisoning/FL00068

Medline Plus. U.S. National Library of Medicine. (2015). *Lead poisoning*. Retrieved from http://www.nlm.nih.gov/medlineplus/leadpoisoning.html

The Merck Manual. (2015). *Lead poisoning*. Retrieved from http://www.merckmanuals.com/professional/injuries_poisoning/poisoning/lead_poisoning.html?qt=lead%20poisoning&alt=sh

United States Environmental Protection Agency. (2015). *Protect your family from lead in your home*. Retrieved from http://www.cpsc.gov/PageFiles/121956/426.pdf

LEUKEMIA

DEFINITION/ETIOLOGY:
Leukemia is the most common childhood cancer, defined as cancer of the white blood cells (WBC). There is an increase in the production of abnormal WBCs in leukemia, which replaces normal bone marrow and spills over into the circulating blood. Leukemic cells may infiltrate any organ: liver, spleen, lymph nodes, kidneys, testes, and the central nervous system (brain and spinal cord).

The initial period of drug therapy is usually 2 ½ - 3 years. After the initial period of drug therapy, the type of medication and length of therapy is individualized.

CAUSES:
The exact cause of leukemia is not fully understood by scientists. Leukemia appears to develop from a combination of genetic and environmental factors.

TYPES:
1. Acute Lymphocytic Leukemia *(ALL)* accounts for approximately 75% of cases. ALL is most common in ages 2-4 years and has the best prognosis during this time period. The survival rate is just under 85%. There are several subtypes of ALL which are identified by bone marrow appearance and other blood tests. Treatment and prognosis depend on age of onset, subtypes of ALL, and other blood factors.
2. Acute Myelogenous Leukemia (AML) is also called acute myeloid leukemia, acute myelocytic leukemia or acute non-lymphocytic leukemia. AML accounts for approximately 20% of cases. AML is most common is the teenage years. The survival rate is 60 – 70%.
3. Chronic Myelogenous Leukemia (CML) is rare in children. Survival rates are 60-80%.

SIGNS AND SYMPTOMS:
- Symptoms are derived from problems in bone marrow
- Onset may be insidious or acute
- Bone and joint pain due to pressure and irritation from infiltration by white blood cells
- Anemia, pallor, fatigue, weakness, lethargy, dizziness, lightheaded (symptoms of low red blood count)
- Increased susceptibility to fevers and recurrent infections due to low white blood cell count and weakened immune system

LEUKEMIA *(continued from previous page)*

SIGNS AND SYMPTOMS: *(continued)*
- Bleeding under the skin; bruising; pinpoint hemorrhages (petechiae) or larger areas; bleeding of nose or gums; blood in stool or urine (symptoms of low platelet count)
- Headache due to infiltration of the brain
- Seizures, balance problems, or abnormal vision
- Vomiting from bleeding in stomach or increased intracranial pressure
- Breathing problems and interference with blood flow to and from the heart
- Enlarged liver, spleen or swollen lymph nodes
- Weight loss

MANAGEMENT/TREATMENT:
- Drug therapy
- Chemotherapy
- Radiation
- Bone marrow or blood stem transplants (required for aggressive ALL)

Side Effects of Treatment:
- Hair loss from drug therapy
- Weight gain from therapy (prednisone)
- High blood pressure
- Breathing problems and interference with blood flow to and from the heart
- One third to 1/2 of survivors have poor short term memory, short attention span, or other learning difficulties (consider referral for Section 504 or special education services)
- Blood stem transplants may affect child's growth
- Emotional and psychological problems (which may affect school work)

FOLLOW UP:
An individualized healthcare plan should be developed and may include:
- Homebound instruction for limited periods.
- Notify teacher of symptoms of possible illness.
- Emphasize that the condition may make the student vulnerable to contagious viral illnesses of others.
- Notify school district registered dietician if child needs dietary accommodations.
- Obtain immunization exemption from healthcare provider if necessary.
- Coordinate with physical education (PE) teacher.

LEUKEMIA *(continued from previous page)*

FOLLOW UP: *(continued)*
- Accommodation of physical/emotional needs (possible Section 504 plan).
- Educate classmates before student returns to school.
- Notify parent/guardian(s) and healthcare providers of unusual symptoms and the occurrence of contagious illnesses, e.g., chickenpox, in the school.
- Continuous follow up care is important and essential for the child diagnosed with leukemia.

NOTES:
- Special treatment is required for exposure to chicken pox.
- A diagnosis of leukemia may be devastating for the family of a child who is newly diagnosed.
- Siblings are "at risk" for contracting leukemia.
- Children treated for leukemia have an increased risk for developing cancer in adulthood.
- Some school districts and hospitals have a school re-entry program.
- Children with Li-Fraumeni syndrome, Down syndrome, and children who have had an organ transplant are on long-term immune suppressing medication are at slightly higher risk of developing leukemia.

Resources
- "Returning to School", Leukemia and Lymphoma Society at http://www.livestrong.org/What-We-Do/Our-Actions/Professional-Tools-Training/For-Educators/Returning-to-School

- "Children Diagnosed With Cancer", American Cancer Society at http://www.cancer.org/treatment/childrenandcancer/whenyourchildhascancer/children-diagnosed-with-cancer-returning-to-school

LEUKEMIA *(continued from previous page)*

References

American Cancer Society. (2015). *How is childhood leukemia diagnosed? Signs and symptoms of childhood leukemia.* Retrieved from http://www.cancer.org/cancer/leukemiainchildren/detailedguide/childhood-leukemia-diagnosis

American Cancer Society. (2015). *Survival rates for childhood leukemias.* Retrieved from http://www.cancer.org/cancer/leukemiainchildren/detailedguide/childhood-leukemia-survival-rates

American Cancer Society. (2015). *What are key statistics for childhood leukemia?* Retrieved from http://www.cancer.org/cancer/leukemiainchildren/detailedguide/childhood-leukemia-key-statistics

American Cancer Society. (2015). *What is childhood leukemia?* Retrieved from http://www.cancer.org/cancer/leukemiainchildren/detailedguide/childhood-leukemia-what-is-childhood-leukemia

Kids Health. (2014). *Leukemia.* Retrieved from http://kidshealth.org/parent/medical/cancer/cancer_leukemia.html

Leukemia & Lymphoma Society. (2015). *Facts and statistics.* Retrieved from http://www.lls.org/http%3A/llsorg.prod.acquia-sites.com/facts-and-statistics/facts-and-statistics-overview/facts-and-statistics

Mayo Clinic. (2015). *Leukemia.* Retrieved from http://www.mayoclinic.com/health/leukemia/DS00351

Medline Plus. U.S. National Library of Medicine. (2014). *Childhood leukemia.* Retrieved from http://www.nlm.nih.gov/medlineplus/childhoodleukemia.html

Merck Manual. (2014). *Acute lymphocytic leukemia (ALL).* Retrieved from http://www.merckmanuals.com/professional/hematology-and-oncology/leukemias/acute-lymphocytic-leukemia-all

Selekman, J., Bobhenek, J. & Lukens, M. (2013).Children with chronic conditions. In J. Selekman (Ed.), *School nursing: A comprehensive text* (2nd ed.) (p. 728). Philadelphia, PA: F.A. Davis.

LICE (HEAD) - Pediculosis humanus capitis

DEFINITION/ETIOLOGY:
Head lice are parasitic insects that can be found in the hair. Head lice feed on human blood so they live close to the human scalp. They lay their eggs which attach to the base of the hair shaft with a glue like substance. Nymphs hatch from the eggs in 7-10 days, and grow to adults capable of reproduction (lay eggs) in 9-12 days, with a life span of 30 days. The female lays about 8-10 eggs per day (more than 200 in a lifetime), attaching them firmly to the hair shaft near the scalp. Head lice move by crawling; they cannot fly or jump. They are spread most commonly by head-to-head contact, for example during play at home or school, slumber parties, sports activities and camp. Although uncommon, it can be spread by contact with clothing such as hats, scarves, combs, brushes or towels. Only lice, not nits, spread the infestation.

Head lice are not dangerous and do not transmit disease but they are contagious until killed from a chemical agent. They most commonly occur in children ages 3-12 years old.

SIGNS AND SYMPTOMS:
- Head lice infestations can be asymptomatic, particularly with a first **infestation or when an infestation is light.**
- Itching (pruritus), the most common symptom of head lice infestation, is caused by an allergic reaction to the saliva associated with louse bites. It may take 4-6 weeks for itching to appear the first time a person has head lice.
- The student may report a tickling feeling or a sensation of something moving in the hair.
- Student irritability and sleeplessness may be present.
- Sores on the head may be caused by scratching. These sores and scabs, caused by scratching, can sometimes become infected with bacteria normally found on a person's skin. These may also be associated with swollen lymph nodes.

The assessment of a child who is suspected of having head lice includes:
- In good lighting, use a wood applicator to separate the hair in small sections. Give particular **attention to the scalp behind the ears and at the nape of the neck, areas of optimal temperature for head lice. Dispose of the applicator after each use.**
- The nurse needs to learn to recognize head lice and nits to avoid misidentification of dandruff and other debris as nits or lice.
- New nits will be found close to the scalp and will not easily be removed from the hair shaft as will dandruff, hairspray droplets and other hair products, dirt particles, other insects (fleas, bedbugs, etc.) and scabs. Magnification may be helpful in making this assessment.

LICE (HEAD) - Pediculosis humanus capitis *(continued from previous page)*

MANAGEMENT/TREATMENT:
Exclusion:

Policies should be based on current scientific evidence and best practice. Administrators, school nurses, local private and public health physicians and concerned parent/guardian(s) can cooperate to develop rational and epidemiologically sound school policies. Policy can be further supported through faculty and staff in-service and parent/community educational programs. School nurse practice includes the dual roles of child advocate and collaboration in policy development.

1. The American Academy of Pediatrics, National Association of School Nurses, Centers for Disease Control and Prevention, and Harvard School of Public Health do not recommend a "no-nit" policy.
2. Children with live head lice should be referred to their parent/guardian(s) for treatment. Data does not support school exclusion for nits (NASN, 2011).
3. The discovery of nits or live lice should not cause the student to be sent home from school or isolated while at school.
4. Notify parent/guardian(s) at the end of the day of the suspected infestation and recommended management.
5. Student may be transported home as usual.
6. Screenings of entire classes or school have not been found to be cost effective and are not recommended.
7. Provide parent with information to increase head lice awareness and prevention to ensure that student's education is not disrupted.
8. **In cases that involve head lice, as in all school health issues, it is vital that the school nurse prevent stigmatizing and maintain the student's privacy as well as the family's right to confidentiality.**

TREATMENT:

Educate and assist families to enable them to be able to effectively and efficiently treat head lice so that the student can return to school the next day.

1. Only students with active infestations need treatment with an over-the-counter (OTC) or prescription medication (pediculicide). Some medications may require 2 treatments (follow manufacturer's recommendation). Some resistance to these products has been reported and may require referral to the healthcare provider.
2. Parents/caregivers should persistently work to remove nits. All nits should be removed to limit newly hatched nymphs (7-10 days).

LICE (HEAD) - Pediculosis humanus capitis *(continued from previous page)*

TREATMENT: *(continued)*

3. "Preventive" use of lice shampoo is NOT advised. Some lice survive sub-lethal doses of residual chemicals and mutate over generations to resist low doses of pediculicide.
4. There is no clear evidence to support the use of food-grade oil, salad dressing, tea tree oil, enzymes, hot air blowers, or other 'remedies.'
5. Parent/guardian(s) should check all household members for lice and treat only those with lice following the instructions.
6. Students with severe or persistent infestation should be referred to their healthcare provider for treatment or to social services to assist with accessing treatment.
7. Supplemental Measures:
   a. Articles such as clothing bedding and other items the infested person wore or used during the 2 days before treatment should be washed at 130° and dried on the hot setting. Items that are not washable can be sealed in a plastic bag for 2 weeks.
   b. Soak combs and brushes in hot water (at least 130°) for 5-10 minutes.
   c. Vacuum carpet, pillows, and furniture where the infested person sat or lay. The risk of being infested by a louse that has fallen onto a rug or carpet or furniture is very small. Head lice survive less than 1-2 days if they fall off a person and cannot feed; nits cannot hatch and usually die within a week if they do not stay at the warm temperature found close to the human scalp. Spending much time and money on housecleaning activities is not necessary to avoid re-infestation by lice or nits that may have fallen off the head or crawled onto furniture or clothing.

FOLLOW UP:
- Monitor progress toward effective eradication of live lice and nits.
- "Treatment failure" may be due to misdiagnosis or misidentification of nits, non-adherence to directions for treatment, a new exposure after treatment, or inadequate or low residual ovicidal (egg-killing) action of the lice medication used.
- Seek information from reliable, current, evidence-based, science-based sources.

POTENTIAL COMPLICATIONS:
- Secondary bacterial infections (impetigo)
- Enlarged lymph nodes

LICE (HEAD) - Pediculosis humanus capitis *(continued from previous page)*

NOTES:
Education/Prevention for Faculty/Staff/Students
- Educate parent/guardian(s), students and staff about prevention, recognition, and treatment of head lice before cases or outbreaks occur.
- Inform staff about appropriate follow-up and dispel myths (e.g., lice fly or hop).
- Ask teachers to observe and refer children who scratch or have visible lice/nits.
- Educate teachers and students to avoid "head-to-head" contact, e.g., during telling secrets, taking "selfie" pictures with a friend, team work, team sports, babysitting, sleepovers, etc.
- Encourage teachers to minimize student use of dress-up hats. Discourage fabric sofas and pillows in classroom. Watch for head contact with fabric items, e.g., daily vacuuming of carpet if students lie on it; keep personal use pillows or blankets for naps stored separately.
- Non-fabric items are low risk. Clean headphones, vinyl bus seat backs, and solid helmets for general hygiene.
- Do not let children pile their winter coats/hats. Although there is no clear evidence of effectiveness, some schools separate coats and back packs on hooks, chair backs. Hats may be tucked into coat sleeves.

Education/Prevention for Parent/Guardian(s) /Students
- Offer clear instructions about effective treatment products and safe actions.
- Utilize multiple instructional strategies that are appropriate for intended audience (parent/guardian(s) /students/staff):
  - Verbal instructions/explanations, and videos.
  - Written head lice information, treatment instructions/directions, policy, pamphlets, letters, and newsletters. Use appropriate reading level and languages for intended audience(s) when developing or selecting print materials.
  - Hands-on strategies include demonstration-return demonstration for scalp inspection, head lice and nit identification, and nit combing technique.
- Assess family needs for treatment assistance and follow-through with nit combing and re-treatment if necessary.

LICE (HEAD) - Pediculosis humanus capitis *(continued from previous page)*

References

Andresen, K., & McCarthy, A.M. (2009). A policy change strategy for head lice management. *The Journal of School Nursing*, 25 (6) 407-416. doi:10.1177/1059840509347316

Devore, C.D., Schutze, G.E., & American Academy of Pediatrics' Council on School Health and Committee on Infectious Diseases. (2015). *Headlice*. Retrieved from http://pediatrics.aappublications.org/content/early/2015/04/21/peds.2015-0746.full.pdf+html

Center for Disease Control and Prevention. (2013). *Parasites-lice-head lice*. Retrieved from http://www.cdc.gov/parasites/lice/head/

National Association of School Nurses. (2011). *Pediculosis management in the school setting* (Position Statement). Retrieved from http://www.nasn.org/PolicyAdvocacy/PositionPapersandReports/NASNPositionStatementsFullView/tabid/462/ArticleId/40/Pediculosis-Management-in-the-School-Setting-Revised-2011

Pontius, D., (2014). Demystifying pediculosis: School nurses taking the lead. *Pediatric Nursing, 40*(5) 226-235.

LYME DISEASE

DEFINITION/ETIOLOGY:

Lyme Disease is a tickborne illness caused by *Borreoia burgdorferi* and is transmitted through the bite of an infected blacklegged tick. Lyme disease is the most common reported vectorborne illness in the U.S. It does not occur nationwide and is concentrated in the northeast and the upper Midwest. It is transmitted by wild rodents (nymph stage) and deer ticks (adult stage).

Erythema migrans (EM) is a round or oval, expanding erythematous skin lesion that develops at the site of the bite and may expand to as much as 20 centimeters in diameter. The over-all appearance of the lesion is that of a bulls-eye. The skin lesion appears 3-31 days after the tick detaches or was removed. The lesion should be at least 5 centimeters in diameter to be diagnostically relevant. Lyme disease occurs in phases.

SIGNS AND SYMPTOMS:

Symptoms are non-specific and frequently found in many conditions, which make Lyme disease difficult to diagnose. Symptoms left untreated, systemic involvement follows that involves the neurologic, cardiac, and musculoskeletal systems.

Early Signs and Symptoms
- Rash
- Flu like symptoms (fever, chills, headache)
- Muscle and joint ache
- Swollen lymph glands

Later Signs and Symptoms
- EM rash on other parts of body
- Severe headache
- Intermittent tendon, muscle joints and bone pain
- Neurological – nerve pain, numbness tingling in and feet
- Shortness of breath/dizziness

LYME DISEASE *(continued from previous page)*

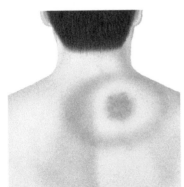
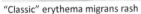
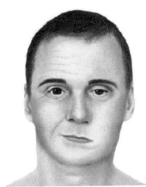
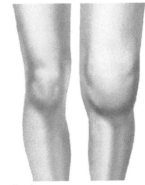

"Classic" erythema migrans rash   Facial palsy   Swollen knee

CDC (2015)

MANAGEMENT/TREATMENT:

1. Prompt removal of the tick with a fine tipped forceps.
2. Grasp the tick as close to the skin as possible.
3. Pull upward with firm, steady pressure. Twisting or jerking may cause some of the mouth-parts to remain in the skin. Attempts to remove the remaining material are unnecessary and may cause further damage to the tissue. Leave it alone and let the skin heal. The risk of Lyme disease is unaffected.
4. After removing the tick thoroughly clean the site and your hands with soap and water.
5. Dispose of the tick by submersing it in alcohol, placing it in a sealed bag or container, wrapping it in tape, or flushing it down the toilet. Never crush a tick with your fingers.
6. Avoid remedies such as covering the tick with nail polish or petroleum jelly, or using heat to make the tick detach. (The goal is to remove the tick as quickly as possible rather than waiting for it to detach.)
7. At the first appearance of flu-like symptoms and/or erythema migrans skin lesion refer to healthcare provider for evaluation.
8. Antibiotic therapy is the treatment of choice for erythema migrans and often prevents later stage Lyme disease.

LYME DISEASE *(continued from previous page)*

FOLLOW-UP:
Persons who have removed ticks themselves should be monitored for 30 days for signs and symptoms of tickborne disease, especially a red round or oval expanding skin lesion (erythema migrans).

POTENTIAL COMPLICATIONS:
1. Neurologic (neuropathy, encelphalitis)
2. Cardiac irregularities
3. Musculoskeletal (pain, arthritis)

NOTES:
1. Prevention strategies are helpful in protecting children include avoiding infested areas and wearing light colored clothing makes it easier to spot ticks.
2. Wear hats or scarves, long sleeves and long pants with the cuffs snuggly secured.
3. Frequent "tick checks" include the scalp, neck, armpits, and groin area are helpful in early detection of a tick.
4. Parents should be alert for the appearance of skin lesions following a visit to an infested area.
5. The use of insect/tick repellents can provide protection, but caution should be used when applying on children. Avoid spray application repellents. Recommend that parents carefully follow label directions. Treated skin should be thoroughly washed once indoors.
6. Lyme disease is unlikely to develop if tick is attached less than 36-48 hours.
7. Resource for Parents and Teachers:
   American Lyme Disease Foundation, Inc.
   P.O. Box 466
   Lyme, CT 06371

See also TICK-BORNE DISEASES AND TICK REMOVAL

LYME DISEASE *(continued from previous page)*

References

Centers for Disease Control and Prevention (CDC). (2015). *Lyme disease*. Retrieved from http://www.cdc.gov/lyme/index.html

Hockenberry, M., Baker, R., and Mondozzi, M. (2013). The child with hematalogic or Immunologic dysfunction. In M. Hockenberry & D. Wilson (Eds.), *Wong's Essentials of Pediatric Nursing* (9th ed.). (pp. 1028-1029). St. Louis, MO: Mosby Elsevier.

Medline Plus/National Library of Health. (2015). *Lyme disease*. Retrieved from https://www.nlm.nih.gov/medlineplus/lymedisease.html

Mayo Clinic. (2015). *Lyme disease*. Retrieved from http://www.mayoclinic.org/diseases-conditions/lyme-disease/basics/definition/con-20019701

Ogle, J.W., & Anderson, M.S. (2014). Infections: Bacterial & spirochetal. In W. Hay, M. Levin, R. Deterding, & M. Abzug (Eds.), *Current diagnosis and treatment pediatrics* (22nd edition) (pp. 1350-1352). New York, NY:McGraw Hill Education, Inc.

MEASLES (Rubeola) and RUBELLA (German Measles)

DEFINITION/ETIOLOGY:

Measles (Rubeola, Seven-Day Measles, Hard Measles, or Old-Fashion Measles)

Measles (Rubeola) is an extremely communicable, viral *(Paramyozvious)* respiratory disease. The measles virus grows in the cells that live in the back of the throat and lungs. Measles are spread by airborne droplets via secretions from the nose, throat, and mouth throughout the prodromal and eruption stages. The measles virus can live up to 2 hours in the air or on surfaces. Infected persons can spread the measles virus up to 4 days before the onset of the virus. A person is contagious 4 days before to 4 days after the appearance of the rash. Incubation for measles is 7-21 days. Clinical evaluation and serological testing confirm diagnosis. Differential diagnosis includes Rubella, drug rashes, and Roseola (Roseola Infectiosum). Measles is a vaccine-preventable disease (see Note below).

Rubella (German Measles, or Three-Day Measles)

Rubella (German Measles) is a communicable disease caused by the *Rubivirus* and is spread by droplets, close contact and through the air. Rubella is less contagious than Rubeola. Transmission can occur 7 days before the rash appears until 14 days after eruption of the rash. The incubation period for Rubella is 14-21 days. Clinical evaluation and serological testing confirm diagnosis. Differential diagnosis includes Measles, Scarlet fever, drug rashes, and erythemus infectiosum. Rubella is a vaccine-preventable disease (see Note below).

MEASLES (Rubeola) and RUBELLA (German Measles) (continued from previous page)

Measles and Rubella---vaccine preventable diseases		
Disease	Measles (Rubeola)	Rubella (German Measles)
Cause	Viral (*Paramyxovirus*)	Viral (*Rubivirus*)
Transmission	Respiratory droplets	Respiratory droplets
Signs and Symptoms	Fever, hacking cough, runny nose, red watery eyes, Koplik's spots/buccal cavity opposite upper 1st & 2nd year molars (resembles white grains of sand surrounded by red areolae). Sore throat. Red blotchy rash begins on face and neck, and spreads head to foot including palms and soles of feet. Fever may exceed 40 C/104 F.	1-5 day prodrome. Low-grade fever (102^0 F or lower). Malaise, headache, stuffy or runny nose, lymph-adenopathy, tender swelling of the suboccipital, post auricular, and posterior cervical glands. Pharyngeal involvement present. Rash begins on the face and neck and spreads to trunk and extremities. Rash begins as blanching, macular erythema and becomes more scarlatiniform with reddish flush. Petechiae form on the soft palate (Forschheimer signs) later spreading into a red blush,
Incubation	7-21 days	14-21 days
Potential Complications	Ear infection, pneumonia, diarrhea, seizures, encephalitis, deafness and even death.	Usually mild, in rare cases can cause ear infections, Thrombocytopenic purpura and encephalitis. Infection during pregnancy can cause spontaneous abortion, stillbirth, and congenital defects.

Rubeola Measles

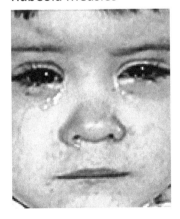

Photo retrieved from
http://www.cdc.gov/measles/about/photos.html

Rubella Measles

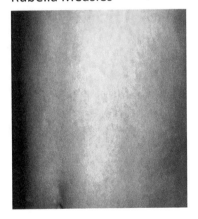

Photo retrieved from
http://www.cdc.gov/rubella/about/photos.html

MEASLES (Rubeola) and RUBELLA (German Measles) (continued from previous page)

MANAGEMENT/TREATMENT:
- Supportive/symptomatic

FOLLOW-UP:
- Both Measles and Rubella are reportable to the local health department.
- Follow state and local health department recommendations for school attendance.
- If an outbreak occurs at school – exclude unvaccinated students and staff from school/ work from the onset of the first diagnosed case through the last confirmed case.

NOTES:
- **Persons with a compromised immune system may not present with a rash.**
- Make susceptible (unvaccinated) pregnant women aware of the presence of Measles and/or Rubella and urge to contact their healthcare provider or obstetrician.
- Check state and local health department's regulations for school exclusion/attendance.

RESOURCES:

Measles and Rubella are vaccine preventable diseases. Check this Center for Disease Control and Prevention website: *http://www.cdc.gov/vaccines/imz-managers/laws/* to view *State Vaccination Requirements* and *School Entry Requirements- By State or By Disease.*

References:

Centers for Disease Control and Prevention. (2015). Measles, for healthcare professionals. Retrieved from *http://cdc.gov/ measles/hcp/index.html*

Center for Disease Control and Prevention (CDC). (2015). Rubella (German Measles: Three-day measles). *Epidemiology and Prevention of Vaccine-Preventable Diseases, the Pink Book: Course Textbook (13th ed.).* Retrieved from *http://www.cdc.gov/rubella/index.html*

Center for Disease Control and Prevention (CDC). (2015). Rubella. *Epidemiology and Prevention of Vaccine-Preventable Diseases, the Pink Book: Course Textbook (13th ed.).* Retrieved from *http://www.cdc.gov/vaccines/pubs/pinkbook/ rubella.html*

Center for Disease Control and Prevention (CDC). (2015). Requirements & laws -State vaccination requirements Retrieved from *http://www.cdc.gov/vaccines/imz-managers/laws/*

Lechtenberg, J. (2015). *Measles (Rubeola): The potential for harm.* Nashville, TN: *School Health Alert.*

Mayo Clinic. (2014). *Measles.* Retrieved from *http://www.mayoclinic.com/health/measles/DS00331*

Mayo Clinic. (2015). *Rubella.* Retrieved from http://www.mayoclinic.com/health/measles/DS00332

Merck Manual. (2014). *Measles (rubeola; morbilli; 9-day measles).* Retrieved from *http://www.merckmanuals.com/ professional/infectious_diseases/other_viruses/measles.html?qt=measles&alt=sh*

Merck Manual. (2014). *Rubella (German Measles; 3-day measles).* Retrieved from *http://www.merckmanuals.com/ professional/infectious_diseases/other_viruses/rubella.html?qt=measles&alt=sh*

MENINGITIS

DEFINITION/ETIOLOGY:
Meningitis is an inflammation of leptomeninges, a covering of the brain and spinal cord. Meningitis may be caused by bacteria, viruses or, rarely, fungi. It is important to know whether meningitis is caused by viral or bacterial infection because the severity of illness and treatment differ depending on the cause.

CAUSES
- **Viral** meningitis is generally less severe and clears up without treatment. The most common viruses causing meningitis are enteroviruses (85-95%).
- **Bacterial** meningitis can be quite severe and may result in brain damage, hearing loss, or learning disabilities. The importance of knowing the type of bacteria causing the meningitis is helpful in providing the appropriate antibiotic treatment to prevent some types from spreading and infecting other people.
  - In children 2 months to 12 years of age, this was traditionally the result of infection with *Streptococcus pneumoniae*, *Haemophilus influenzae* or *Neisseria meningitides*.
  - In those who are 9 years old or older, common causes have traditionally been *Streptococcus pneumoniae* or *Neisseria meningitides.*
  - Recent advances immunizations have led to decrease of disease associated with *Streptococcus pneumoniae* and *Haemophilus influenza.*
  - In children who have ventriculoperitoneal (VP) shunt, meningitis is the result of *Staphylococcus epidermidis* and, less commonly, *Staphylococcus aureus.*
- **Fungal and Mycobacterium** tuberculosis: uncommon, but should be considered in immuno-compromised host.

SIGNS AND SYMPTOMS:
- Classic triad for suspicion (these findings are most common in children less than 2 years of age):
  - Sudden high fever
  - Severe headache
  - Stiff neck (neck typically can be rotated but not flexed).
- Signs of brain dysfunction such as altered mental status or consciousness, seizures.
- Signs of increased of intracranial pressure (ICP) including headache, vomiting or papilledema
- May have rash (meningococcal meningitis)
- Photosensitivity

251

MENINGITIS *(continued from previous page)*

MANAGEMENT/TREATMENT:

1. **Meningitis is an emergency condition** and REQUIRES diagnosis and appropriate treatment as soon as possible to prevent serious complications.

2. Suspected cases should be referred to a healthcare provider with concomitant notification of parents/guardians.

3. Closely monitor vital signs and physical findings, especially neurological findings such as level of consciousness.

4. Specific treatment of meningitis depends on confirmed diagnosis:
   - For suspected viral meningitis: supportive care may be done as an outpatient, *except* herpes meningitis (for which antiviral therapy occurs with close supervision in hospital setting). Most children with non-herpetic viral meningitis recover completely.

   - For suspected bacterial meningitis, treatment is initially directed to the most common pathogens based on child's age and setting. All children need to be admitted for close monitoring. Delay in treatment may result in brain damage or death.

5. Chemoprophylaxis of close contacts are considered, and based on the type of pathogen that was cultured (*Haemophilus influenzae* or *Neisseria meningitides*), age, and other aspects of the situation surrounding exposure. Contact Public Health Department with details.

6. Work closely with health department and school officials to reduce public anxiety.

7. Follow local and/or state public health officials' decisions regarding outbreak control and management.

MENINGITIS *(continued from previous page)*

POSSIBLE COMPLICATIONS:

Poor prognosis is associated with young age, long duration of illness before effective antibiotic therapy, late onset seizure, coma, shock, and immuno-compromised status. Those with bacterial meningitis may sustain complications such as:

- Hearing loss
- Kidney damage
- Seizures
- Brain damage
- Learning disabilities
- Blindness
- Ataxia
- Hydrocephalus
- Limb loss
- Death

FOLLOW UP:

- All children with meningitis should have a hearing evaluation before hospital release and follow-up visit.
- After hospitalization, children need to be transitioned to rehabilitation at home until there is complete recovery.
- When children return to school: monitor for mental, social, and functional alterations that may be present and provide planning with a multi-disciplinary team, e.g., Section 504 plan.
- Monitor side effects of medical therapy (i.e., anticonvulsant drugs).
- Risk of contracting meningitis increases if not up-to-date on vaccinations. Vaccines to prevent some types of meningitis include:
  - Haemophilus Influenza Type B (Hib)
  - Meningococcal Conjugate vaccine

NOTES:

Following good hygiene practices is effective in reducing the spread of infection causes by viruses. Proper hand hygiene and respiratory etiquette can reduce the spread of viral infections such as viral meningitis. Cleaning contaminated surfaces, avoid sharing items with sick people, and obtaining childhood vaccinations can reduce the chances of becoming infected with a virus or spreading infection to others.

MENINGITIS *(continued from previous page)*

References

American Academy of Pediatrics. (2013). *Meningitis*. In S. Aronson, & T. Shope (Eds.), *Managing infectious diseases in child care and schools (2nd ed.)* (pp. 119-120). Elk Grove Village, IL: American Academy of Pediatrics.

Atkinson, W., Wolfe, S., Hamborsky, J., & McIntyre, L. (Eds.) (2015). *Epidemiology and prevention of vaccine-preventable diseases (*12th ed.). Washington DC: Public Health Foundation/ Centers for Disease Control and Prevention. Retrieved from http://www.cdc.gov/vaccines/pubs/pinkbook/downloads/mening.pdf

Centers for Disease Control and Prevention (CDC). (2015). *Meningitis*. Retrieved from http://www.cdc.gov/meningitis/index.html

Centers for Disease Control and Prevention (CDC). (2015). *Vaccines and immunizations*. Retrieved from http://www.cdc.gov/vaccines/vpd-vac/mening/default.htm

Mayo Clinic. (2015). *Meningitis*. Retrieved from http://www.mayoclinic.org/diseases-conditions/meningitis/basics/definition/con-20019713

Merck Manual. (2013). Overview of meningitis. Retrieved from http://www.merckmanuals.com/professional/neurologic-disorders/meningitis/overview-of-meningitis

Selekman, J. & Coates, J. (2013). Disease prevention. In J. Selekman (Ed.), *School nursing: A comprehensive text* (2nd ed.) (pp. 509-510). Philadelphia, PA: F.A. Davis.

MENSTRUAL DISORDERS

DEFINITION AND ETIOLOGY:

Term	Definition
Amenorrhea	Absence of menstruation.
Dysmenorrhea	Defined as "difficult menstrual flow" and can cause painful menstruation (cramps). Primary dysmenorrhea is the result of increased prostaglandin production (in the absence of pelvic pathology). Secondary dysmenorrhea is painful uterine contractions related to an identified cause, e.g. endometriosis, pelvic inflammatory disease. Typically occurs in the first three years after initial menstruation.
Hypermenorrhea	Excessive bleeding in amount and duration, at regular intervals (also called *menorrhagia*).
Intermenstrual	Not excessive bleeding, occurring between otherwise regular menstrual periods.
Menarche	Onset of menses. Average age of onset is 12, but may occur from 8-15 years. Menstrual periods are often irregular during first six months to two years.
Menometrorrhagia	Excessive and prolonged bleeding, frequent and irregular intervals.
Metrorrhagia	Not excessive bleeding, but intervals are irregular.
Mittelschmerz	Intermenstrual pain and/or bleeding, lasting a few hours to 3 days. Pain is usually associated with ovulation.
Oligomenorrhea	Infrequent, irregular episodes of bleeding, usually occurring at intervals greater than 40 days.
Polymenorrhea	Frequent but regular episodes of bleeding, occurring at intervals of 21 days or less.
Dysfunctional Uterine Bleeding	Irregular, painless bleeding that is prolonged and excessive.

MENSTRUAL DISORDERS *(continued from previous page)*

SIGNS AND SYMPTOMS:

Dysmenorrhea

- Primary dysmenorrheal - pain, usually the first day or two of menses
- Suprapubic pain radiating to the thigh and lower back
- Associated nausea, vomiting, and diarrhea
- Breast tenderness
- Headache, fatigue, sleep disturbances
- Dizziness, nervousness, syncope

Amenorrhea

Requires evaluation when:

- Menarche delayed beyond age 15
- No secondary sexual characteristics develop by age 14 (breasts, pubic and axillary hair)
- Three years after developing secondary sexual characteristics if menstruation has not begun

Persons at risk:

- Runners, gymnasts, ballet dancers (excessive exercise)
- Girls with too little body fat, e.g. anorexia nervosa, extreme dieters such as vegan vegetarians
- Possible development of osteoporosis due to lack of estrogen (female hormone)

Note: Amenorrhea is part of the female athlete triad which is a concern among competitive athletes: amenorrhea, anorexia, and osteoporosis

Excessive Uterine Bleeding

- It is helpful to divide cases in to mild, moderate or severe to determine treatment.
- Hemoglobin < 8 gm/dL with tachycardia, pallor would indicate a severe case.
- Hemoglobin between 9-11 gm/dL would indicate moderate hemorrhage.
- In mild cases, there is no anemia.

MENSTRUAL DISORDERS *(continued from previous page)*

MANAGEMENT/TREATMENT:

Anovulatory cycles where there is a lack of a progesterone peak, are present in the majority of girls within 24 months of menarche and are responsible for irregular menses. Irregular cycles after 24 months post menarche should be evaluated.

1. **Primary dysmenorrhea**
   - Analgesic medication specifically NSAIDS (non-steroid anti-inflammatories) which reduce prostaglandin level.
   - Educate on proper use of NSAIDS to avoid stomach irritation or overdose.
   - Warm pad to lower abdomen and position of comfort.
   - Encourage physical exercise and balanced diet.
   - Refer severe disorders for medical evaluation.
   - Hormonal contraception can be used to treat dysmenorrhea when NSAIDS are ineffective.

2. **Amenorrhea**
   - Refer for medical evaluation girls who should have begun menstruating or have stopped.
   - Consider the possibility of pregnancy.

3. **Excessive Uterine Bleeding**
   - For severe cases, hospitalization and transfusion may be necessary.
   - Oral hormonal therapy may be used to regulate cycles and decrease bleeding.
   - Reassurance, a high iron diet, and the use of a multivitamin with iron should be encouraged.

MENSTRUAL DISORDERS *(continued from previous page)*

POTENTIAL COMPLICATIONS:

Refer to healthcare provider if:
- Menstruation has not begun by the age of 15.
- Menstruation has not begun within 3 years after breast growth began, or if breasts have not started to grow by age 13.
- Period suddenly stops for more than 90 days.
- Periods become very irregular after having had regular, monthly cycles.
- Periods occurs more often than every 21 days or less often than every 35 days.
- Bleeding for more than 7 days.
- Bleeding is heavier than usual or using more than 1 pad or tampon every 1 to 2 hours.
- Bleeding occurs between periods.
- There is severe pain during period.
- Sudden fever and feel sick after using tampons.

NOTES:
- Educate students to keep diary of menstrual cycles to share with parent/guardian and healthcare provider.
- Encourage students to keep sanitary napkins/tampons at school. An emergency supply of sanitary napkins and tampons should be kept in health room.
- Students may keep medication for discomfort at school following school policy and guidelines for medication at school.
- Be alert to history and signs that suggest pregnancy or secondary dysmenorrhea, e.g., PID (pelvic inflammatory disease).
- Irregular menstrual cycles in a girl within two years of menarche can usually be observed before an extensive work up. Provide reassurance.

References

Carey, A. & Murray, P. (2014). Menstrual disorders: Dysmenorrhea and premenstrual syndrome. In M. Fisher, E. Alderman, R. Kreipe, W. Rosenfeld, W.(Eds.). *Textbook of adolescent health care* (pp. 589-610). Elk Grove Village, IL: American Academy of Pediatrics.

Mayo Clinic. (2014). *Menstrual cramps*. Retrieved from http://www.mayoclinic.org/diseases-conditions/menstrual-cramps/DS00506

Medline Plus, U.S. National Library of Medicine. (2014). *Menorrhagia (heavy menstrual bleeding)*. Retrieved from http://www.mayoclinic.org/diseases-condfitionsa/menorrhagia/CON-2021959?p=1

Kollar, L., Jordan, K., & Wilson, D. (2013). Health problems of school-age children and adolescents. In M. Hockenberry, E. In I. Chg, & D. Wilson (Eds.). *Wong's Essentials of Pediatric Nursing,* (9th ed.), (p. 508-509). St Louis, MO: Elsevier/Mosby.

MOSQUITO-BORNE DISEASES

DEFINITION/ETIOLOGY:
A mosquito-borne disease is a transmitted from a mosquito infected from a virus or parasite. Mosquitoes become infected by feeding off of birds, mammals or people who are carriers of diseases. Most people infected with a mosquito-borne disease do not become ill except with Malaria. However, the potential for them to become ill fluctuates from mild, flu like symptoms to severe illness and even death.

Types

Eastern Equine Encephalitis (EEE)	A rare illness in humans and only a few cases are reported in the United States each year. EEE is considered the most serious mosquito-borne disease in the United States. Most cases occur in the Atlantic and Gulf Coast states.
Western equine encephalitis	Most cases of Western equine encephalitis occur in the eastern and central states.
La Crosse encephalitis	Most cases of La Crosse encephalitis occur in the southeastern states, upper mid-Western, and mid-Atlantic states. Children under the age of 16 usually have the most severe cases.
West Nile Virus (WNV)	Most cases of WNV occur in the summer to fall months in North America. Risk highest July through September. Mosquitoes infect people, horses, and mammals with the virus. Although the risk is very low, WNV has been known to spread through organ transplants, blood transfusions, breast-feeding and during pregnancy from mother to baby.
Dengue	Dengue is uncommon in United States, but has been seen in Texas, Florida, and Hawaii. Suspect Dengue fever if individual suddenly develops symptoms and has recently travelled to Puerto Rico, Southeast Asia and/or the Caribbean. Dengue is vaccine preventable.
Malaria	A small amount of malaria cases exist in the United States. Those infected typically become ill.

MOSQUITO-BORNE DISEASES *(continued from previous page)*

SIGNS AND SYMPTOMS:
- Range from none to severe
- Depends on the virus or parasite transmitted
- Mild, flu like (fever, body aches, headache, vomiting, nausea)
- Stiff neck
- Rash
- High fever
- Altered mental status
- Swollen lymph glands
- Convulsions
- Encephalitis
- Meningitis
- Coma, paralysis, death

MANAGEMENT/TREATMENT:
- No specific treatment – supportive care
- Based on symptoms
- Pain control
- OTC medications to alleviate flu like symptoms
- Avoid ibuprofen, naproxen sodium which may increase bleeding disorders
- Close medical monitoring is required for severe symptoms

PREVENTION /CONTROL:
Educate students, families, staff, and the community on prevention:
- Wear protective clothing (long pants, long sleeves and socks).
- Use insect repellents (containing diethyltoluamide, amount used is determined by number of hours of protection needed) – follow manufacturer's directions.
- Install screens on windows and doors.
- Remove standing water around your home (flower pots, buckets, pool cover, bird baths, pet dishes, etc.).
- Avoid shaded and wooded areas.
- Limit outdoor exposure between dusk and dawn.
- Community-wide mosquito prevention programs.

MOSQUITO-BORNE DISEASES *(continued from previous page)*

NOTES:
- Report sick or dead bird, or mammal to local health department.

References

American Academy of Pediatrics. (2013). Mosquito-borne diseases. In S. Aronson, & T. Shope (Eds.), *Managing infectious diseases in child care and schools (2ⁿᵈed.)* (p. 125). Elk Grove Village, IL: American Academy of Pediatrics.

Centers for Disease Control and Prevention. (2015). *Division of vector-borne diseases.* Retrieved from http://www.cdc.gov/ncezid/dvbd/index.html

Centers for Disease Control and Prevention. (2015). *Malaria facts.* Retrieved from http://www.cdc.gov/malaria/about/facts.html

Centers for Disease Control and Prevention. (2015). *West nile virus.* Retrieved from http://www.cdc.gov/Features/WestNileVirus/

Mayo Clinic. (2012). *West nile virus.* Retrieved from http://www.mayoclinic.com/health/west-nile-virus/DS00438/DSECTION=symptoms

Merck Manual. (2014). *Dengue.* Retrieved from http://www.merckmanuals.com/professional/infectious-diseases/arboviridae-arenaviridae-and-filoviridae/dengue

Oakland County Health Department. (2015). *West nile virus what you need to know.* Retrieved from https://www.oakgov.com/health/information/Documents/Fact%20Sheets/fs_west_nile_virus.pdf

MONONUCLEOSIS (Glandular Fever, Infectious Mono)

DEFINITION/ETIOLOGY:

An acute viral infection caused by the Epstein-Barr virus (EBV). Incubation period is 4-6 weeks. The virus is present in pharyngeal secretions and is spread by saliva. The virus can be excreted for some months after infection and can even occur intermittently throughout life. It can occur at any age, but is most common in adolescents.

SIGNS AND SYPMTOMS (COMMON):

- Milder and often undiagnosed in young children, more severe in high school and college age
- Fever, malaise, nausea, headache, and fatigue
- Sore throat and enlarged, red, exudative tonsils. Occasionally strep infection is associated with the sore throat
- Lymph nodes swollen in axilla, groin, above elbow, and especially in neck (post cervical)
- Enlarged spleen
- Maculopapular confluent rash if treated with penicillin
- Fever may last 1-2 weeks; fatigue and malaise may last 4-6 weeks
- Periorbital edema (25% cases)
- Jaundice (approximately 10% cases)

MANAGEMENT/TREATMENT:

Treatment is aligned with supporting the symptoms; most patients recover in 4-6 weeks without medication.

1. Refer to healthcare provider; laboratory tests are needed for diagnosis; strep throat may accompany. Healthcare provider may prescribe oral steroids if symptoms are severe.
2. Symptomatic support for sore throat (gargle), fever (fluids) and fatigue (rest).
3. Return to school on advice of healthcare provider.
4. May be in school during illness if temperature is below 100° and able to tolerate activity.
5. Rest and contact sports restrictions may be needed for a month or longer.

FOLLOW UP:

- Monitor 1-2 weeks after return to school for full recovery.

MONONUCLEOSIS (Glandular Fever, Infectious Mono) *(continued from previous page)*

POTENTIAL COMPLICATIONS:

- Complications are rare and can include: encephalitis, Guillain-Barré syndrome, anemia, myocarditis.
- Danger of ruptured spleen. Must be asymptomatic before return to activity. Protect from contact sports for 1 month or until splenomegaly has resolved.
- Liver issues such as hepatitis (liver inflammation) or jaundice.

NOTES:

Health education:

- Transmitted person-to-person via saliva. Virus may remain in saliva several weeks during and after convalescence.
- Avoid kissing on the mouth and sharing food from the same container and/or by sharing things like eating utensils, glasses, toothbrushes and lipstick or lip gloss.
- Use good handwashing techniques at all times.

References

American Academy of Pediatrics. (2013). Mononucleois. In S. Aronson, & T. Shope (Eds.), *Managing infectious diseases in child care and schools. (2nded.)* (p.123). Elk Grove Village, IL: American Academy of Pediatrics.

American Academy of Pediatrics, Committee on Infectious Diseases. (2015).Epstein-Barr virus infections. In D.W. Kimberlin, M. T. Brady, M.A. Jackson, & S.S. Long (Eds.), *Red Book: 2015 report of the committee on infectious diseases* (30th ed.) (pp. 336-340). Elk Grove Village, IL: American Academy of Pediatrics.

Centers for Disease Control and Prevention (CDC), National Center for Infectious Diseases. (2014). *Epstein-Barr Virus and Infectious Mononucleosi.* Retrieved from CDC website at http://www.cdc.gov/epstein-barr/about-ebv.html

Mayo Clinic. (2015). *Mononucleosis.* Retrieved from http://www.mayoclinic.com/health/mononucleosis/DS00352

MedlinePlus. (2014). *Mononucleosis.* Retrieved from http://www.nlm.nih.gov/medlineplus/ency/article/000591.htm

MUMPS

DEFINITION/ETIOLOGY:

Mumps an acute viral illness characterized by swelling of one or more of salivary glands, usually the parotid glands.

Mumps is caused by *Rubulavirus* that infects the respiratory tract. The virus is spread by direct contact with respiratory droplets and saliva. The incubation period is generally 16-18 days (range 12-25 days) from time of exposure to onset of symptoms. Mumps virus has been isolated from saliva from between 2 and 7 days before symptom onset until 9 days after onset of symptoms. Interactions of students during sporting or other inter-collegiate events and mass mobilization of students during holidays are opportunities for transmission among students from geographically diverse parts of the country and world.

Mumps is a vaccine preventable disease (VPD).

SIGNS AND SYMPTOMS:
- Non-specific prodrome, which includes myalgia, anorexia, malaise, headache, and fever
- Unilateral or bilateral tender swelling of parotid or other salivary glands
- 30%-70% of mumps infections are associated with typical acute parotitis (most common manifestation)
- Nearly 50% are associated with non-specific or primarily respiratory symptoms, with or without parotitis

MANAGEMENT/TREATMENT:
- Rapidly identify infected and susceptible persons and report to public health department.
- If a case of mumps is identified, educate school staff on signs and symptoms and how to prevent the spread of the virus.
- There is no specific treatment for mumps. The healthcare provider may recommend that parent/guardian(s) apply ice or heat packs to the neck and the administration of non-aspirin analgesics (e.g. Tylenol®). Do not give aspirin to children with a viral illness because of the risk of Reye's Syndrome.
- Use soft diet if pain with chewing.
- Infected student should be excluded for 5 days from onset of parotid glands swelling.

MUMPS *(continued from previous page)*

MANAGEMENT/TREATMENT: *(continued)*

- Anyone born in 1957 or after, without evidence of immunity, should have at least one dose of MMR vaccine. A second dose should be given, at least 28 days later, to school children and adults at high risk of mumps exposure. (e.g. healthcare personnel, students at post high school educational institutions and international travelers). The routine use of vaccine is not advised for people born before 1957, however immunization is not contraindicated in those people having unknown serologic status.
- Mumps vaccine has not been effective in preventing of infection after exposure; however, immunization will provide protection to subsequent exposures.
- Recommend that unimmunized, pregnant females exposed to mumps consult with their healthcare provider. Pregnant women who are infected with mumps may be at risk for complications.
- Follow local and/or state public health officials' decisions regarding outbreak control and management.

Potential Complications:
- Aseptic meningitis
- Orchitis (in post-pubertal males)
- Nerve deafness
- Encephalitis
- Pancreatitis
- Mastitis
- Oophoritis (inflammation of the ovaries)
- Mumps during pregnancy

MUMPS *(continued from previous page)*

NOTES:

PREVENTION
- Mumps is a vaccine preventable disease.
- Mumps immunization status should be assessed. Mumps vaccine is given as an MMR for students and staff who have not already had mumps or mumps vaccine.
- In children the first MMR is given on or after first birthday. Second dose is given between ages four and six.
- The effectiveness of MMR against mumps is approximately 80% after one dose and approximately 90% after two doses.
- Because the vaccine is not 100% effective, some cases can occur in vaccinated persons.
- Students should be kept home until 9 days after the onset of paratoid swelling.

References

American Academy of Pediatrics. (2013). Mumps. In S. Aronson, & T. Shope (Eds.), *Managing infectious diseases in child care and schools (2nd ed.)* (pp. 131-132). Elk Grove Village, IL: American Academy of Pediatrics.

American Academy of Pediatrics, Committee on Infectious Diseases. (2015). Mumps. In D.W. Kimberlin, M. T. Brady, M.A. Jackson, & S.S. Long (Eds.), *Red Book: 2015 report of the committee on infectious diseases* (30th ed.) (pp. 564-568). Elk Grove Village, IL: American Academy of Pediatrics.

Centers for Disease Control and Prevention. (2015a). *Mumps.* Retrieved from http://cdc.gov/mumps/index.html

Center for Disease Control and Prevention (CDC). (2015b). Mumps. In J. Hamborsky, A. Kroger, & S. Wolfe (Eds.), *Epidemiology and prevention of vaccine-preventable diseases, the pink book: Course textbook (13th ed.).* Washington D.C. Public Health Foundation. Retrieved from http://www.cdc.gov/vaccines/pubs/pinkbook/mumps.html

Levin, M.J., & Weinberg, A. (2014). Infections: Viral & rickettsial. In W. Hay, M. Levin, R. Deterding, & M. Abzug (Eds.), *Current diagnosis and treatment pediatrics* (22nd edition) (pp. 1265-1266). McGraw Hill Education, Inc.

Merck Manual. *Mumps* (epidemic parotitis). (2014). Retrieved from http://www.merckmanuals.com/professional/pediatrics/miscellaneous_viral_infections_in_infants_and_children/mumps.html?q=mumps&alt=sh

Selekman, J., & Coates, J. (2013). Disease prevention. In J. Selekman (Ed.), *School nursing: A comprehensive text (2nd ed.)* (p. 503). Philadelphia, PA: F.A. Davis.

MUSCULAR DYSTROPHY

DEFINITION/ETIOLOGY:
Muscular dystrophy is a group of genetic, degenerative diseases primarily affecting voluntary muscles. Muscles become progressively weaker. In the late stages of muscular dystrophy, fat and connective tissue often replace muscle fibers. Some types of muscular dystrophy affect heart muscles, other involuntary muscles, and organs. The most common types of muscular dystrophy appear to be due to a genetic deficiency of the muscle protein dystrophin. There is no cure for muscular dystrophy. Supportive care, therapy, and medications can prolong functionality and slow the course of the disease.

SIGNS AND SYMPTOMS:
Duchenne Muscular Dystrophy
- Most common and most severe form of muscular dystrophy.
- Occurs mostly in males. Typically affects the legs first. Child may experience delay in walking, usually evident by age 3 and obvious by 5-6.
- May exhibit language delays.
- Early symptoms are clumsiness, toe walking, swayback, frequent falling, difficulty with stairs and getting up from floor, weakness in lower leg muscles resulting in difficulty running and jumping, waddling gait, and constipation.
- Always progressive, leading to need for leg braces, wheelchair dependency, contractures, obesity, respiratory complications (may progress to need for oral suctioning, tracheostomy and ventilator) and cardiac symptoms. Some may exhibit curvature of the spine (scoliosis).
- Calf and some other muscles enlarge due to fatty infiltration.
- Intellectual impairment is often present.
- Life expectancy age 20-30s, often from pneumonia, respiratory muscle weakness, or cardiac complications.

Other forms of muscular dystrophy
Becker's muscular dystrophy
- Signs and symptoms similar to Duchenne Muscular Dystrophy
- Milder form of muscular dystrophy
- Affects older boys and young men with onset around age 11, but may not occur until mid-20s or later. Most are able to walk through their teens and into adulthood.

MUSCULAR DYSTROPHY *(continued from previous page)*

Myotonicdystrophy (Steinert's Disease), Facioscapulohumeral muscular dystrophy (Landouzy-Dejerine dystrophy), Emery-Dreifuss muscular dystrophy, Limb-Girdle muscular dystrophy, Congenital muscular dystrophy, Oculopharyngeal muscular dystrophy, are other forms of muscular dystrophy. All vary in age onset, severity, rapidity of progression, associated intellectual impairment, and years of life.

MANAGEMENT/TREATMENT:

1. **Medication** - Corticosteroids, immunosuppressive drugs, anticonvulsants, skeletal muscle relaxants and antiarrhythmic drugs may be used improve muscle strength and delay progression for muscle weakness, delay the damage to dying muscle cells and to manage the muscle spasms, rigidity and affected cardiac muscles in certain types of muscular dystrophy.
2. **Physical therapy** keeps joints flexible and delays the progression of contractures.
3. **Assistive devices** such as braces, walkers, canes, and wheel chairs improve mobility and independence. Ventilators assist with oxygenation if muscles used to facilitate respiration become weakened.
4. **Surgery** may be necessary to relieve painful contractures. Curvatures of the spine, significant enough to compromise respiratory function may warrant surgical consideration. Consider homebound school services while recovering after surgery.
5. Cardiac muscle may become compromised; treated with medication or pacemaker.
6. When swallowing is affected, the family may opt for gastrostomy tube placement for nutrition.
7. As respiratory muscles weaken, respiratory support in the form of Nocturnal Nasal Intermittent Positive Pressure Ventilation (NNIPPV) or a ventilator may be used.
8. Altered cough secondary to neuromuscular weakness may require manual or mechanical cough assist.
9. May require oral suctioning to clear the airway.

FOLLOW-UP:

- Continually monitor for progress toward goals and watchful for signs and symptoms of complications.
- Update the Individualized Healthcare Plan (IHP) as necessary and update appropriate faculty and staff of changes in the care plan.
- Individualized Education Plan (IEP) or Section 504 plan for special services and accommodations, if needed.

MUSCULAR DYSTROPHY *(continued from previous page)*

POTENTIAL COMPLICATIONS:
- Breathing difficulties
- Obesity
- Contractures and spinal curvature
- Diminished fine motor skills
- Compromised skin integrity
- Urinary tract infections
- Constipation
- Respiratory infections
- Decline in independence with ADL's
- Swallowing difficulties
- Cardiac inefficiency
- Emotional/mental health issues secondary to condition itself, medications, or living with a chronic illness
- Sense of helplessness and hopelessness (depression)

Role of the School Nurse
- Child and family advocate
- To partner with the healthcare provider, parents/guardians and other members of the school health team to develop the Individualized Healthcare Plan (IHP)
- To assemble and lead the school's child care team. The team and their focus may include:

  School physician
  - Coordinate medical management plan with the student's healthcare provider, parent/guardian(s), and support services
  - Monitor immunization, influenza, and pneumonia status

  School nurse
  - Case management
  - Health education and health counseling
  - Staff development/in-service
  - Monitor respiratory status, early intervention can decrease severity of respiratory illness and prevent hospitalization
  - Monitor growth

MUSCULAR DYSTROPHY *(continued from previous page)*

Role of the School Nurse *(continued)*

Physical therapist
- o Assess range of motion and ambulation abilities
- o Develop a plan for both active and passive range of motion, stretching exercises, ambulation, transfer (to chair, toilet, positioning blocks/devices, etc.), and positioning needs

Occupational therapist
- o Assess activities of daily living skills, large motor skills, and fine motor skills
- o Develop a plan for work surfaces, note taking/adapted technology, dietary assistance (special utensils, lunch tray set-up, food served to meet mastication needs [bite size pieces], may need assistance with feeding or to be fed, feeding tube)

Speech/language therapist
- o Assess mastication/swallowing abilities and needs and coordinate plan with school food service personnel
- o Assess speaking abilities for students with tracheostomies/ventilators and develop a communication plan

School dietitian
- o Coordinate special dietary needs with occupational therapist and speech therapist
- o Coordinate with school physician to develop an appropriate nutritional plan for caloric intake, sodium intake/steroid therapy, vitamins and minerals, and antioxidants

School counselor/social worker
- o Assess mental health status
- o Plan for appropriate student, sibling, friends, and family supports

Director of transportation
- o Coordinate special transportation needs with physical therapist and occupational therapist

Education specialists
- o Develop appropriate educational plans and may include:
  - ✓ Special education
  - ✓ General education
  - ✓ Adapted physical education

MUSCULAR DYSTROPHY *(continued from previous page)*

NOTE: As the disease progresses the student may be followed by a palliative care team or hospice. Often these students wish to continue to attend school. Accommodations can be made to make the child comfortable and have optimal quality of life while at school. See **Do Not Attempt Resuscitation (DNAR)** for further information, if needed.

Resources

Education Matters: A Teacher's Guide to Duchenne Muscular Dystrophy. Downloadable from: http://www.parentprojectmd.org/site/DocServer/EdMatters-TeachersGuide.pdf

Learning and Behavior in Duchenne Muscular Dystrophy for Parents and Educators. Downloadable from: http://www.columbia.edu/cu/md/Learning_and_Behavior_Guide.pdf

Muscular Dystrophy Association: Research, information, support at http://mda.org

Parent Project Muscular Dystrophy: 1-800-714-5437

References

Centers for Disease Control. (2015). *Muscular dystrophy*. Retrieved from http://www.cdc.gov/ncbddd/musculardystrophy/

Mayo Clinic. (2014). *Muscular dystrophy*. Retrieved from http://www.mayoclinic.com/health/muscular-dystrophy/DS00200

Muscular Dystrophy Association (MDA). (2014). Duchenne muscular dystrophy: Medical management. Retrieved from http://www.mda.org/disease/duchenne-muscular-dystrophy/medical-management

National Institute of Neurological Disorders and Stroke. (2015). *NINDS muscular dystrophy information page*. Retrieved from http://www.ninds.nih.gov/disorders/md/md.htm

Selekman, J., Bochenek, J., & Lukens, M. (2013). Muscular dystrophy. In J. Selekman (Ed.), *School nursing: A comprehensive text* (2nd ed.) (pp. 751-755). Philadelphia, PA: F.A. Davis.

NOROVIRUS

DEFINITION/ETIOLOGY:
Norovirus is an acute highly contagious virus that causes acute inflammation of the stomach and intestines (gastroenteritis). It is the most common cause of acute gastroenteritis in the United States. It spreads easily through contact with an infected person, contaminated food or water or by touching contaminated surfaces.

SIGNS AND SYMPTOMS:
Symptoms typically begin 12 – 48 hours after exposure and may include:
- Diarrhea
- Vomiting
- Nausea
- Stomach pain/cramps
- Fatigue/malaise
- Low grade fever

MANAGEMENT/TREATMENT:
There is no treatment for norovirus. Treatment is support for symptoms. Norovirus symptoms in most people resolve without treatment in 1-3 days.
- Rehydrate with oral rehydration fluids, sport drinks and broths. Avoid liquids with a lot of sugar as this can make diarrhea worse.
- Infected persons should wash hands frequently to prevent spreading virus to others.
- Wash fruits and vegetables before eating them.
- Wash hands before preparing food.
- Clean contaminated surfaces with bleach based cleansers. Exclusion from school until symptoms are completely resolved (children should not go to daycare or school while they have diarrhea or vomiting)
- Norovirus can be found in the stool for at least 2 weeks after symptoms resolve.

FOLLOW-UP:
- Any outbreak of norovirus in the school should be reported to the local health department for surveillance purposes and for guidance in school procedure and student exclusion.
- Practice universal precautions when changing diapers or any contact with stool.

NOROVIRUS *(continued from previous page)*

POTENTIAL COMPLICATIONS:
Young children, older adults and those immunocompromised are at greater risk for dehydration, malnutrition and even death.

NOTES:
The way to prevent getting norovirus is to practice good hand washing in every situation. Norovirus spreads quickly and easily when people are in close proximity such as hotels, resorts, cruise ships, nursing homes, schools (especially with dormitories) and childcare cent

References

American Academy of Pediatrics, Committee on Infectious Diseases. (2015). Norovirus and other human calicivirus infections . In D.W. Kimberlin, M. T. Brady, M.A. Jackson, & S.S. Long (Eds.), *Red Book: 2015 report of the committee on infectious diseases* (30th ed.) (pp. 573-574). Elk Grove Village, IL: American Academy of Pediatrics.

Centers for Disease Control and Prevention (CDC). (2013). *Norovirus.* Retrieved from http://www.cdc.gov/norovirus/about/overview.html

Kids Health/Nemours. (2015). *A to Z: Norovirus*. Retrieved from https://secure02.kidshealth.org/parent/dictionary/n/az-norovirus.html

Mayo Clinic. (2014). *Norovirus Infection*. Retrieved from http://www.mayoclinic.org/diseases-conditions/norovirus/basics/definition/con-20029968

Michigan Department of Health and Human Services. (n.d.) *Norovirus fact sheet*. Retrieved from http://michigan.gov/documents/emergingdiseases/General_Noro_Fact_Sheet_173589_7.pdf

National Institute of Allergy and Infections. (2014). Norovirus overview. Retrieved from http://www.niaid.nih.gov/topics/norovirus/Pages/default.aspx

NOSEBLEED (Epistaxis)

DEFINITION/ETIOLOGY:
A nosebleed can be caused by trauma, scratching the nose, picking the nose; repeated nose blowing that irritates the mucous membranes. It may start with sudden temperature change, dry air, mucosal infection, inflammation associated with allergic rhinitis, or upper respiratory infections. Students with nosebleeds may also have a foreign body in the nose. Most nosebleeds come from blood vessels in the front of the nose.

SIGNS AND SYMPTOMS:
- Blood coming from the nose
- Complaint of tasting blood or swallowing blood

MANAGEMENT/TREATMENT:
1. Instruct person to breathe through their mouth. Reassure the young or anxious child that he can still breathe through the mouth.
2. Have the person sit down and lean forward. This minimizes the amount of blood swallowed that may cause nausea and/or hematemisis.
3. Assist the student to firmly pinch anterior nose (nostrils closed) below the bone continuously for 5 minutes (timed by clock).
4. If bleeding continues, hold nose closed an additional 10 minutes. If bleeding continues for more than 15 to 20 minutes, contact the parent/guardian to refer for medical care, e.g., vasoconstricting nose drops.
5. Additionally, a cold compress or ice applied to the bridge of the nose may help.
6. Seek medical help if the person is dizzy, light-headed, pale, has a rapid heart rate, or is taking anticoagulant or aspirin therapy (blood thinner).

FOLLOW UP:
- Restrict excessive physical exertion remainder of that day.
- For the rest of the day, avoid blowing, sniffing, probing/picking the nose and dislodging the clot.
- Inquire about any clotting abnormalities and use of aspirin or anticoagulants.
- Repeated nosebleeds: refer to healthcare provider.
- Assess if family history of bleeding disorders.
- Assess if there is possible substance abuse by nasal snorting.
- Assess if history of other types of frequent or excess bleeding, for example with menstruation.
- Assess if history of blood in stool (black or tarry appearance).

NOSEBLEED (Epistaxis) *(continued from previous page)*

POTENTIAL COMPLICTIONS:
- Choking on blood
- Vomiting from swallowed blood
- Anemia with frequent nosebleeds

NOTE:
- Young children have more nosebleeds because the blood vessels are more fragile.
- Most nosebleeds that occur in children are not serious and usually stop within a few minutes.
- High blood pressure does not cause nosebleeds, but it may increase the severity.
- Frequent heavy, hard to stop nose bleeds may be due to an absence of clotting factors, possible Von Willebrand's disease.

References

Friedman, N.R., Scholed, M.A., & Yoon, P.J. (2014). Ear, nose, & throat. In W.W. Hay, R.R. Deterding, M.J. Levin, & M.J. Abzug (Eds.), Current diagnosis and treatment pediatrics (22nd edition)(pp. 521-522). New York, NY: McGraw Hill Education.

Hockenberry, M., Baker, R., & Mondozzi, M. (2013). The child with hematalogic or immunologic dysfunction. In M. Hockenberry (Ed.), Wong's essentials of pediatric nursing (9th ed.) (p. 888). St. Louis, MO: Mosby Elsevier.

Mayo Clinic. (2014). Nosebleeds: First aid. Retrieved from http://www.mayoclinic.org/first-aid/first-aid-nosebleeds/basics/art-20056683

Medline Plus, U.S. National Library of Medicine. (2013). Nosebleeds. Retrieved from http://www.nlm.nih.gov/medlineplus/ency/article/003106.htm

Merck Manual. Epistaxis. (2012). Retrieved from http://www.merckmanuals.com/professional/ear_nose_and_throat_disorders/approach_to_the_patient_with_nasal_and_pharyngeal_symptoms/epistaxis.html?qt=nosebleeds&alt=sh

PANDAS /PANS

DEFINITION/ETIOLOGY:

PANDAS/PANS are acronyms that refer to a Pediatric Autoimmune Neuropsychiatric Disorders Associated with Strep A (PANDAS) and Pediatric Acute-Onset Neuropsychiatric Syndrome (PANS) which are neuro-psychiatric disorders triggered by an underlying autoimmune response <u>not associated with Strep infections.</u>

In PANDAS the student generally has a dramatic and quite sudden onset of symptoms after a strep infection. In PANS, sudden symptoms may be caused by other bacterial or viral infections. PANDAS/PANS are rare conditions. The symptoms generally affect students between the ages 4-10.

SIGNS AND SYMPTOMS: (Sudden, Dramatic and Often Episodic)
- Motor or vocal tics
- Obsessions and/or compulsions (obsessive-compulsive disorder[OCD] like behaviors)
- Heightened anxiety
- Increased urinary frequency
- Impulsivity, inattention, poor concentration
- Handwriting changes and deterioration in school performance
- Sensory issues

There is no test to diagnose for PANDAS or PANS. It is a clinical diagnosis based on the following diagnostic criteria:
- A pediatric onset of symptoms
- The presence of obsessive-compulsive disorder and/or tics
- An episodic course of symptom severity
- A positive throat culture for strep A or a history of Strep A or Scarlet Fever for PANDAS (Anti-streptococcal antibody titers may be drawn to determine evidence of a previous strep infection)
- An association with neurological abnormalities

MANAGEMENT/TREATMENT:

The best treatment for PANDAS is to eradicate the strep infection with a single course of antibiotics with the hope that the PANDAS symptoms will subside. Cognitive behavioral therapy and the use of medications to treat OCD and TIC disorders may be used. In addition, anti-inflammatory medication as well as steroids or intravenous immunoglobulin (IVIG) may be helpful.

PANDAS /PANS *(continued from previous page)*

FOLLOW-UP:
- School nurses can be essential in assisting families of children with sudden behavioral changes in the identification of a possible PANDAS/PANS case. The nurse may also be the first one to link the behavior to a recent strep case.
- Educating school staff on PANDAS/PANS is an important role of the school nurse.
- Positive behavioral classroom supports should be put in place.
- Academic accommodations such as extended time and frequent breaks may be needed.

POTENTIAL COMPLICATIONS:
Exacerbations and times of remissions may occur, the longer the student remains untreated the greater the effects of the symptoms.

References

National Institute of Mental Health. (n.d.). *Information about PANDAS*. Retrieved from http://www.nimh.nih.gov/labs-at-nimh/research-areas/clinics-and-labs/pdnb/web.shtml

Pandas Network.org. (2015). *PANS/PANDAS fact sheet*. Retrieved from http://pandasnetwork.org/wp-content/uploads/2015/09/2015-PNETWORK-fact.pdf

Perlstein, D. (2015). *What causes PANDAS?* Retrieved from http://www.medicinenet.com/pandas/page2.htm#what_are_symptoms_and_signs_of_pandas

PERTUSSIS (WHOOPING COUGH)

DEFINITION/ETIOLOGY:

Pertussis is a highly contagious bacterial infection caused by *Bordetella pertussis*. Pertussis is a vaccine preventable disease (VPD) that is increasing in incidence. Incubation period for *Bordetella pertussis* is from 4-21 days, usually 7-10 days and is spread from person to person through airborne droplets in close contact (coughing and sneezing).

SIGNS AND SYMPTOMS:
- Pertussis is divided in 3 stages:
  1. The catarrhal stage lasts 1-2 weeks, may not be recognized or non-specific symptoms such as rhinorrhea (runny nose), sneezing, mild cough, slight sore throat, sinus congestion, and low-grade fever. Pertussis is most contagious from catarrhal stage until 2 weeks after onset of cough, without appropriate treatment.

  2. The paroxysmal stage lasts 2-4 weeks or longer, characterized by paroxysmal cough or whooping cough. Vomiting during or after coughing fits. Exhaustion.

  3. The convalescent stage lasts 1-2 weeks as cough becomes milder and less often. Cough can persist for several months.

- The duration of classic pertussis is 6-10 weeks or longer.

MANAGEMENT/TREATMENT:
1. Refer to healthcare provider for diagnosis and appropriate treatment. Diagnosis is made on history and possible nasopharyngeal culture.
   a. Treatment includes antibiotics. They are most effective in shortening the length of infection when given in the catarrhal stage. After the catarrhal stage, antibiotics cannot shorten the duration of the illness, but reduce the amount of time an infected person can transmit the bacteria to others.

2. Implement state health regulations/ school policy for control measures.
   a. Students and staff with pertussis should be excluded from school and may return 5 days after they begin appropriate therapy.
   b. Those who do not receive antimicrobial therapy should be excluded from school for 21 days after onset of symptoms (coughing).
   c. School-wide or classroom chemoprophylaxis generally has *not* been recommended because of the delay in recognition of outbreak.

PERTUSSIS (WHOOPING COUGH) *(continued from previous page)*

MANAGEMENT/TREATMENT (continued)

    d. People who have been in contact with an infected person should be monitored closely for respiratory tract symptoms for 21 days after last contact.

    e. Surveillance for community health reporting.

For household contacts: Immunization recommended according to schedule for adolescents 11 – 18, adults 19 and older and children 7-10 who are not fully vaccinated against pertussis (fewer than 4 doses).

3. A course of antibiotics may be recommended to be administered to close contacts with three weeks of exposure.

4. Cough medicine will <u>not</u> likely help and should not be given unless instructed by the healthcare provider.

5. A cool mist vaporizer may help to loosen secretions.

6. Encourage good handwashing.

7. Encourage fluids.

FOLLOW-UP:
Monitor nutritional status. To avoid vomiting after coughing, eat smaller, more frequent meals instead of larger meals.

POTENTIAL COMPLICATIONS:
- Pertussis causes disease in every age group, but has the most significant impact on un-immunized young children, particularly infants.
- Major complications are most common among infants and young children. Complications include bacterial pneumonia, seizure, encephalopathy, and death. Most deaths occur among unvaccinated children or children too young to be vaccinated.
- Other complications may include difficulty sleeping, urinary incontinence, syncope, pneumonia and rib fracture during violent coughing.
- Previously immunized adolescents can become susceptible when immunity wanes, but they can receive a booster (Tdap) if they previously received only the tetanus-diphtheria toxoids (Td) booster at age 11-13 years. Secondary schools, in most states, require a Tdap, for this age group.

PERTUSSIS (WHOOPING COUGH) *(continued from previous page)*

References

American Academy of Pediatrics. (2015). Whooping cough (pertussis). Retrieved from http://kidshealth.org/parent/infections/lung/whooping_cough.html#

American Academy of Pediatrics. (2013). Whooping cough (pertussis). In S. Aronson, & T. Shope (Eds.), *Managing infectious diseases in child care and schools (2nd ed.)* (pp. 173-174). Elk Grove Village, IL: American Academy of Pediatrics.

American Academy of Pediatrics, Committee on Infectious Diseases. (2015). Pertussis. In D.W. Kimberlin, M. T. Brady, M.A. Jackson, & S.S. Long (Eds.), *Red Book: 2015 report of the committee on infectious diseases* (30th ed.) (pp. 608-621). Elk Grove Village, IL: American Academy of Pediatrics.

Centers for Disease Control and Prevention. (2015a). *Pertussis outbreak trends*. Retrieved from http://www.cdc.gov/pertussis/outbreaks/trends.html

Centers for Disease Control and Prevention. (2015b). Recommended *immunization schedules for persons aged 0 through 18 years — United States, 2013*. Retrieved from http://www.cdc.gov/vaccines/schedules/downloads/child/0-18yrs-schedule.pdf

Center for Disease Control and Prevention (CDC). (2015c). *Pertussis*. In J. Hamborsky, A. Kroger, & S. Wolfe (Eds.), *Epidemiology and prevention of vaccine-preventable diseases, the pink book: Course textbook (13th ed.)*. Washington D.C. Public Health Foundation. Retrieved from http://www.cdc.gov/vaccines/pubs/pinkbook/pert.html

Immunization Action Coalition. (2015). *State Information*. Retrieved from http://www.immunize.org/laws/tdap.asp

Merck Manual. (2014). *Pertussis*. Retrieved from http://www.merckmanuals.com/professional/infectious_diseases/gram-negative_bacilli/pertussis.html?qt=pertussis&alt=sh

PINWORM INFECTION (Enterobiasis)

DEFINITION/ETIOLOGY:
Pinworms are the most common of all roundworm infections. They are small thread-like roundworms measuring about 1/4 to 1/2 inch in length. The ova of the parasite transfers from the perineal area to fomites, are picked up by a new host, transferred to the mouth, and swallowed. The lifecycle of the pinworm - egg, larva (immature stage), and mature worm takes place inside the colon and requires 3-6 weeks to complete. Eggs can be carried to the mouth by contaminated food, drink, or fingers and are capable of clinging to bedding, clothes, toys, doorknobs, furniture, or faucets for up to two weeks. Pinworms are found more commonly among people living in crowded conditions, day-care facilities, and schools.

SIGNS AND SYMPTOMS:
- More common in children
- Many people have no symptoms at all
- Itching around the anus and vagina
- Intense itching that may interfere with sleep
- Irritability from lack of sleep
- Intermittent abdominal pain and nausea

MANAGEMENT/TREATMENT:
- Eggs may be collected with a strip of sticky, clear tape and identified by a healthcare provider.
- Mild infections may not need medication.
- If medication (Mebendazole, Pyrantel Pamaoate, or Albendazole (Albenza) is indicated, the entire household should be treated.
- Medication works by keeping the worm from absorbing sugar (glucose) causing the death of the worm or by causing sudden contraction, followed by paralysis, of the parasite, causing the worm to "lose its grip" on the intestinal.
- Children that are infected are likely to become re-infected outside the home; therefore, major efforts to eliminate eggs from the home are of little help.
- Antipruritic creams and ointments may be recommended to relieve anal itching.

FOLLOW UP:
Monitor for sleepiness and weight loss.
Clean classroom as indicated - pinworm eggs can survive for two to three weeks on surfaces.

PINWORM INFECTION (Enterobiasis) *(continued from previous page)*

POTENTIAL COMPLICATIONS:
- Infection of the female genitalia and reproductive system
- Abdominal pain
- Weight loss

NOTES:
Prevention
- Bathe after waking.
- Wash nightclothes and bedding often.
- Frequent hand washing, especially after using the bathroom or changing diapers, and before eating.
- Change underclothes each day.
- Avoid nail biting.
- Avoid scratching anal area.

References

Centers for Disease Control and Prevention. (2013). Parasites- enterobaisis (also known as pinworm infection). (2013). Retrieved from http://www.cdc.gov/parasites/pinworm/treatment.html

Drug,com. (2015). Pyrantel pamoate. Retrieved from http://www.drugs.com/cdi/pyrantel-pamoate.html

Mayo Clinic. Pinworm infection. (2015). Retrieved from http://www.mayoclinic.com/health/pinworm/DS00687

Mayo Clinic. (2015). Mebendazole (oral route). Retrieved from http://www.mayoclinic.org/drugs-supplements/mebendazole-oral-route/before-using/drg-20064631

Medline Plus. U.S. National Library of Medicine. (2013). Pinworms. Retrieved from http://www.nlm.nih.gov/medlineplus/pinworms.html

Merck Manual. Pinworm infestation. (2013). Retrieved from http://www.merckmanuals.com/professional/infectious_diseases/nematodes_roundworms/pinworm_infestation.html?qt=pinworms&alt=sh

National Institute of Allergy & Infectious Diseases, National Institute of Health. (2014). Pinworm infection. Retrieved from http://www.niaid.nih.gov/topics/pinworm/Pages/default.aspx

PNEUMONIA

DEFINITION/ETIOLOGY:

Pneumonia is an infection of the lungs and may occur in one or both lungs. When pneumonia occurs, the air sac of one or both lungs become inflamed. During the pneumonia infection, the air sacs may fill with fluid or pus, causing cough with phlegm or pus, fever, chills and difficulty breathing. Pneumonia may be caused by bacteria, viruses, and fungi.

Pneumonia can range from mild to life-threatening and is most serious for infants and young children, as well as adults older than 65 years of age. Also, people with underlying health problems or weakened immune systems are at increased risk of pneumonia complications. Antibiotics and antiviral medications are used to treat many common forms of pneumonia.

CAUSES OF PNEUMONIA

Pneumonia may be caused by many small germs. There are five main causes of pneumonia:

- Bacteria
- Viruses
- Mycoplasmas
- Fungi and other infectious agents
- Various chemicals

TYPES OF PNEUMONIA

Pneumonia is classified according to the location where the infection is acquired. Below are four types of pneumonia based on the specific acquired location and the specific organisms associated with the cause.

- Community-acquired pneumonia – most common type and may be caused by the following:
  - Bacteria: Streptococcus pneumoniae
  - Bacteria-like organisms: Mycoplasma pneumoniae produces milder signs and symptoms. The term "Walking Pneumonia" may result from Mycoplasma pneumoniae.
  - Viruses: Most common cause of pneumonia in children younger than two years of age. Usually mild and can become severe when caused by certain influenza viruses such as sudden acute respiratory syndrome (SARS).
  - Fungi: Common in people with chronic health problems or weakened immune systems, as well as those who have inhaled large doses of organisms. The fungi that cause it can be found in soil or bird droppings.

283

PNEUMONIA *(continued from previous page)*

TYPES OF PNEUMONIA *(continued)*
- Hospital-acquired pneumonia –bacterial infection; occurs within 48 hours after being hospitalized for another condition.
  - Bacteria causing this type of pneumonia may be resistant to antibiotics.
  - People who are assisted by a ventilator for breathing are at higher risk for hospital-acquired pneumonia.
- Healthcare-acquired pneumonia – bacterial infection; general occurs among people when living in a long-term care facility or if treated by an outpatient center/clinic.
  - Bacteria may be resistant to antibiotic treatment.
- Aspiration pneumonia - occurs when food, drink, vomit, or saliva are inhaled into the lungs.
  - May occur if the normal gag reflex is disturbed by brain injury, swallowing problems, or excessive use of drugs and alcohol

SIGNS AND SYMPTOMS OF PNEUMONIA:
- Fever and shaking chills
- Sweating and clammy skin
- Lower than normal temperature in people with weakened immune system or poor health
- Cough - which may produce phlegm
- Chest pain with deep breathing and coughing
- Shortness of breath
- Wheezing (may be more common in viral pneumonia)
- Muscle aches and muscle fatigue
- Nausea, vomiting, and diarrhea
- Headache

POTENTIAL RISKS AND COMPLICATIONS:
- Chronic health conditions (asthma, - COPD, heart disease, etc.)
- Tuberculosis
- Chronic diseases such as asthma, chronic obstructive pulmonary disease (COPD), and heart disease
- Weak, compromised or suppressed immune system
- Smoking because it damages the body's natural defenses against bacteria and viruses causing pneumonia
- Using ventilator assistance for breathing while hospitalized

PNEUMONIA *(continued from previous page)*

Complications:
- Bacteremia – bacteria in the bloodstream can cause organ failure.
- Abscess in the lung due to formation of pus in the lung cavity.
- Pleural effusion – fluid accumulation around the lungs; chest tube may be necessary to drain infected fluid.
- Difficulty breathing.

MANAGEMENT/TREATMENT:
General Information
- Hospitalization is recommended for severe cases of pneumonia.
- Immunizations provide protection against pneumonia, e.g. pertussis, influenza and pneumococcal vaccines.
- Adequate nutrition helps to improve the natural immunity of children.
- Promote good hygiene practices, e.g. handwashing.

Bacterial Pneumonia
- Treated with oral antibiotics.
- Proper diet.
- Oxygen as needed.
- Other medications for chest pain and coughing as needed.

Viral Pneumonia
- May be treated with antiviral medication.
- Usually improves in one to three weeks.

Mycoplasma Pneumonia
- May be weak for extended period of time.
- Adequate rest is important for progression toward full recovery.

References

American Lung Association. (2015). *Pneumonia*. Retrieved from http://www.lung.org/lung-disease/pneumonia/

Centers of Disease Control and Prevention (CDC). (2014). *Pneumonia can be prevented – Vaccines can help*. Retrieved from http://www.cdc.gov/Features/Pneumonia/

Mayo Clinic. (2015). *Pneumonia*. Retrieved from http://www.mayoclinic.org/diseases-conditions/pneumonia/basics/definition/con-20020032

World Health Organization (WHO). (2014). *Pneumonia factsheet*. Retrieved from http://www.who.int/mediacentre/factsheets/fs331/en/

POISON IVY/OAK (Contact Dermatitis)

DEFINITION/ETIOLOGY:

Poison ivy/oak is a skin reaction (contact dermatitis) due to the allergen, urushiol, which is found in all parts (stem, flowers, berries, and roots) of the poison ivy, oak and sumac (rhus) plant. Poison ivy/oak grows as a low-lying shrub and a short or high trailing vine. Leaves appear in groups of three with white berries and greenish flowers. A rash only occurs in people sensitive to these plants when the skin directly touches the urushiol from the plant, contaminated objects or smoke from burning plants. A reaction is most commonly seen on the hands, forearms, and face.

SIGNS AND SYMPTOMS:

Reaction typically begins 12-48 hours after exposure but can also take as long as a week.

- Red, itchy rash
  - Small papules and vesicles
  - Rash may have a linear appearance were the plant brushes against the skin
- May have large blisters and generalized weeping of skin
- Localized swelling
- Dryness, crusting and gradual shedding of crusts and scabs is a sign of healing which may take 2-3 weeks

MANAGEMENT/TREATMENT:

1. Wash skin and fingernails thoroughly with a degreasing detergent (dishwashing soap) and cool water within 10 minutes of exposure or with a commercial product (e.g., Tecnu® or Zanfel® cleansers) as soon as possible to prevent or decrease a reaction.
2. Continue to rinse the area frequently to prevent wash solutions from drying on the skin and the spread of urushiol.
3. To relieve itching, apply cool packs (every 15-20 minutes, 3-4 times daily), and/or a warm baking soda or colloidal oatmeal bath. Avoid hot water that will exacerbate the symptoms.
4. Plain calamine lotion may be applied to dry lesions. (Follow OTC medication guidelines.)
5. Topical corticosteroid cream may be used to reduce inflammation.
6. Healthcare provider may prescribe oral steroids for extensive cases.
7. Oral antihistamines are usually not helpful for itch, but hydroxyzine (Atarax®) may be prescribed.
8. Applying a loose dressing may help discourage scratching.
9. Refer to healthcare provider if itching is distracting child from attention to tasks, rash is extensive, or involving eye, face, genitals or mucous membranes.

POISON IVY/OAK (Contact Dermatitis) *(continued from previous page)*

FOLLOW UP:
- Observe for infection and treat as needed.
- Wear disposable rubber gloves to:
  - Promptly wash contaminated clothing such shoes, shoelaces, socks, pants, and shirts in detergent and hot water.
  - Clean additional contaminated objects used outdoors such as garden tools and jewelry with hot water and detergent.
- Educate regarding how to identify poison ivy/oak and to avoid re-exposure.
- If on school or public play property, report location for safe removal (without burning).

POTENTIAL COMPLICATIONS:
Scratching the rash with dirty fingernails can cause a secondary infection.

NOTES:
- Do not exclude from school; educate staff on transmission of urushiol.
- Contents of blisters and weepy skin CANNOT cause rash in another individual or even in another location on patient.
- Inhaling smoke from burning poison ivy/oak plants may cause a severe respiratory reaction. A reaction if burning particles land on your skin.
- To prevent a potential exposure, an over the counter barrier cream containing bantoquatam may be used. However, avoidance is the best protection.
- Urushiol can remain active for five (5) years. If contaminated objects are not cleaned, contact with them at a later date may cause a reaction.
- Consider pet fur as possible source of exposure.

POISON IVY/OAK (Contact Dermatitis) *(continued from previous page)*

References

American Academy of Dermatology. (n.d.). *Poison ivy, oak, and sumac.* Retrieved from http://www.aad.org/dermatology-a-to-z/diseases- http://www.aad.org/dermatology-a-to-z/diseases-and-treatments/m---p/poison-ivy and-treatments/m---p/poison-ivy

Mayo Clinic. (2015). *Poison ivy rash.* Retrieved from http://www.mayoclinic.com/health/poison-ivy/DS00774

Morelli, J.G., & Prok, L.D. (2014). Skin. In W.W. Hay, R.R. Deterding, M.J. Levin, & M.J. Abzug (Eds.), *Current diagnosis and treatment pediatrics* (22nd edition)(p. 441). New York, NY: McGraw Hill Education.

Renzi, L. & Clark Graham, M. (2013). Skin disorders. In J. Selekman (Ed.), *School nursing: A comprehensive text* (2nd ed.) (p. 693). Philadelphia, PA: F.A. Davis.

National Institute for Occupational Safety & Health, Centers for Disease Control and Prevention. (2014). NIOSH *fast facts: Protecting yourself from poisonous plants* (Publication No. 2010-118). Retrieved from http://www.cdc.gov/niosh/docs/2010-118/

Vernon, P., Brady, M., & Starr, N.B. (2013). Dermatologic diseases. In C. Burns, M. Brady, A. Dunn, N.B. Starr, C. Blosser, L. Garzon (Eds.), *Pediatric primary care* (5th ed.) (pp. 974-975). Philadelphia, PA: Saunders Elsevier.

Hockenberry, M., Baker, R., & Mondozzi, M. (2013). The child with integumentary dysfunction. In M. Hockenberry (Ed.), *Wong's essentials of pediatric nursing* (9th ed.) (p. 1022). St. Louis, MO: Mosby Elsevier.

PUBERTAL GROWTH AND DEVELOPMENT

DEFINITION/ETIOLOGY:
Puberty is a sequence of stages affecting the skeletal, muscular, reproductive, and almost every other body system. The normal age of onset of puberty is considered to be between 8 and 13 years in the general population of girls and between the ages of 9 and 14 years in the general population of boys. The sequences of body changes are visible and predictable. The onset of these changes is influenced by nutritional status, genetics and environmental factors and can vary greatly from person to person. Tanner staging, also recognized as the Sexual Maturity Rating (SMR) system, provides a means to document a child's progression through puberty Separate scales are used for breast size and shape (female), genitalia size and shape (male) and pubic hair development and distribution (both sexes). There are five stages of puberty for both males and females. A pubertal assessment includes a physical assessment in addition to any information provided by the child or parent.

STAGES OF NORMAL DEVELOPMENT:

A. **Females - Pubic hair development**
   Tanner Stage 1- pre-pubertal, pubic hair is absent
   Tanner Stage 2- fine sparse, straight hair along the vulva
   Tanner Stage 3-darker, coarser, and slightly curly that extends over the mid pubis
   Tanner Stage 4-adult type hair that covers the eternal genitalia but does not extend to the thighs
   Tanner Stage 5-adult type hair that extends to the medial thighs

B. **Females - Breast Development**
   Tanner Stage 1- flat appearance with only the papilla (nipple) raised
   Tanner Stage 2- a breast "bud" under the enlarging areola
   Tanner Stage 3- further enlargement of the breast tissue beyond the margins of the areola
   Tanner Stage 4- formation of a secondary mound of the widening and darkening areola above the breast tissue (considered sexual maturity)
   Tanner Stage 5- recession of the areola to the same level of skin overlying breast tissue and projection of the papilla beyond the areola and breast (some normal adult women only reach stage 5 in pregnancy)

PUBERTAL GROWTH AND DEVELOPMENT *(continued from previous page)*

C. **Males - Pubic Hair Development**
Tanner Stage 1- pre-pubertal pubic hair is absent
Tanner Stage 2-fine sparse straight hair at the base of the penis
Tanner Stage 3-darker, coarser, slightly curly hair over the mid pubis
Tanner Stage 4- thicker, more curled adult like hair but covers eternal genitalia but not thighs
Tanner Stage 5-adult like hair that extends to the medial thigh

D. **Males – Genitalia**
Tanner Stage 1 – pre-pubertal, testes, scrotum and penis are the same as early childhood
Tanner Stage 2 – enlargement of testes and scrotum but no enlargement of the penis
Tanner Stage 3 – continued enlargement of the testes and scrotum along with penile growth
Tanner Stage 4 – continued growth of testes, scrotum and penis, with enlargement of the glans
Tanner Stage 5 – mature genitalia

NOTES:

FEMALES
- Breast development in non-Hispanic African American and Mexican American girls is considered normal during the seventh year (about 15% experience thelarche or breast Stage 2 by 8 years of age).
- The pubertal growth spurt in girls begins at breast and pubic hair Stage 2. Approximately, 99% of girl's growth is complete at a bone age of 15 years. Girls experience a pubertal growth spurt approximately one year after the onset of breast development.
- Menstruation usually starts about 18 months to two years after the onset of puberty. Menarche occurs at an average age of 12.6 years in white girls, 12.1 years in African American girls of normal weight and Mexican girls are intermediate.
- Obesity advances the onset of puberty in girls. Excess adiposity contributes to the trend of an earlier age of puberty onset in girls by an average of about 0.5 years.

PUBERTAL GROWTH AND DEVELOPMENT *(continued from previous page)*

FEMALES *(continued)*
- Asymmetric breast development is a normal variation in pubertal progression.
- About 50% of menstrual cycles are anovulatory or have attenuated ovulation during the first two years after menarche.
- Bone health is very important for girls entering puberty and has a great effect for later in life bone health.

MALES
- The pubertal growth spurt for boys begins an average of two years later than girls, generally by age 15. Linear growth accelerates beginning at genital and pubic hair Stage 2. Growth in boys is approximately 99% complete at a bone age of 17 years.
- Testicular enlargement is the first clinically significant pubertal event in boys.
- Currently, there is a debate about the trend and effect of obesity in boys.
- Approximately one half to one third of boys develop gynecomastia (visible or palpable development of breast tissue in males) during mid- puberty that may last 12 to 18 months.
- Generally, with pubertal maturation there are also changes in cognition and social development.
- Boys with chronic illnesses such as inflammatory bowel disease, sickle cell disease or cystic fibrosis may mature later.
- Boys can add 13-14 inches and forty pounds in 3-4 years.
- Voice changes, wet dreams, involuntary erections, breast enlargement and having one testicle lower than the other are all part of the normal growth process.

PUBERTAL GROWTH AND DEVELOPMENT *(continued from previous page)*

POTENTIAL COMPLICATIONS:

- The absence of menses after a female has achieved breast development to Stage 4 and has completed a growth spurt may be a cause for concern and indicates a referral to a healthcare provider.
- The onset of vaginal bleeding without a growth spurt or breast development may be a cause for concern and indicates a referral to a healthcare provider.
- Breast development in a boy before puberty is abnormal.
- Delayed puberty is defined as a lack of breast development by age 13 years in girls and a lack of pubertal testicular development (genital Stage 2) by age 14 in boys. If puberty does not begin by age 18 in boys, it is pathologic.
- Girls are vulnerable to the reproductive effects of undernutrition and stress. Decreased body fat is a major cause of pubertal delay in girls. It can be seen in girls who are very athletic or in girls with anorexia nervosa.
- Missing a menstrual cycle for 90 or more days or having an average cycle length less than 21 days is abnormal for a girl of any age. An average cycle length of more than 45 days by 2 years after menarche is a risk factor.
- Breast masses may present in about 3.2% of the population and may be caused by a variety of etiologies but malignancy is very rare.
- Abrupt testicular pain should be an immediate referral for evaluation of potential testicular torsion.
- Gynecomastia that is unresolved or resembles the breasts of a female in Stage 3-5 of development should be evaluated for a potential pathological condition.
- The physical and psychological changes of puberty add to the challenges of diabetes management. Throughout puberty, the response to insulin decreases in all children and declines 25% -30% in those with diabetes, causing insulin requirements to rise.

PUBERTAL GROWTH AND DEVELOPMENT *(continued from previous page)*

References

American Academy of Pediatrics. (2015). *Concerns boys have about puberty.* Retrieved from https://www.healthychildren.org/English/ages-stages/gradeschool/puberty/Pages/ Concerns-Boys-Have-About-Puberty.aspx

American Academy of Pediatrics. (2015). *Concerns girls have about puberty.* Retrieved from https://www.healthychildren.org/English/ages-stages/gradeschool/puberty/Pages/ Concerns-Girls-Have-About-Puberty.aspx

American Academy of Pediatrics. (2015). *Delayed puberty in boys: Information for parents.* Retrieved from https://www.healthychildren.org/English/ages-stages/gradeschool/puberty/Pages/Delayed-Puberty.aspx

American Academy of Pediatrics. (2015) *Delayed puberty in girls*: Information for parents. Retrieved from https://www.healthychildren.org/English/ages-stages/gradeschool/puberty/Pages/ Delayed-Puberty-in-Girls-Information-for-Parents.aspx

American Academy of Pediatrics. (2015). *Physical changes during puberty.* Retrieved from https://www.healthychildren.org/English/ages-stages/gradeschool/puberty/Pages/ Physical-Development-of-School-Age-Children.aspx

American Academy of Pediatrics. (2015). *Physical development: What's normal? What's not?* Healthychildren.org. Retrieved from https://www.healthychildren.org/English/ages-stages/gradeschool/puberty/Pages/ Physical-Development-Whats-Normal-Whats-Not.aspx

Bordini, B., & Rosenfield, R.L. (2011). Normal pubertal development: Part II: Clinical aspects of puberty. *Pediatrics in Review, 32* (7), 281-292. doi: 10.1542/pir.32-7-281

Bowden, V.R., & Greenberg, C. S. (2014). Principles and physiologic basis of growth and development. In V. R. Bowden, & C.S. Greenberg (eds.), *Children and their families: The continuum of care* (3rd edition) *(p. 103). Philadelphia, PA: Lippincott Williams and Wilkins.*

Fisher, M. M., & Alderman, E., Kreipe, R., & Rosenfeld, W. (Eds.). (2011). Growth and development. In *Textbook of adolescent health care* (pp. 23-31). Elk Grove Village, IL: American Academy of Pediatrics.

Trast, J. (2014). Diabetes and puberty: A glycemic challenge. *American Journal of Nursing, 111*(7), 26-35. doi: 10.1097/01.NAJ.0000451674.51200.6e

Rasmussen, A.R., Wohlfahrt-Veje, C., Tefre de Renzy-Martin, K., Hagen, C.P., Tinggaard, J., Mouritsen, A., Mieritz, M. G., & Main, K.M. (2015). Validity of self-assessment of pubertal maturation. *Pediatrics 135*(1), 86-93. doi: 10.1542/peds.*2014-0793*

PUBERTAL GROWTH AND DEVELOPMENT *(continued from previous page)*

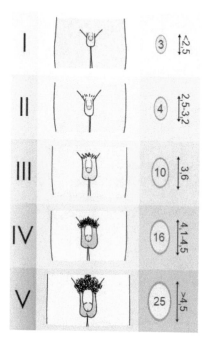

Illustration of Tanner scale for males.
Lawrence Neinstein, MD, Children's Hospital of LA

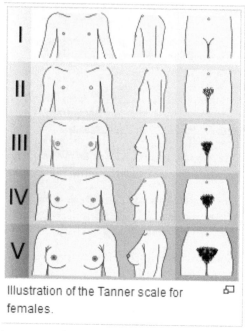

Illustration of the Tanner scale for females.

Lawrence Neinstein, MD, Children's Hospital of LA

PUNCTURE WOUNDS

DEFINITION/ETIOLOGY:
Small but deep hole produced by penetrating object. Sharp pointed objects such as nails, tacks, pencils, knife and teeth can cause puncture wounds. Most often occurs in hands and feet but can be any body surface area. Object may penetrate the skin and leave a hole or remain partially or completely in wound. Puncture wounds are typically deeper than lacerations or abrasions.

SIGNS AND SYMPTOMS:
If small object:
- Small hole at puncture site
- Little to no bleeding
- Potential for retained foreign body
- History of injury

If larger object:
- May be medical emergency
- May cause heavy bleeding and injury to areas beneath puncture site

> **Puncture wounds to the eye, neck, chest or abdomen are serious. Seek medical treatment. If necessary, call 911.**

MANAGEMENT/TREATMENT:
1. Use standard precautions.
2. Apply pressure with a clean cloth or bandage for several minutes to stop bleeding.
3. Once bleeding has stopped, wash around the wound with soap and water.
4. Irrigate the wound with water to remove debris.
5. If debris remains in wound after irrigation with water, do not probe or pull debris from a wound as it may splinter and leave pieces; refer to healthcare provider for follow-up care.
6. If embedded object in wound, minimize movement and leave object in place.
7. Do not try to clean a major wound as it may cause heavy bleeding.
8. Do not clean the wound with *Hydrogen peroxide*. *Hydrogen peroxide is not appropriate for fresh wounds; it damages tissues and interferes with healing.*
9. Apply antibiotic ointment and bandage per school district policy. Do not seal the hole with non-porous bandage.
10. Determine cause of puncture, e.g., nail, glass, wood, human or animal bite, etc.

PUNCTURE WOUNDS *(continued from previous page)*

MANAGEMENT/TREATMENT: *(continued)*

11. Seek medical treatment if puncture wound is caused by an animal bite. Contact animal control.
12. Determine date of last tetanus booster and refer to healthcare provider if booster is needed. Should have tetanus booster within 48 hours of injury,
13. Seek emergency medical services if wound is deep, bleeding heavily or a large object is embedded in the wound.

FOLLOW-UP:

- Monitor of signs of infection. Signs and symptoms of infection that require a visit to healthcare provider include:
  - o Early signs and symptoms of infection include: increased pain, redness around the edge of wound, swelling and tenderness
  - o Late signs and symptoms of infection include: fever, purulent drainage and lymphangitis (infection of the lymph vessel caused by a bacterial infection); look for red streak from infected area to armpit or groin

POTENTIAL COMPLICATIONS:

- Puncture wounds are hard to clean resulting in increased risk of infection.
- Wounds can often be deep with little bleeding so there is an increased risk of infection because germs are imbedded deeply and not washed out by the flow of blood.
- Tetanus is a danger with puncture wound because tetanus bacteria (*Clostridium tetani*) grow well in a deep wound with little oxygen.
- Puncture wounds obtained by stepping on a nail has increased risk of contracting a pseudomonas infection.
- Wounds resulting from an animal or human bite are at increased risk of becoming infected.

NOTES:

- Pencils are not made of lead but nontoxic graphite. Pencil lead is rarely embedded after puncture but more likely the "tattoo" from the graphite leaving a mark.

PUNCTURE WOUNDS *(continued from previous page)*

References

Boston Children's Hospital. (n.d.) *Treatments for puncture wounds in children.* Retrieved from
http://www.childrenshospital.org/conditions-and-treatments/conditions/p/puncture-wounds/treatments

John, R., & Chewey, L. (2013). *Common complaints.* In J. Selekman (Ed.), *School nursing: A comprehensive text* (2nd ed.) (pp.578-640). Philadelphia, PA: F. A. Davis.

Mayo Clinic. (2015*). Puncture wounds: First aid*. Retrieved from http://www.mayoclinic.com/health/first-aid-puncture-wounds/FA00014

MedlinePlus. U.S. National Library of Medicine. (2013). *Cuts and puncture wounds.* Retrieved from
http://www.nlm.nih.gov/medlineplus/ency/article/000043.htm

WebMD. (2014*). First aid & emergencies*. Retrieved from http://firstaid.webmd.com/tc/cuts-topic-overview

RASHES

Differential Diagnosis of Common Childhood Disease Associated with Rash

	Rubeola (measles)	Rubella (German measles)	Roseola	Scarlet Fever (scarlatina)	Fifth Disease	Varicella (chicken pox)
Etiology	Viral Herpes virus 6 Herpes Virus 7 Paramyxovirus	Viral Rubivirus	Viral, Human Herpes virus 6 & herpes 7	Streptococcus Bacteria	Human Parvovirus B19	Varicella zoster virus
Characteristics of Rash	Generalized dusky red blotchy maculopapular rash begins on day 3-7 and last 4-7 days	Large, light pink or light red flat blotches that often flow into one another Rash usually follows 5-10 days after infection occurs May resemble measles, scarlet fever, or fifth disease Approximately ½ of infections do not have a rash	Small flat pink spots or patches not usually itchy Last 2-3 days	Bright red rash, feels like sandpaper lasts 2-5 days Tongue may appear strawberry-like When rash fades, skin peels from tips of fingers and toes	Red, patchy facial rash ("slapped cheek") Cold-like symptoms may precede rash May be asymptomatic Not contagious before development of rash	Consists of maculopapular rash for a few hours, then fluid filled vesicles for 3-4 days drying and crusting over "New" vesicles can continue to appear for 4-7 Rash is itchy and scratching can produce skin abrasions and lead to secondary infection
Part of body rash first appears on	Behind the ears or on forehead/ face	Face	Chest and back	Neck, face, palms of hands and tips of fingers and toes	Face, cheeks and trunk	Face, abdomen and back
Spreads to	Arms, trunk, thighs, legs, and feet Small white spots (Koplik's spots) are inside mouth	Trunk, arms legs and then disappearing in the same order	Abdomen, neck and arms	Chest, back, and rest of body	May spread to rest of body in lace-like pattern	Rest of the body including the mouth, arms, genitals and scalp

RASHES *(continued from previous page)*

	Rubeola (measles)	Rubella (German measles)	Roseola	Scarlet Fever (scarlatina)	Fifth Disease	Varicella (chicken pox)
Progression and time intervals for diagnosis	Usually 8-12 days from exposure to onset of symptoms Average interval between appearance of rash after exposure is 7-14 days; range 7-18 days	Usually 16-18 days; range 14-23 days	Usually 10 days; range 5-15 days	1-3 days, can be up to 5 days	Variable, 4-20 days	Usually 14-16 days from exposure to rash, but may range from 10-21 days
Severity of illness	Usually severe	Usually mild	Mild , but moderate mild to high mild	Mild to moderate	Mild, resolves on its own	Severe in older adolescents and adults
Associated symptoms other than rash	Sudden onset of chills followed by sneezing, runny nose, conjunctivitis, photophobia, low-grade fever (102° F or lower), though Fever may exceed 40 C/104 F., dry cough, Koplik's spots, sore throat	Mild illness with low fever, mild rash, usually associated with enlargement of nodes on the back of the neck, headache, stuffy nose, inflamed red eye	Cough, runny nose, sore throat before sudden onset of high fever greater than 103 degrees which may last 3-5 days	Fever and sore throat/tonsillitis with tender, enlarged lymph nodes, abdominal pain, vomiting, headache	Fever, headache, runny nose Joint swelling and pain is more common is adults	Slight to moderate fever and itching
Complications	Otitis media, bronchitis, croup, pneumonia, seizures, encephalitis, low platelet count, pregnancy loss	Usually none. Women sometimes have arthritis in knees, fingers and wrist. Complications to an unborn can be severe	Usually none Can cause febrile seizures in children and is a risk for those with weak immune system	Rheumatic fever, carditis, painful joints, otitis media, sinus infection, kidney infection, meningitis, sepsis and pneumonia	Usually none Can cause Pneumonia Can be serious with weak immune system, anemia, cancer or pregnancy	Occasional arthritis encephalitis arthritis, recurrent breakthrough infections later on in life (shingles, Cerebellar ataxia)

RASHES *(continued from previous page)*

	Rubeola (measles)	Rubella (German measles)	Roseola	Scarlet Fever (scarlatina)	Fifth Disease	Varicella (chicken pox)
Period of Infectivity	Contagious in nose or throat 4 days before rash to 4 days after appearance of the rash Immuno-compromised children can be contagious for the duration of the illness	Maximal communicability is from 10 days before rash to 1-2 weeks days after onset of rash Children with congenital rubella syndrome may be infectious for up to 1 year. Highly communicable	Unknown Contagious even if no rash is present.	Infectious for 10-21 days if untreated or until 24 hours after start of antibiotic treatment	Most infectious before the onset of rash; not contagious after rash appears	From 1-2 days before rash appears, to when all lesions are completely crusted over Persons who are susceptible to varicella should be considered to be infectious from 10- 21 days after exposure NOTE: Persons with weakened immune systems may be communicable for longer periods
Additional information	Vaccine preventable More likely to contract measles if diet if deficient in Vitamin A Do not use aspirin	Vaccination is the key preventive measure	No specific control or preventive measures indicated	Curable with Penicillin. Control measures: Emphasize respiratory etiquette ("cover your cough") and frequent hand washing Common in 5-15 year olds	No Vaccine or medicine to available Proper hand hygiene encouraged	Vaccine is key preventive measure. Some children who have had the vaccine may still develop a mild case of chickenpox. Do not use aspirin or ibuprofen to treat symptoms Most cases are < 10 years old

RASHES *(continued from previous page)*

NOTES:

Infection control measures should be considered in regards to the anticipated contact to prevent the spread of communicable diseases. In general, children may be excluded from school for medical reasons related to communicable diseases or due to program or staffing requirements.

Follow local health department or school policy in regards to exclusion from school. In general, exclusion should be considered based on the following criteria:

- If children are not able to fully participate in the program,
- If elevated temperature,
- When the level of care during and illness is not able to be met without jeopardizing the safety of other children, or
- When the risk or spread of disease to other children cannot be avoided with the appropriate environmental or individual management.

NOTE: Vaccine preventable rashes (Rubeola, rubella, varicella) - If an outbreak occurs at school – unvaccinated students and staff must be excluded from school/work per health department guidelines.

RASHES *(continued from previous page)*

References

Indiana Department of Health, Epidemiology Resource Center. (2015). *Communicable disease reference guide for schools: 2012 edition.* Retrieved from http://www.state.in.us/isdh/23291.htm

Mayo Clinic. (2014). *Measles.* Retrieved from http://www.mayoclinic.com/health/measles/DS00331/DSECTION=complications

Mayo Clinic. (2015). *Rubella.* Retrieved from http://www.mayoclinic.com/health/rubella/DS00332/DSECTION

Mayo Clinic. (2015). *Roseola.* Retrieved from http://www.mayoclinic.com/health/roseola/DS00452/DSECTION=complications.

Mayo Clinic. (2011). *Scarlet fever.* Retrieved from http://www.mayoclinic.com/health/scarlet-ever/DS00917/DSECTION=complications.

Medline Plus. (2013). *Fifth Disease.* Retrieved from https://www.nlm.nih.gov/medlineplus/fifthdisease.html

Medline Plus. (2015). *Scarlet fever.* Retrieved from https://www.nlm.nih.gov/medlineplus/ency/article/000974.htm

Medline Plus. U.S. National Library of Medicine. (2013). *Chicken pox.* Retrieved from http://www.nlm.nih.gov/medlineplus/ency/article/001592.htm

Medline Plus. U.S. National Library of Medicine. (2013). *Roseola.* Retrieved from http://www.nlm.nih.gov/medlineplus/ency/article/000968.htm

Medline Plus. (2015). *Acute cerebellar ataxia.* Retrieved from https://www.nlm.nih.gov/medlineplus/ency/article/001592.htm

RINGWORM – TINEA

DEFINITION/ETIOLOGY:
Ringworm is caused by a fungus which can affect the skin, nails and hair.

Tinea corporis:	Ringworm of the body
Tinea capitis:	Ringworm of the scalp
Tinea cruris:	Ringworm of the groin area (also called jock itch)
Tinea pedis:	Ringworm of the feet (also called athlete's foot)
Onychomycosis:	Ringworm of the nails
Tinea faciei:	Ringworm of the face

Ringworm on the skin of a child is considered infectious as long as the fungus stays present in the skin lesion. Ringworm can be spread as long as lesions are present and viable fungus persists on contaminated materials and surfaces. The fungus is considered eradicated when the lesion begins to shrink. The fungi that cause ringworm thrive in warm, moist environments. Pets can be carriers of the fungus. Cats are an especially common carrier.

SIGNS AND SYMPTOMS:
Tinea pedis: Maceration and fissuring, scaly lesions, between toes and on plantar surface of foot. Itchy, vesiculo-papular (blisters or tiny pimples) or scaly lesions on sides of the feet. Lesions may become infected due to scratching. It is most commonly seen in adolescents, especially adolescent males.

Tinea cruris: Discolored areas (sharply demarcated scaling patches, may be pruritic, and usually itchy) between upper thighs extending onto groin buttocks and may involve scrotum in males. Also referred to as "jock itch". Frequently involve males and especially obese males. It is rarely seen in females.

Tinea corporis: Small (1-3 cm) red bump or papule on the body or face that spreads outward so that each affected area takes on the appearance of a red, scaly outer ring with a clear central area. The lesions are usually unilateral, frequently itchy and can become infected if scratched. There may be single or multiple lesions. Tinea corporis is not uncommon in student wrestlers and more often seen in warm climates.

RINGWORM – TINEA *(continued from previous page)*

SIGNS AND SYMPTOMS *(continued)*

<u>Tinea capitis</u>: In early stages, asymptomatic, but the scalp or back of the neck may itch. A tender, boggy lesion called a kerion may form which is from a hypersensitivity reaction to the fungus. A flaky scalp that resembles dandruff may be present. Round, oval or confluent patches of alopecia on be present on the scalp. Patches may be a small as 1-2 cm up to 10 cm. with hairs broken off in the center of the patch. Lesion will generally appear as an itchy, bald patch of scaly skin. This form of ringworm is most common in children.

<u>Onychomycosis:</u> thick and yellowed nails (rare in children).

<u>Tina faciei</u>: Presents as a rash that the face, the ears, or both with borders that may be indistinct. The rash often resembles dermatosis and a delayed or missed diagnosis may result. The rash may get worse after being in the sun. Rashes or patches that appear with an active border are composed of papules, vesicles, and/or crusts. Most commonly, the lesions are only located on the cheeks, the nose, periorbital area, chin, and forehead. In men, tinea faciei is known as tinea barbae as the infection appears on the bearded surface of the face.

MANAGEMENT/TREATMENT:
1. Keep skin and feet clean and dry.
2. When used as directed, over-the-counter (OTC) anti-fungal medications (creams) can effectively treat mild cases of ringworm. More severe cases or cases that do not respond in 2-4 weeks with OTC medications should be referred to the healthcare provider for additional medication.
3. Topical antifungal medications are not effective for the treatment of tinea capitis. Systemic antifungal medication is required for up to 4-8 weeks and should be used for 2 weeks after resolution.
4. Students with tinea capitis should be instructed not to share combs, hats, hair ribbons, or brushes.
5. Avoid contact sports, such as wrestling, for at least 48 hours after treatment was started.
6. Haircuts, shaving of the head, or wearing a cap for tinea capitis during treatment is unnecessary.
7. Students with tinea cruris, tinea corporis, or tinea pedis should be excluded at the end of the school day and be readmitted once treatment is initiated.

RINGWORM – TINEA *(continued from previous page)*

MANAGEMENT/TREATMENT: *(continued)*

8. Students with tinea pedis should be excluded from swimming pools, and from walking barefoot on locker room and shower floors until treatment has been initiated.
9. Siblings and household contacts should be evaluated.

FOLLOW-UP:

- Refer cases with scalp and nail lesions to healthcare provider.
- Refer severe cases (those which do not improve within 2-4 weeks of starting treatment) or for a secondary bacterial infection which may require an antibiotic.
- Inform parent/guardian to check contacts, family members, and pets.
- Work with maintenance personnel, teachers, and coaches to assure proper cleaning of headphones, swimming pool and locker areas, PE mats, wrestling headgear, and other equipment with which skin contact is common.

POTENTIAL COMPLICATIONS:

Secondary bacterial infections

NOTES

- Wash hands thoroughly and often.
- Keep skin dry and clean.
- Shampoo hair regularly, especially after haircuts.
- Do not share clothing, shoes, towels, hairbrushes, combs, headgear, or other personal care items.
- Avoid walking barefoot in public places.
- Wear waterproof shoes or "flip-flops" in public showers and swimming pool areas.
- Change wet socks.
- Use powder on feet to absorb moisture.
- Check pets for areas of hair loss. Consult a veterinarian. Avoid touching pets with bald spots.
- Keep all clothing and bed clothing clean.
- Stay cool and dry.
- Change clothing that becomes sweaty or wet.
- Make sure safety mats and other surfaces that might be home to infectious bacteria, such as MRSA, ringworm and impetigo, are disinfected often (preferably daily).
- Cleaning and draining the school shower areas should be done frequently.

RINGWORM – TINEA *(continued from previous page)*

References

American Academy of Pediatrics, Committee on Infectious Diseases. (2015). Summaries of infectious disease – tinea capitis, tinea corporis, tinea cruris, tinea pedis and tinea unguium. In D.W. Kimberlin, M. T. Brady, M.A. Jackson, & S.S. Long (Eds.), *Red Book: 2015 report of the committee on infectious diseases* (30th ed.) (pp. 778-786). Elk Grove Village, IL: American Academy of Pediatrics.

American Academy of Pediatrics. (2013). Ringworm. In S. Aronson, & T. Shope (Eds.), *Managing infectious diseases in child care and schools (2ⁿᵈ ed.)* (p.p. 141-142). Elk Grove Village, IL: American Academy of Pediatrics.

Cole, G.W., Manifold, C.A. (2015). *Jock itch overview.* Retrieved from http://www.emedicinehealth.com/jock_itch/article_em.htm

Cunha, J.P. *(2015). Ringworm on the body.* Retrieved from http://www.emedicinehealth.com/ringworm_on_body/article_em.htm

Denehy, J. (2013). Athlete health promotion. In J. Selekman (Ed.), *School nursing: A comprehensive text (2ⁿᵈ ed.),* (pp. 565-585). Philadelphia, PA: F.A. Davis.

Emedicine Health. (2014). *Slideshow pictures: Ringworm -- causes, types, symptoms and treatment.* Retrieved from http://www.emedicinehealth.com/slideshow_ringworm_pictures/article_em.htm

Mayo Clinic. (2014). *Athlete's foot.* Retrieved from http://www.mayoclinic.com/health/athletes-foot/DS00317

Mayo Clinic. (2013). *Ringworm (body).* Retrieved from http://www.mayoclinic.com/health/ringworm/DS00489

Mayo Clinic. (2014). *Ringworm (scalp) definition.* Retrieved from http://www.mayoclinic.com/health/ringworm/DS00892

Oishi, M. L., & Irizarry, L. (2014). *Ringworm on scalp.* Retrieved from http://www.emedicinehealth.com/ringworm_on_scalp/article_em.htm

ROTAVIRUS

DEFINITION/ETIOLOGY:
Rotavirus is the most common cause of gastroenteritis and severe diarrhea among infants and children worldwide. Most children experience rotavirus at least one time by the age of two or three. The incubation period for rotavirus ranges from 1-3 days. The name rotavirus is derived from the Latin word *rota* meaning "wheel." When a rotavirus is viewed under an electron microscope, the virus has a characteristic wheel-like appearance. Rotaviruses are non-enveloped double-shelled viruses and are stable in the environment.

CAUSES
Rotavirus is present in an infected person's stool several days before symptoms appear and up to 10 days after symptoms subside. The virus spreads very easily through hand to mouth contact. There are many types of rotaviruses and it is possible to be infected more than once.

The primary mode of transmission is fecal-oral, although low titers of the virus have been reported in respiratory tract secretions and other body fluids. Laboratory testing of stool specimens is necessary to diagnose rotavirus infection. Because of the rotavirus stability in the environment, transmission can occur through ingestion of contaminated food and water and contact with contaminated surfaces. In the United States, the disease has a winter seasonal pattern and epidemics generally occur from November through April.

SIGNS AND SYMPTOMS:
- Fever
- Watery diarrhea and vomiting (for three to eight days)
- Abdominal pain
- Pale skin
- Dry lips
- Sunken eyes

The healthcare provider should be called if the child has:
- Severe or bloody diarrhea
- Frequent episodes of vomiting for more than three hours
- Temperature of 102°F or higher
- Seems lethargic, irritable, or in pain
- Has signs or symptoms of dehydration, e.g. dry mouth, crying without tears, little or no urination, unusual sleepiness or unresponsiveness

ROTAVIRUS *(continued from previous page)*

MANAGEMENT/TREATMENT:
- There is no specific treatment for rotavirus infection as antibiotics are not effective for viral infections.
- Rotavirus infections generally resolve in three to eight days. Prevention of dehydration during rotavirus infection is the most important concern.
- Drinking plenty of fluids, e.g. clear liquids, while rotavirus infection runs its course will help prevent dehydration.
- Oral rehydration such as Pedialyte® for infants and a rehydration fluid for children replace lost electrolytes more effectively than water or other liquids.
- Severe dehydration may require hospitalization for intravenous fluids.

FOLLOW UP:
The Advisory Committee on Immunization Practices (ACIP) recommends routine vaccination of infants in the United States. Two different rotavirus vaccines, RotaTeq® (RV5) and Rotarix® (RV1), are currently licensed for infants in the United States.

Both vaccines are live oral vaccines recommended for infants (6-24 months) to prevent subsequent disease later.

COMPLICATIONS:
- Severe dehydration.
- Intussusception is an uncommon type of bowel obstruction that occurs when the bowel folds on itself. Intussusception is most common in young children and can occur with viral infections.

NOTES:
Prevention
- Proper hand hygiene can reduce the spread of rotavirus infection. Hands should be washed often and thoroughly after use of toilet or in assisting child in use of toilet or after diapering.
- Surfaces should be cleaned with soap and water.
- Approved vaccinations for rotavirus are offered to infants 6 to 24 months for the prevention of rotavirus infection.

ROTAVIRUS *(continued from previous page)*

References

American Academy of Pediatrics, Committee on Infectious Diseases. (2015). Rotavirus infection. In D.W. Kimberlin, M. T. Brady, M.A. Jackson, & S.S. Long (Eds.), *Red Book: 2015 report of the committee on infectious diseases* (30th ed.) (pp. 684-688). Elk Grove Village, IL: American Academy of Pediatrics.

Centers for Disease Control and Prevention. (2014). Rotavirus *(Rotavirus Infection)*. Retrieved from http://www.cdc.gov/rotavirus/

Centers for Disease Control and Prevention. (2015). Vaccine safety: Rotavirus. Retrieved from http://www.cdc.gov/vaccinesafety/vaccines/rotavsb.html

Centers for Disease Control and Prevention (CDC). (2014). *Rotavirus vaccine (Rotashield) and Intussusception*. Retrieved from http://www.cdc.gov/vaccines/vpd-vac/rotavirus/vac-rotashield-historical.htm

Immunization Action Coalition. (2015). *Vaccine information for the public and health professionals: Vaccine information statement Rotavirus VIS*. Retrieved from http://www.immunize.org/vis/vis_rotavirus.asp

Mayo Clinic. (2013). *Rotavirus*. Retrieved from http://www.mayoclinic.com/health/rotavirus/DS00783

SCABIES

DEFINITION/ETIOLOGY:

Scabies is caused by a tiny, eight-legged burrowing mite called *Sarcoptes scabiei var hominis*. It is a highly contagious infection spread through direct, prolonged, skin-to-skin contact and shared clothing or linen of someone who has scabies. A person infected for the first time may not exhibit symptoms for 2-6 weeks and can transmit scabies to another person during that time. A person previously infected with scabies may exhibit symptoms as early as 1-4 days after exposure. In addition, the mite can survive 48-72 hours without human contact.

SIGNS AND SYMPTOMS:

- The most common symptom is intense itching, especially at night and the appearance of rash.
- Typical lesion is a "burrow" which is a tiny, pale, irregular line that marks the path of the scabies mite.
- Rash: tiny (1-2 mm) erythematous papules, vesicles, pustule and scabs, sometimes with tiny, linear dark scabs (0.5-1 mm long).
- Location: webbing between the fingers, flexor surface of wrist and elbow, axillary – skin folds, waist, and thighs and can also spread to breasts and penis.
- **The face, neck, palms and soles** may be involved in infants and very young children **(a good assessment clue).**
- Frequently found in other family members.
- Secondary skin infections (pustules) are frequent due to scratching.
- Itching is related to an allergic reaction to mites and may persist a month after successful treatment until top layers of skin are shed.

Diagnostic hints:
1) Appearance and distribution of rash and the presence of burrows.
2) Color suspected burrow and surrounding skin with purple felt marker and wipe off with alcohol. Burrow will be outlined in purple.
3) Microscopic examination of skin scrapings for mites, eggs or fecal matter.

MANAGEMENT/TREATMENT:

- Exclude from school for prompt treatment. May return 8 hours/next day after proper treatment.
- Steroid ointments or lotions are contraindicated.
- Instruct parent/guardian to wash clothes, towels, and bed linen used by the infected person within the previous 2 days at 130 º F or hotter, and dry in hot dryer.

SCABIES *(continued from previous page)*

MANAGEMENT/TREATMENT *(continued)*

- MEDICATIONS:
  - Over the counter (OTC) products have not been approved to treat human scabies.
  - Scabacides are available by prescription from the healthcare provider. Follow label directions.
  - The usual prescription product is permethrin 5% cream (Elimite®). Crotamiton 10% cream (Eurax®) for scabies nodules is approved only for adults. Lindane 1% lotion is available, but is rarely used due to side effects.
  - Apply scabacide lotions should to the entire body (chin-line to toes.) NEVER ON THE FACE. The lotions should be left on as recommended on the package insert and then washed off thoroughly with soap and water.
  - Use anti-scabetic lotions/creams no more than twice in a month.
  - Oral antihistamine helps itching that may persist up to one month after treatment.

FOLLOW-UP:
- Assess each day or two after first treatment.
- Watch for new lesions. A second treatment may be necessary.
- Watch for secondary infection and refer accordingly.
- Check siblings in school.
- Educate staff about scabies and transmission.

POTENTIAL COMPLICATIONS:
Vigorous scratching can cause breaks in the skin, potentially leading to secondary bacterial infections.

NOTES:
May be asymptomatic the first two to six weeks of an **initial** infection of scabies. However, even though the person is asymptomatic, they remain contagious during this time period.

SCABIES *(continued from previous page)*

References

American Academy of Dermatology. (n.d.). *Scabies.* Retrieved from http://www.aad.org/dermatology-a-to-z/diseases-and-treatments/q---t/scabies

American Academy of Pediatrics. (2013). Scabies. In S. Aronson, & T. Shope (Eds.), *Managing infectious diseases in child care and schools (2nd ed.)* (p. 151). Elk Grove Village, IL: American Academy of Pediatrics.

American Academy of Pediatrics, Committee on Infectious Diseases. (2015). Scabies. In D.W. Kimberlin, M. T. Brady, M.A. Jackson, & S.S. Long (Eds.), *Red Book: 2015 report of the committee on infectious diseases* (30th ed.) (pp. 702-704). Elk Grove Village, IL: American Academy of Pediatrics.

Ball, J., Binder, R., & Cowen, K. (Eds.). (2012). Alterations in skin integrity. *Principles of Pediatric Nursing: Caring for Children (5th ed.)* (p. 1052). Upper Saddle River, NJ: Pearson Education, Inc.

Center for Disease Control and Prevention. (2010). *Scabies.* Retrieved from http://www.cdc.gov/parasites/scabies/

Mayo Clinic. (2015). *Scabies.* Retrieved from http://www.mayoclinic.com/health/scabies/DS00451

Medline Plus, U.S. National Library of Medicine. (2014). *Scabies.* Retrieved from http://www.nlm.nih.gov/medlineplus/scabies.html

Merck Manual. *Scabies.* (2014). Retrieved from http://www.merckmanuals.com/professional/dermatologic_disorders/parasitic_skin_infections/scabies.html?qt=scabies&alt=sh

SEIZURES - EPILEPSY

A seizure results from abnormal and excessive electrical activity in cerebral neurons that lead to a change of consciousness, motor activity, behavior, and/or sensation. Most seizures last a minute or two typically followed by confusion and sleepiness. Triggers include stress, sleep patterns, hormone changes, light sensitivity or drugs. A seizure can be a one-time episode from a fever or brain injury or occur with frequency.

People may have one or more types of seizures, but most people with epilepsy will have a similar pattern with each seizure. Seizures are divided into types; generalized seizures (absence, atonic, tonic-clonic, myoclonic), partial (simple and complex), non-epileptic and status epilepticus.

A seizure is not a diagnosis but a symptom of a diagnosis. Epilepsy is a seizure disorder and is a chronic condition of recurrent seizures without an identifiable cause.

SIGNS AND SYMPTOMS:
ALL TYPES
- Signs and symptoms are dependent on where the problem in the brain is located
- Distinct beginning and rapid cessation
- Amnesia of seizure, sometimes including events that occurred a few seconds to minutes prior to seizure (retrograde amnesia)
- EEG not always abnormal

GENERALIZED: ABSENCE (PETIT MAL)
- Very brief (10-20 seconds) period of cessation of motion
- Brief loss of consciousness
- May drop glass or pencil
- May appear to be staring into space
- Occasional brief muscular twitches
- Chewing motion or blinking of eyes
- Usual onset between 4-10 years of age, may occur several times a day
- Most children will outgrow

SEIZURES - EPILEPSY *(continued from previous page)*

GENERALIZED: CLONIC-TONIC
- Generalized, violent muscle contractions
- Affects most of the body
- Loss of consciousness
- Incontinence of urine/stool
- Tongue or cheek biting
- Sometimes seizure is preceded by aura of light, noise or odor
- Dusky facial skin color
- Post-convulsive state; drowsy to deep sleep
- Awakened to confusion, headache or speech difficulty
- Frequency varies from daily, to monthly, to annually
- Generally last 1-3 minutes

FOCAL SEIZURES
A. Simple Partial
- Seizure of one part of body, usually on one side only; hand, arm, face, tongue, foot, or leg
- May "spread" to other muscle groups
- Usually no loss of consciousness

B. Complex Partial: (Psychomotor)
- Purposeful but inappropriate motor acts, often repetitive; running, chewing, swallowing
- Arm extension with slow turn of body
- Usually no tonic or clonic activity
- Consciousness is impaired
- May be disorientated or confused
- Often sleepy after seizure

NON-EPILEPTIC (Psychogenic Seizures)
- Rarely injures self
- Incontinence rare
- Consciousness regained quickly
- Often preceded by anxiety
- Cyanosis absent or momentary

SEIZURES - EPILEPSY *(continued from previous page)*

STATUS EPILEPTICUS
- Definition: Seizure lasting 30 minutes or a 30 minute period of serial seizures without regaining consciousness
- Follow medical order and the individualized healthcare plans for students with a history of seizures.
- Typically, emergency help should be called after a seizure lasting more than 5 minutes.

MANAGEMENT/TREATMENT:

PHARMCOLOGICAL TREATMENT
- Antiepileptic drugs are the most common treatment for epilepsy.
- Drug treatment varies with the type of seizure, age of person, and effectiveness.
- Medication must be taken consistently.
- Diazepam or Midazolam (rectal, buccal and intranasal) may be administered according to the healthcare provider instructions, state nursing practice guidelines and school district policy.

NON-PHARMACEUTICAL TREATMENTS
KETOGENIC DIET
- High fat (80%) diet that works by burning stored fat versus glucose for energy.
- Ketosis prevents seizures.
- Important side effects include dehydration, increased cholesterol blood levels, constipation, kidney or gallstones, menstrual irregularities, pancreatitis, and decreased bone density.
- OTC medication may interfere with diet, check with healthcare provider for sugar free medication substitutes.
- Supervised by a dietician.

SEIZURES - EPILEPSY *(continued from previous page)*

VAGAL NERVE STIMULATOR (VNS)
- Currently approved for people over age 12.
- Battery-operated device (similar in concept to a pacemaker), about the size of a silver dollar, that is implanted in the chest wall or sometimes in the lower abdominal area.
- Small wires are threaded under the skin and wound around the vagus nerve in the neck.
- The device works by sending regular small pulses of electrical energy to the brain.
- When a person feels a seizure coming on, they can activate the discharge of electrical energy by passing a small magnet over the battery to stop the seizure.
- It is also possible to turn the device off by holding the magnet over it.
- Side effects include hoarseness, voice alteration, coughing and increased salivation.

SURGICAL INTERVENTION
- Removes affected area of the brain.
- Is done when other options are not successful.
- Can significantly reduce or stop seizures.
- Can result in decline in memory or defect in visual field.

FIRST AID FOR SEIZURE
- Keep calm and reassure other people who may be nearby. Keep onlookers away.
- Do not hold person down or try to stop movements.
- Time the seizure.
- Gently lower person to the floor.
- Position on side with mouth toward floor to prevent aspiration of salvia or vomitus.
- Clear area around person of sharp objects or items that may lead to secondary injury.
- Loosen anything around neck that may interfere with breathing.
- Place something soft under the head.
- DO NOT stimulate by rubbing chest, face, or arms or loosening clothing on body.
- DO NOT try to force mouth open; DO NOT insert any padded object into the mouth.
- Reassure person as consciousness returns.
- Allow to rest following seizure.
- Remain with student until entirely awake.

SEIZURES - EPILEPSY *(continued from previous page)*

FIRST AID FOR SEIZURE IN A WHEELCHAIR
- Do not remove the person from the wheelchair unless totally necessary.
- Secure the wheelchair to prevent movement.
- Loosely fasten the seatbelt.
- Protect the head.
- Pad the wheelchair to prevent injuries to the limbs.

WHEN TO SEEK IMMEDIATE MEDICAL ATTENTION:
- First time seizure
- Generalized tonic-clonic seizures lasting more than 5 minutes unless otherwise instructed by healthcare provider
- Repeated seizures without regaining consciousness between seizures
- A change in seizure pattern or an increase in seizures
- Seizure in the water
- Injury occurs during seizure
- Some students will have a healthcare provider order for rectal valium for a seizure lasting a specific amount of time (this may vary for individuals, but often it is ordered given for seizures lasting over 3-5 minutes)
- Seek medical attention if person has:
  - Diabetes (follow emergency healthcare plan)
  - Brain infection
  - Heat exhaustion
  - Pregnancy
  - Poisoning
  - Head injury

FOLLOW UP:
- Obtain accurate detailed history.
- Develop an Individualized Healthcare Plan.
- Emergency plan should be available for classroom and EMS personnel.
- Assess school environment for triggers.
- Monitor student for medication effectiveness and untoward side effects Obtain necessary releases of information.
- Educate all staff including bus drivers on all aspects of seizures.
- Record current body weight, medications and typical seizure episodes.
- Become familiar with quality of life issues; emotional issues, driving, cognitive abilities and employment.

SEIZURES - EPILEPSY *(continued from previous page)*

NOTES:
- Most seizures are not considered medical emergencies.
- The most frequent cause of breakthrough is failure to take prescribed seizure medication.
- Febrile seizures are common in young children.
- About 70% of children using one or more treatment mentioned above become seizure free.
- Some individuals are able to stop medication after remaining seizure free for a lengthy period of time.
- Epilepsy can cause death. The most common reason is from SUDEP (Sudden Unexpected Death in Epilepsy).
- Lack of attention (e.g., staring out the window) is often mistaken for petit mal.

References

Blair, J. (2013). Seizures and epilepsy. In J. Selekman (Ed.), *School nursing: A comprehensive text (2nd ed.)* (pp. 1003-1027). Philadelphia, PA: F.A. Davis.

Epilepsy Foundation. (2014). *What is epilepsy?* Retrieved from http://www.epilepsy.com/learn/epilepsy-101/what.epilepsy

Medline Plus/ U.S. National Library of Medicine. (2014). *Seizures*. Retrieved from http://www.nlm.nih.gov/medlineplus/seizures.html#skip

National Institute of Neurological Disorders and Stroke. (2015). *NINDS Epilepsy Information Page*. Retrieved from http://www.ninds.nih.gov/disorders/epilepsy/epilepsy.htm

Smith, G., Wagner, J. L. & Edwards, J.C. (2015, May). CE: Epilepsy update, part 1: Refining our understanding of a complex disease. *American Journal of Nursing, 115*(5), 40–47. doi: 10.1097/01.NAJ.0000465030.89975.e8

Smith, G., Wagner, J. L. & Edwards, J.C. (2015, June). CE: Epilepsy update, part 2: Nursing care and evidence-based treatment. *American Journal of Nursing, 115*(6), 34-44. Retrieved from http://www.nursingcenter.com/ovidws/_PDF_.aspx?an=00000446-201506000-00026&Journal_ID=&Issue_ID=

SELF-INJURY, NON-SUICIDAL SELF-INJURY (NSSI)

DEFINITION/ETIOLOGY:
School nurses have become increasingly aware of NSSI, especially at the middle and high school level. In fact, schools are often a common site for identification, referral and intervention for students with mental health concerns. NSSI can be defined as the deliberate, self- inflicted destruction of body tissue without suicidal intent for the purposes not socially sanctioned (Mayo Clinic, 2012). It has been referred to as self-injury, self- harm and commonly "cutting" although the self- injurious behaviors often encompass more than cutting behaviors. It is important that school nurses understand intentional self- harm and know how to respond.

Although cutting is the most common form of NSSI, burns, placing objects under the skin, rubbing the skin raw with erasers or using any other method such as razor blades or paper clips can be included. Individual may persistently pick at wound to interfere with the healing process.

 A student who engages in self-injury has a different intent than a student engaging in suicide-related behaviors. NSSI is considered a coping mechanism that provides relief to the student and is often considered a form of self- soothing. Students describe it as a quick fix to address loneliness, hurt anger and pain. Intentional self- injury is not a suicide attempt but often students who do commit suicide have a past injury of self -harm.

Students are often referred to the school nurse by other students, or by faculty who have witnessed the event. It may also be noted during a physical assessment or a student may self-disclose to the school nurse or other staff.

SIGNS AND SYMPTOMS:
- Unexplained markings or injuries on the skin
- Long sleeved clothing during warm weather
- Constant use of wrist coverings or wrist bands
- Signs of depression or anxiety
- Refusal to participate in things such as swimming due to unwillingness to expose skin

SELF-INJURY, NON-SUICIDAL SELF-INJURY (NSSI) *(continued from previous page)*

MANAGEMENT/TREATMENT:
- Identify students who may be engaging in NSSI behaviors.
- Assess injuries, noting old scars or injuries, and provide first aid as needed.
- Identify any injuries that may require immediate attention or more advanced medical care.
- Assess the student in a calm, kind, non-judgmental manner, asking questions in a direct and honest way about a student's self-harm behaviors and history.
- Involve the school crisis team and/or counselors or psychologists to illicit counseling supports in the school itself as appropriate.
- Refer to psychiatrist and/or psychologist who have experience in treating individuals with self-injury behaviors.
- Provide parents with the relief of information forms to communicate with any outside providers.

FOLLOW-UP:
- Schools should develop protocols to help all school staff responds appropriately to NSSI in the school setting. School nurses can be integral in not only developing protocols but also in educating staff and being a resource for parents and the community.
- Although NSSI is not generally associated with suicide, a suicide assessment should be completed by trained staff if there is any indication the student may be suicidal.
- A list of referral sources or contact information should be maintained.
- Students should be encouraged to call his/her parents/caregivers to make them aware of what has occurred. A point person in the school may be utilized to help the student in disclosing this to the parent and assisting the parent in obtaining outside assistance.
- State and local laws may differ in response to parental/guardian notification and each school nurse should be aware of these laws as well as specific district policy.

POTENTIAL COMPLICATIONS:
1. Life threatening wounds
2. Wound infection
3. Scarring/disfigurement
4. Worsening of potential underlying mental health condition
5. Death

SELF-INJURY, NON-SUICIDAL SELF-INJURY (NSSI) *(continued from previous page)*

References

American Psychological Association. (2015). *Who self-injures?* Retrieved from http://www.apa.org/monitor/2015/07-08/who-self-injures.aspx

Burrick, K., Goodwin, J., & Whitlock J. (n.d.). *Non –suicidal self-injury in schools: Developing and implementing school protocol.* Retrieved fromhttp://www.selfinjury.bctr.cornell.edu/documents/schools.pdf

Hayes, R.A. (n.d.). *Self-harm*. Retrieved from http://www.isbe.state.il.us/spec-ed/np_handouts/2010/session11.pdf

Kerr, P., Mueblenkamp, J., & Turner, J. (2010). Nonsuicidal self-injury: A review of current research for family medicine and primary care physicians. *Journal of the American Board of Family Medicine, 23*(2), 240-259. doi: 10.3122/jabfm.2010.02.090110

Mayo Clinic. (2012). *Self-injury/cutting*. Retrieved from http://www.mayoclinic.org/diseases-conditions/self-injury/basics/definition/con-20025897

Merck Manual Professional. (2014). *Suicidal behavior in children and adolescents.* Retrieved from http://www.merckmanuals.com/professional/pediatrics/mental-disorders-in-children-and-adolescents/suicidal-behavior-in-children-and-adolescents

SEXUALLY TRANSMITTED DISEASES/INFECTIONS

DEFINITION/ETIOLOGY:

Sexually transmitted infections (STI), sometimes referred to as sexually transmitted diseases (STD) are infections acquired by sexual contact. STIs can be passed to a person anytime they have unprotected sex with a partner who is already infected. It can be spread during vaginal, anal or oral sex. The organisms that cause STIs may pass from person to person through blood, semen, or vaginal fluids. Human Papillomavirus and Herpes Simplex Virus can be spread by contact in the area of the skin not covered by a condom (skin to skin).

Over twenty (20) diseases are classified as sexually transmitted and are reportable to the local health department. Sexually transmitted diseases commonly seen in the adolescent population will be reviewed in this document.

Chlamydial Infections

Chlamydia is the most frequently reported infectious disease in the United States and prevalence is highest among those under 25 years of age. It is caused by the organism *C. trachomatis*. Adolescent women are at a particular risk for C. trachomatis. Annual screening of all sexually active adolescents is recommended.

Gonococcal Infections

Gonorrhea is the second most commonly reported bacterial STI and is caused by *N. gonorrhoeae*. Symptoms usually develop 2-21 days after having sex. Genital GC generally causes local infection of the urethra, vagina, rectum and cervix, but may ascend into the upper genital tract in women or infect the testicles or prostate in men.

SIGNS AND SYMPTOMS (for chlamydia and gonorrhea):
- Asymptomatic infection is common
- Vaginal, penile, rectal and cervical discharge
- Pain/burning with urination
- Unusual vaginal bleeding, between periods or after sex
- Abdominal pain, sometimes with fever or nausea
- Enlarged inguinal or femoral lymph nodes
- Swollen testicles
- Rectal pain or discharge

SEXUALLY TRANSMITTED DISEASES/INFECTIONS *(continued from previous page)*

MANAGEMENT/TREATMENT (for chlamydia and gonorrhea):

- Students with possible chlamydial and gonococcal infections should be referred to a healthcare provider for testing and treatment.
- Chlamydial and gonococcal infections or suspected infections should be treated with antibiotics.
- C. trachomatis is generally treated with a single dose of oral azithromycin.
- Often presumptive treatment of chlamydial infection for students with gonococcal infections is indicated.
- Uncomplicated gonorrhea is treated with a one-time intramuscular dose of ceftriaxone.
- Students should be re-tested in 3-4 months.
- Students should be instructed to refer their sex partners to a healthcare provider if they have had sexual contact within 60 days of onset of the symptoms.

Genital Herpes Simplex Virus

Genital herpes is a chronic, life- long viral infection. Two types have been identified, HSV-1 and *HSV-2*. Most cases of genital herpes are caused by *HSV-2*. Many persons have mild or asymptomatic infection but shed the virus intermittently in the genital tract. Herpes episodes may be characterized as primary, first episode of infection, or re-current in a student with a past history of symptomatic HSV infection.

SIGNS AND SYMPTOMS (for genital herpes simplex):

- A flu-like feeling
- Small painful blisters on the genitals, rectum or mouth
- Itching or burning before the symptoms occur
- Inguinal lymphadenopathy
- Blisters may last 1-3 weeks
- Blisters may return

MANAGEMENT/TREATMENT (for genital herpes simplex):

- Anti-viral medication may be ordered by the healthcare provider for initial and episodic infections and for suppression.
- Warm baths may be helpful.
- Students should understand that although it can be treated, herpes cannot be cured.
- Daily suppression therapy may also decrease the risks of transmission.

SEXUALLY TRANSMITTED DISEASES/INFECTIONS (continued from previous page)

Genital Human Papillomavirus (HPV)

HPV is the most common sexually transmitted infection in the U.S today. Over half of sexually active women and men are infected at some point in their lives. More than 100 different types of HPV commonly affect the mucosal surfaces of the genital area. The virus is transmitted through skin-to-skin contact. It is associated with genital warts and cervical cancers although most infections do not result in cancer.

SIGNS AND SYMPTOMS (for HPV):

- Many people have no symptoms.
- Genital warts in the genital area.
- Warts may be alone or in groups, flat or rounded, pink or skin colored.
- Abnormal cervical cytology.

MANAGEMENT/TREATMENT (for HPV):

- Students with genital warts should be referred to their healthcare provider.
- Although there is no cure for genital warts, they can be treated.
- Genital warts may spontaneously resolve without treatment.
- Warts can be treated with ointments, surgical or laser removal.
- Warts may recur after treatment.
- Sexually active students should be referred for pap smears as abnormal cervical cytology can progress to invasive cervical cancer.
- Vaccines for the prevention of HPV are available and approved for both males and females 10-25 years.

POTENTIAL COMPLICATIONS of untreated STIs:

- Infertility
- Neurological or cardiovascular problems occur with some infections
- Pelvic Inflammatory Disease (PID)
- Ectopic pregnancy
- Reactive arthritis (Reiter Syndrome) as a complication of chlamydia
- Many STIs may be transmitted to newborns during birth or have an adverse effect on pregnancy
- Epididymitis, prostatitis

If a student had sexual contact with someone who had or has any of the above symptoms related to STI, it is important to **see a healthcare provider immediately**.

SEXUALLY TRANSMITTED DISEASES/INFECTIONS *(continued from previous page)*

FOLLOW-UP:
- Encourage student to continue full course of prescribed treatment and obtain necessary tests.
- Abstinence from sexual activity for 7 days is encouraged following treatment.
- Encourage student to cooperate in locating sexual contacts.
- Educate students in regard to prevention, re-infection, and complications.
  - HIV is easier to acquire if one already has another sexually transmitted disease.
  - Many infections are asymptomatic in boys but may cause serious infection in girls (e.g. chlamydia).
- Latex condom use has been shown to prevent transmission of most bacterial infections and is helpful in limiting some transmission of HSV and HPV.
- Students should be aware that abstinence is the only way to prevent a STI with 100% accuracy.
- Most state laws permit treatment of a minor without parental consent or notification.
- Nurses should be aware of their own state laws and regulations regarding confidentiality.
- Students should be encouraged to involve a parent or responsible adult in the process.

NOTES:
According to the CDC, the reporting of STIs in an accurate and timely manner is important for assessing morbidity trends, targeting limited resources, and assisting local health authorities in partner notification and treatment. Cases related to STI, HIV, and acquired immune deficiency syndrome (AIDS) should be reported in accordance with state and local statutory requirements. Additionally, Syphilis, Gonorrhea, Chlamydia, Chancroid, HIV infection, and AIDS are reportable diseases in every state. The reporting requirements for other STIs differ by state, thus clinicians should be familiar with state and local reporting requirements.

SEXUALLY TRANSMITTED DISEASES/INFECTIONS (*continued from previous page*)

NOTES: (*continued*)

Adolescents ages 15-24 account for nearly half of the 20 million new cases of STD's each year (CDC, 2014). Minor consent laws may vary from state to state. With a few exceptions, all adolescents in the United States can legally consent to confidential diagnosis and treatment of STIs. In all 50 states and the District of Columbia, adolescents can receive medical care for STIs without parental consent or knowledge. Additionally, adolescents can consent to HIV counseling and testing in the majority of states. According to the CDC (2014), the consent laws for vaccination of adolescents differ by state. However, some states consider provision of vaccine similar to treatment of STI and provide vaccination services without parental consent. Healthcare providers should follow policies which provide confidentiality and comply with state laws for STI services.

The management of children with STIs requires the close cooperation clinicians, laboratory technicians, and child protective services authorities. Prompt initiation of official investigations is important when needed. Specific diseases, e.g. Gonorrhea, Syphilis, and Chlamydia, if acquired after the neonatal period, are indicative of sexual contact. Other diseases, e.g. HPV infections and vaginitis, do not have a clear association with sexual contact.

References

Centers for Disease Control and Prevention. (2015). Sexually transmitted diseases treatment guidelines, 2015. Retrieved from http://www.cdc.gov/std/tg2015/

Centers for Disease Control and Prevention. (2014). *Reported STDs in the United States*. Retrieved from http://www.cdc.gov/nchhstp/newsroom/docs/STD-Trends-508.pdf

Fisher, M., Alderman, E., Kreipe, R., & Rosenfeld, W. (Eds.). (2011). *Textbook of adolescent health care* (pp. 477-501). Elk Grove Village, IL: American Academy of Pediatrics.

Mayo Clinic. (2014). Sexually *transmitted diseases (STDs)*. Retrieved from http://www.mayoclinic.com/health/sexually-transmitted-diseases-stds/DS01123

Reirden, D.H., & Nyquist, A. (2014). Sexually transmitted infections. In W.Hay, M. Levin, R. Deterding, & M. Abzug (Eds.), *Current diagnosis and treatment pediatrics* (22nd edition) (pp. 1400-1422). McGraw Hill Education, Inc.

U.S. Department of Health and Human Services, Office of Adolescent Health. (2015). *Sexually transmitted diseases*. Retrieved from http://www.hhs.gov/ash/oah/adolescent-health-topics/reproductive-health/stds.html

SHINGLES (VZV) - also called Herpes Zoster (HZV), Postherpetic neuralgia (PHN)

DEFINITION/ETIOLOGY:

Shingles is a disease caused by varicella-zoster virus the same virus that causes chickenpox. The virus of clinical chickenpox remains dormant in the body and can reactivate years later causing shingles.

1. Shingles can develop in any age group. Most often shingles occur in people over 60 years old, but anyone who has had chickenpox is at risk. Even children can get shingles.
2. Many who have chicken pox the case is so mild that they may not be aware that they have the varicella zoster virus.
3. Persons who had chickenpox before the age of 1 year are at greater risk.
4. Those with weakened immune systems are more susceptible.
5. The virus spreads through direct contact with the rash (transmission of the shingle virus is not airborne).
6. An adult or child, who has direct contact with the shingles rash and did not have chickenpox as a child or did not receive the chickenpox vaccine, can develop chickenpox, not shingles.

SIGNS AND SYMPTOMS:

- Characteristically, the first symptoms of shingles are burning or shooting pain and tingling or itching, usually on one side of the body.
- The pain and burning can be mild to severe.
- A rash or blisters appear one to 14 days later and usually involves a narrow area from the spine around to the front of the abdomen of chest.
- The blisters break, forming small lesions that begin to dry and form crusts. The crusts fall off in two to three weeks.
- Scarring is rare.
- The pain of shingles may last for weeks, months, or even years.

Other symptoms may include:

- General feeling of "not well", headache, fever and chills, enlarged lymph nodes, and/or joint pain.
- With pain, there may be accompanying muscle weakness, and a rash involving different parts of the face.
- If the shingles virus affects a nerve in the face, some of the following symptoms may occur: difficulty moving some of the muscles in the face, drooping eyelid (ptosis), loss of eye motion and other vision problems, hearing loss, taste problems.

SHINGLES *(continued from previous page)*

MANAGEMENT/TREATMENT:
The healthcare provider may prescribe an oral antiviral drug to reduce the pain, prevent complications, and shorten the course of the disease. The medication should be started within 72 hours of first appearance of pain and itching and it is best to begin the antiviral treatment before the blisters appear.

Other management and treatment measures to follow during the course of shingles infection include:
- Following the healthcare provider's instructions for home care.
- The application of cool, wet compresses to reduce pain and soothing baths and resting in bed until the fever subsides.
- A person with shingles infection should stay away from others while the lesions are oozing to avoid infecting those who have never had chickenpox or chickenpox vaccine, especially pregnant women and those with compromised immune systems.
- Isolate/exclude the affected child from other children in the school setting.

FOLLOW-UP: Refer to healthcare provider if:
- Signs and symptoms suggest shingles.
- Symptoms worsen.
- Alert those with a compromised immune system (i.e. chemotherapy, HIV, other, immune-suppressed) and recommend they seek advice from their healthcare provider.
- Identify those who have not had chickenpox or the chickenpox vaccine.
- Women who are pregnant or might become pregnant should contact their healthcare provider.
- Shingles that affect the eye may result in permanent vision loss. These persons should be referred to immediate/emergency medical services.

POTENTIAL COMPLICATIONS:
Recurrences of shingles, bacterial skin infections, permanent vision loss (if shingles occur in the eye), permanent healing loss (if shingles occur in the ear), infections that include encephalitis or sepsis in those with compromised immune systems, and if shingles virus affects the face or ear the infection could result in Ramsay Hunt Syndrome. Posthepetic pain does not occur in children.

SHINGLES *(continued from previous page)*

PREVENTION:
Do not touch the rash or blisters on a person with shingles if you have never had chickenpox or the chickenpox vaccine.

Herpes zoster vaccine is available. This is a different vaccine than chickenpox vaccine. CDC recommends that people over 60 years old get the shingles vaccine to prevent shingles or PHN.

References

Centers for Disease Control and Prevention. (2014). *Shingles (Herpes Zoster).* Retrieved from http://www.cdc.gov/shingles/index.html

Centers for Disease Control and Prevention. (2015). *Shingles vaccination: What everyone should know.* Retrieved from http://www.cdc.gov/vaccine/vpd-vac/shingles/vacc-need-know.htm

Hockenberry, M., Baker, R., & Mondozzi, M. (2013). The child with integumentary dysfunction. In M. Hockenberry (Ed.), *Wong's Essentials of Pediatric Nursing,* (9th Ed). (p. 1019). St. Louis, MO: Elsevier/Mosby

Levy, D., Zieve, D., & Ogilvie, I. (2015). *Shingles.* Retrieved from https://www.nim.nih.gov/medlineplus/ency/article/000858.htm

McCarthy, K. (2013). Health problems of toddlers and preschoolers. In M. Hockenberry (Ed.), *Wong's Essentials of Pediatric Nursing,* (9th Ed). (p. 431). St. Louis, MO: Elsevier/Mosby

Medline Plus. (2015). *Shingles.* Retrieved from https://www.nim.nih.gov/medlineplus/shingles.html

SICKLE CELL DISEASE

DEFINITION/ETIOLOGY:

Sickle cell disease (SCD) is a hereditary disorder present at birth that affects the red blood cells. Symptoms appear around 5 months of age. The term *sickle cell disease* refers to a group of genetic disorders where Hemoglobin S is more prevalent than the normal Hemoglobin A in the blood. The red blood cells take on a sickle shape, become sticky and hard, and fail to function well. The sickle cells die early causing chronic anemia. As they travel through small blood vessels, they often get stuck due to their sticky composition. The blocked flow of blood is called vaso-occlusive crisis (VOC). If the student develops a fever, dehydration or a decreased oxygen level, the sickling will become enhanced. A trauma or infection (viral or bacterial) may precipitate a sickle cell episode.

There are several types of sickle cell disease but the most severe form is sickle cell anemia and when the sickle cell gene is inherited from both parents.

Sickle cell disease is most common among those of African descent but also affects children from Central America, the Mediterranean, South America, and the Caribbean. It rarely affects white children.

SIGNS AND SYMPTOMS:
- Hand and foot syndrome, swelling of the hands and feet (may be the first sign)
- Pain episode or "crisis" caused by the sickle cells obstructing the circulation (the hallmark sign). Pain may be severe and include joint pain, chest pain, headache, abdominal pain, nausea or vomiting
- Frequently occurring infections
- Anemia
  - Fatigue
  - Pallor
  - Tachycardia
  - Delayed growth
  - Irritability
- Mild jaundice
- Leg ulcers
- Vision loss
- Hematuria

SICKLE CELL DISEASE (continued from previous page)

MANAGEMENT/TREATMENT:

1. Treatment measures for the pain crisis should include prevention of an episode with plenty of fluids, avoiding hot and cold temperatures, avoiding high altitudes or extreme exercising.
2. Pain management with strong narcotic analgesics may be necessary to provide relief during an acute episode.
3. Fluid therapy is initiated during a crisis to restore circulating blood volume.
4. At the first sign of an infection, it is important for children to see a healthcare provider.
5. Prophylactic antibiotics are often given to prevent infection.
6. Blood transfusions are sometimes needed for severe anemia.
7. During the school day, the child should receive extra fluids and rest periods during times of physical activity.
8. Monitor immunization status. Refer to healthcare provider as necessary to ensure that student is up-to-date on vaccine preventable diseases.
9. Children who have experienced splenic sequestration may subsequently have an elective splenectomy.

POTENTIAL COMPLICATIONS

- Impaired growth and development.
- Acute Splenic Sequestration: Because the sickle cells are trapped, a large amount of blood accumulates in the spleen. This usually occurs in the young child as the spleen commonly stops functioning in early childhood.
- Aplastic Crisis: Episodes of bone marrow suppression that cause the red blood cell production to be decreased. Often occurs after a viral or bacterial infection including *parvovirus B19*.
- High risk for sepsis, meningitis, pneumonia, and other severe infections.
- Possible damage to internal organs.
- Acute chest syndrome: Similar to pneumonia with sudden onset of chest pain, difficulty breathing and fever. It should be treated in the hospital. Occurs most often in children.
- Cerebral stroke: Can occur in 10% of children with SCD due to the clogged blood flow to the brain.
- Pulmonary emboli/Deep vein thrombosis: Sickling of the red blood cells increases the risk of forming blood clots.
- Priapism – painful erection of the penis - occurs most often in young men.

SICKLE CELL DISEASE (continued from previous page)

FOLLOW UP:

- The child with SCD should be managed by an interdisciplinary medical team with ongoing maintenance and regular visits to the healthcare provider.

NOTES:

- Newborn screening for sickle cell is mandated in the United States. All infants should undergo testing between 24 and 72 hours of age. If sickle cell is suspected in an older child, hemoglobin electrophoresis is used to confirm the diagnosis.
- Children with SCD should have their eyes examined yearly to check for retinal damages.
- The school nurse can assist the child and family by providing information to the staff about the child and the condition. The staff should be aware of the need for prompt medical care in the event of a "crisis" or infection.
- An Individualized Healthcare Plan (IHP) should be developed for the child with sickle cell disease.

References

Bowden, V. Greenberb, C. (Eds.). (2014). The child with altered hematologic status. In *Children and their families: The continuum of care (3rd ed.)* (pp. 1172-1227). Philadelphia, PA: Lippincott Williams and Wilkins.

Cosby, M.F., Miller, N.B., & Youngman, K. (2013). Acute measures for emergent problems. In J. Selekman (Ed.), School *nursing: A comprehensive text (2ⁿᵈ ed.)* (pp. 548-549). Philadelphia, PA: F.A. Davis.

Centers for Disease Control and Prevention (CDC), National Center for Infectious Diseases. (2015). Sickle *cell disease (SCD)*. Retrieved from http://www.cdc.gov/ncbddd/sicklecell/treatments.html

Merck Manual. (2013). Sickle cell disease. Retrieved from http://www.merckmanuals.com/professional/hematology-and-oncology/anemias-caused-by-hemolysis/sickle-cell-disease

Selekman, J., Bochenek, J. & Lukens, M. (2013). Children with chronic conditions. In J. Selekman (Ed.), School *nursing: A comprehensive text (2ⁿᵈ ed.)* (pp.734-737). Philadelphia, PA: F.A. Davis.

SINUSITIS

DEFINITION/ETIOLOGY:
Sinusitis is inflammation of the mucous membranes that line the paranasal sinuses, and is commonly referred to as **rhino-sinusitis.**

Acute sinusitis: abrupt onset of infection of one or more of the paranasal sinuses with resolution following therapy usually within 30 days.

Subacute bacterial sinusitis: persistent occurrence of purulent nasal discharge, despite treatment with symptoms lasting less than 3 months.

Chronic sinusitis: episodes of prolonged inflammation or may be repeated acute infection. Clinical symptoms last more than 90 days.

CAUSES:
Predisposing factors for acute bacterial sinusitis:
Any condition that blocks the flow of secretions can lead to sinusitis. Mucous stasis creates a good environment for pathogens to grow.
- 80% associated with acute viral rhino-sinusitis.
- 20% from allergic inflammation.
- Other factors that increase risk of sinusitis include:
  o smoke exposure,
  o swimming,
  o school aged siblings,
  o astroesophageal reflux,
  o cystic fibrosis,
  o immunodeficiency,
  o ciliary dyskinesia, and
  o anatomical abnormalities.
- Sinusitis is more commonly seen in adults or older children.

Common pathogens:
- *Streptococcus pneumoniae* (about 30% of cases)
- *Haemophilus influenzae* (about 20% of cases)
- *Moraxilla catarrhalis* (about 20% of cases)

SINUSITIS *(continued from previous page)*

SIGNS AND SYMPTOMS:
- Cough (worsening at night)
- Fever
- Purulent rhinorrhea (runny nose) usually yellow or green
- Postnasal secretions (purulent drainage)
- Halitosis (bad breath) or loss of smell
- Headache/face pain/toothache
- Head pain with bending over of sudden movements
- Snoring
- Earache
- Nasal speech
- Facial swelling

A clinical diagnosis is generally made after upper respiratory signs and symptoms are present for greater than 10-14 days and with symptoms such as facial swelling, facial pain and fever.

CLASSIFYING SEVERITY:

Mild persistent symptoms: Nasal or postnasal discharge and cough (which may be worse at night); symptoms last longer than 10-14 days,

Severe symptoms include high temperature, at least 102° F (39°C); purulent nasal discharge for at least 3 to 4 consecutive days.

MANAGEMENT/TREATMENT:
1. If student has fever or looks ill, notify parent/guardian(s) and refer to healthcare provider.
2. A cool compress on the forehead may make the student more comfortable.
3. Encourage fluids.
4. Monitor returning students to be sure they complete the antibiotics regimen and for any side effects.
5. If recommended by healthcare provider, normal saline nose drops to assist with drainage and ventilation that can be done both at home and at school.
6. Monitor for complications such as orbital cellulitis, exacerbation of asthma, cavernous sinus thrombosis and optic neuritis.
7. Prevention: avoid allergens and treat allergies when appropriate.

SINUSITIS *(continued from previous page)*

FOLLOW UP:

Because of the close proximity of the paranasal sinuses to the brain, intracranial complications can result and progress rapidly. Symptoms of intracranial complications include acute headache, fever, lethargy, change in mental status, seizure, and coma. Sinus infections are usually curable with medical treatment and self-care measures. Recurrent sinus attacks require follow up with a healthcare provider to assess for underlying causes such as nasal polyps or allergies.

School nurses can help with prevention by encouraging hand washing, use and disposal of tissues and cough etiquette.

NOTES:

Risk factors include:

    1) attendance at day care,

    2) antimicrobial treatment within past 90 days, and

    3) under 2 years of age.

References

Drtbalu's otolaryngology. (n.d.) . *CNS complications of frontal sinusitis*. Retrieved from https://sites.google.com/site/drtbalusotolaryngology/rhinology/cns-complications-of-frontal-sinusitis

Hogate, S., Giel, J. & Selekman, J. (2013). Allergy. In J. Selekman (Ed.), *School nursing: A comprehensive text (2nd ed.)*(p. 798). Philadelphia, PA: F.A. Davis.

Pappas, D., Hendley, O. (2016). Sinusitis. In R.M. Kliegman, B.S. Stanton, J. St. Geme, & N.F. Schor (Eds.), *Textbook of pediatrics: Expert consult (20th ed.)* (p. 2014-2017). Philadelphia, PA: Elsevier.

Mayo Clinic. (2013). *Chronic sinusitis*. Retrieved from http://www.mayoclinic.com/health/chronic-sinusitis/DS00232

Medline Plus/ U.S. National Library of Medicine. (2014). *Sinusitis*. Retrieved from http://www.nlm.nih.gov/medlineplus/ency/article/000647.htm

SKIN AND SOFT TISSUE INFECTION (Boils, Cellulitis, Lymphangitis, and MRSA)

DEFINITIONS/ETIOLOGY:

Acute infection of the skin and soft tissues (subcutaneous tissue, fascia, and muscles). The infection may occur secondary to a wound, abrasion, bug bite, impetigo, pustule, furuncle and/or carbuncle. Skin and soft tissue infections are classified as uncomplicated or complicated. Uncomplicated skin and soft tissue infections respond well to oral antibiotics and local wound care. Uncomplicated skin infections can become a complicated skin infection. Complicated skin and wound infections do not respond to conventional antibiotic therapy. A complicated skin and wound infection typically involves deeper tissue (subcutaneous tissue, fascia, and/or muscle). Complicated skin infections may require multiple antibiotics and surgical intervention.

Types of skin and soft tissue infections include:

A furuncle (boil) is a skin infection, consisting of a walled off, puss filled mass that is most commonly staph (*S. aureus*), involving the entire hair follicle and the adjacent subcutaneous tissue. They occur most commonly on sites of friction and swelling such as under the belt, groin, armpit, buttocks, and thighs. Some people are afflicted with many, with little success at prevention. Boils can be a small bump to an abscess filled with pus.

Cellulitis – acute infection of skin and soft (subcutaneous) tissue. Cellulitis indicates an acute spreading infection of the dermis and subcutaneous tissues. *Staphylococcal aureus* and *Group A Streptococus* are the most common causes of cellulitis.

Lymphangitis is a bacterial infection in the lymphatic vessels. Most often results from *Group A Streptococus* infection of the skin, less frequently from *Staphylococcal aureus*. Lymphangitis may be an indication that a skin infection is worsening. This should raise concern that bacteria may have spread into the bloodstream which can cause life-threatening problems.

Methicillin-resistant *Staphylococcus aureus* (MRSA) is a type of *staphylococcus aureus* (staph) infection that is resistant to beta-lactams antibiotics (such as methicillin, penicillin, and amoxicillin). MRSA is usually transmitted by direct skin-to-skin contact or contact with shared items or surfaces that have come into contact with someone else's infection (e.g., towels, used bandages). MRSA skin infections can occur anywhere.

SKIN AND SOFT TISSUE INFECTION (Boils, Cellulitis, Lymphangitis, and MRSA)
(continued from previous page)

SIGNS AND SYMPTOMS:

Boils
- Pain, swelling, and redness
- May be about the size of a marble (1-2 cm) or larger
- May be firm or fluctuant
- Redness progresses to yellowish center of pus

Cellulitis
- First appears as a tiny edge of redness encircling a primary lesion.
- Redness spreads in circular fashion, indicating that local body defenses are not limiting the infection. There is pain or tenderness, redness, warmth, and/or swelling at the site.
- The sore or rash (macule) appears suddenly, grows quickly in the first 24 hr., and usually has sharp borders.
- If the infection is around a skin wound, there may be swelling and drainage.
- There may be enlarged lymph nodes near the cellulitis.
- May be seen in children on the face, genital area or involving a joint or an extremity.

Lymphangitis
- Painful, red streak below the skin surface leading away from primary lesion to the axilla or to the groin
- Lymph nodes or red streaks above the area (elbow, axilla, or groin) may be enlarged or painful
- May have chills, fever (100°-104°), and malaise

MRSA
- Abscess, pimple, boil, or area on skin
- Redness/swelling around lesion
- Painful around lesion
- Warm to touch
- Lesion may be full of pus or other drainage
- Fever

SKIN AND SOFT TISSUE INFECTION (Boils, Cellulitis, Lymphangitis, and MRSA)
(continued from previous page)

MANAGEMENT/TREATMENT:

1. Gentle skin cleansing of new wounds.
2. May apply warm, moist compresses to reduce inflammation and discomfort.
3. Refer to healthcare provider.
4. Refer to healthcare provider immediately if circle or redness is 1/2 cm (dime size) or larger, over a joint, or on the face.
5. Antibiotic ointment is not generally considered effective but may help eradicate a carrier state. A healthcare provider may recommend an antibiotic for eradicating nasal carriage of staphylococcus.
6. Lesion may require incision and drainage for healing.
7. To prevent recurrence, the role of good hygiene should be stressed to student and family.
8. Washing with an antibacterial soap may be helpful in the event of frequent episodes.
9. Healthcare provider may prescribe oral antibiotics for the infection and an analgesic for pain.
   - If antibiotic is prescribed, contact healthcare provider if condition worsens or there is no improvement after 3 days on antibiotic.
   - **Cellulitis – if no improvement or condition worsens may need hospitalization and intravenous antibiotic therapy; refer to healthcare provider for immediate follow-up.**
10. **Refer suspected lymphangitis to healthcare provider for emergency care immediately.**
    - Prompt treatment with antibiotics typically result in complete recovery.
11. **Contact healthcare provider immediately if suspect MRSA.**
    - Most MRSA infections are treated with oral antibiotics.
    - May be treated by draining the abscess or boil; this is done by a healthcare professional.
    - If indicated, provide wound care per healthcare provider's orders (may include topical antibiotic).
    - Cover the wound with an appropriate bandage.
    - MRSA infections may reoccur.
      - Prevention steps are necessary to avoid reoccurrence of infection (avoid sharing towels or athletic gear, etc.)

SKIN AND SOFT TISSUE INFECTION (Boils, Cellulitis, Lymphangitis, and MRSA)
(continued from previous page)

FOLLOW UP:
- MONITOR CAREFULLY!
- If antibiotic is prescribed, all doses must be completed unless otherwise directed by the healthcare provider to stop medication.
- MRSA – the decision to close a school for any communicable disease should be made by school officials in consultation with local and/or state public health officials.
  - Generally, students with MRSA should not be excluded from school unless the wound is draining and cannot be covered.
  - In most cases, it is not necessary to close schools because of a MRSA infection in a student.

POTENTIAL COMPLICATIONS:
- Methicillin-resistant *Staphylococcus aureus* (MRSA).
- Lymphangitis (abscess, cellulitis, sepsis)
- Meningitis (if cellulitis is on the face)
- Gangrene
- Sepsis

NOTES:
Prevention
- Keep skin clean and hydrated (use lotions) to prevent cracking.
- Give meticulous attention to cuts and wounds (cleaning, bandaging, and observing for signs of infection).
- Give special attention to foot care (trimming nails and wear properly fitted shoes).
- Wear protective clothing for work and sports.
- MRSA transmission can be prevented by simple habitual measures such as good handwashing hygiene, avoid sharing of personal items, and athletic gear.
- Discuss and monitor preventive measures if student participates in any contact sport, or sports that use mats (gymnastics, wrestling, martial arts).

SKIN AND SOFT TISSUE INFECTION (Boils, Cellulitis, Lymphangitis, and MRSA)
(continued from previous page)

References

American Academy of Pediatrics, Committee on Infectious Diseases. (2015). Staphylococcal infections. In D.W. Kimberlin, M. T. Brady, M.A. Jackson, & S.S. Long (Eds.), *Red Book: 2015 report of the committee on infectious diseases* (30th ed.) (pp. 715-732). Elk Grove Village, IL:

Center for Disease Control. (2015). *Methicillin-resistant* Staphylococcus Aureus *(MRSA) infections.* Retrieved from http://www.cdc.gov/mrsa/

Mayo Clinic. (2015). *Cellulitis.* Retrieved from http://www.mayoclinic.com/print/cellulitis/DS00450/DSECTION=all&METHOD=print

Medline Plus. U.S. National Library of Medicine. (2014). *Boils.* Retrieved from http://www.nlm.nih.gov/medlineplus/ency/article/001474.htm

Merck Manual. (2013a). *Cellulitis.* Retrieved from http://www.merckmanuals.com/professional/dermatologic_disorders/bacterial_skin_infections/cellulitis.html?qt=mrsa&alt=sh

Merck Manual. (2013b). *Overview of bacterial infections.* Retrieved from http://www.merckmanuals.com/professional/dermatologic_disorders/bacterial_skin_infections/overview_of_bacterial_skin_infections.html

Morelli, J.G., & Prok, L.D. (2014). Skin. In W. Hay, M. Levin, R. Deterding, & M. Abzug (Eds.), *Current diagnosis and treatment pediatrics* (22nd edition) (pp. 426-446). McGraw Hill Education, Inc.

Ross, L. & Graham, M. (2013). Skin disorders. In J. Selekman (Ed.), *School nursing: A comprehensive text* (2nd ed.) (pp. 578-697). Philadelphia, PA: F. A. Davis.

Singhal, H. (2014). *Skin and soft tissue infections - incision, drainage, and debridement.* Retrieved from http://dx.doi.org.proxy1.cl.msu.edu/10.3928/00904481-20111209-07 pediatric annals

SORE THROAT (PHARYNGITIS) (including Streptococcal Infection)

DEFINITION/ETIOLOGY:
Pharyngitis is defined as inflammation of the pharynx and the surrounding lymph tissue which is often caused by a viral (influenza or common cold) or bacterial (streptococcus) infection, and/or non- infectious causes such as an irritation (air pollution, allergens, sinus drainage). The most common causes are viruses that cause upper respiratory infections. The viruses are spread by oral and respiratory secretions and occur more commonly in fall, winter or spring.

SIGNS AND SYMPTOMS OF VIRAL PHARYNGITIS:
- Dry, scratchy throat
- Complaints of pain with swallowing
- Frequent swallowing and sniffing (from sinus drainage)
- Presence/absence of fever and signs of systemic illness
- Appearance of tonsils and tympanic membrane
- Irritability in the younger child
- Increased drooling
- Symptoms associated with the common cold such as runny nose , cough, and congestion

SIGNS AND SYPMTOMS OF STREP THROAT:
"Strep" throat is due to *Group A Streptococcus*.
- Sudden onset of sore throat
- Fever (often > 101°F)
- Headache, nausea, abdominal pain, occasionally vomiting
- Marked inflammation of throat and tonsils; bright red tonsils may have thin white exudate
- Petechiae on the soft palate and posterior pharynx
- Initially a white swollen tongue which may progress to a "strawberry tongue"
- Enlarged cervical lymph nodes
- Absence of diarrhea or coryza, cough, and conjunctivitis
- Does not usually result in a cough or runny nose

341

SORE THROAT (PHARYNGITIS) (including Streptococcal Infection)
(continued from previous page)

Scarlet Fever is a vascular response usually associated with streptococcal pharyngitis.

UNIQUE FINDINGS OF SCARLET FEVER:
- Diffuse redness of cheeks and upper chest on "goose flesh" skin, the sensation of fine sandpaper.
- The rash spreads and, in 5-10 days, skin peels. Most cases are mild, lasting a few days, but severe cases occur.
- Two major complications: acute rheumatic fever (joints, heart) occurs in 1% of Group A strep cases, and acute self-limiting glomerulonephritis (kidney disease) can be serious.

Primary oral herpes simplex virus may cause a sore throat due to the presence of ulcerating vesicles throughout the anterior pharynx and the lips. High fever and difficulty taking fluids are common and may last up to 14 days.

MANAGEMENT/TREATMENT OF MINOR, VIRAL, AFEBRILE SORE THROAT:
1. Warm, salty (1/2 teaspoon to 1 glass water) gargles
2. Warm fluids (broth; hot water with melted lemon drop or warm lemonade)
3. Over-the-counter lozenges (some do not advise lozenges or drops at school for safety reasons)
4. Analgesics such as Tylenol® or Advil®
5. May attend school if feeling well enough unless other exclusion criteria are present such as fever

MANAGEMENT/TREATMENT (Streptococcal Infection):
1. Refer for diagnosis by rapid strep test and culture. Some school clinics are equipped to provide the rapid strep test. If positive, it confirms Group A strep infection. If the test result is negative, a regular culture (read in 12-24 hours) is still required to rule out strep, so many prefer to refer all suspected cases directly.
2. Encourage adequate fluid to keep mucus thin.
3. Treatment of choice is penicillin; untreated cases (milder sore throat, low fever) treated symptomatically risk complications. Treatment is aimed at preventing complications such as Rheumatic fever.
4. Return to school after 24 hours on antibiotic treatment and fever-free. For many children, 3-5 days absence may occur.
5. Treatment of scarlet fever is no different from the treatment of streptococcal infection.

SORE THROAT (PHARYNGITIS) (including Streptococcal Infection)
(continued from previous page)

FOLLOW-UP (Strep and Scarlet Fever):
- Monitor for a completed course of antibiotic therapy to prevent complications and carrier state.
- Encourage student to replace toothbrush.
- Monitor for complications (high fever, joint pain, blood in the urine) and refer immediately.

POTENTIAL COMPLICATIONS:
- Ear infection
- Glomerulonephritis
- Rheumatic fever
- Sinusitis
- Tonsillitis
- Peritonsillar abscess

NOTE:
Avoid giving aspirin under the age of eighteen. Aspirin can play a role in causing Reye's Syndrome.

References

American Academy of Pediatrics. (2013). Strep throat (streptococcal pharyngitis). In S. Aronson, & T. Shope (Eds.), *Managing infectious diseases in child care and schools (2nd ed.)* (pp. 157-158). Elk Grove Village, IL: American Academy of Pediatrics.

Mayo Clinic. (2013). *Sore throat.* http://www.mayoclinic.com/health/sore-throat/DS00526

Medline Plus, U.S. National Library of Medicine. (2015). *Sore throat.* Retrieved from http://www.nlm.nih.gov/medlineplus/sorethroat.html

John, R. & Chewey, L. (2013). Common complaints. In J. Selekman (Ed.), *School nursing: A comprehensive text* (2nd ed.) (pp. 578-640). Philadelphia, PA: F.A. Davis.

Tanz, R. (2015). *Acute pharyngitis.* In R.M. Kliegman, B.F. Stanton, J.W. St. Geme, & N.F. Schor *(Eds.), Nelson textbook of pediatrics* (20th ed.) (p.p. *2017-2021* (2017). Philadelphia, PA: Elsevier Saunders.

SPIDER BITE (Brown Recluse, Black Widow, and Hobo)

DEFINITION/ETIOLOGY:

Brown Recluse spider bites produce poisonous venom that contains both a toxin and an enzyme that spreads the toxin through tissue. Ten species, six of which are poisonous, live in the United States. The spiders are non-hairy, yellowish-tan to dark brown, and have a violin pattern on their back. They prefer dark, dry spaces (under porches, attic, closet, woodpiles). They are not aggressive but bite defensively.

Black Widow spiders produce potent, protein venom that attacks the central nervous system. The Southern species are about ½-inch long, shiny, black, globular shape with distinctive red hourglass shape on the underside. The Northern species have a row of red spots down the middle of the upper surface of the abdomen and two cross bars on the underside. The Black Widow spider is nocturnal, prefers dark corners and crevices, and bites defensively.

Hobo spider bites may go unnoticed until a moderate to severe, slow healing wound develops. Hobo spiders do not have banded legs and have distinct, yellow markings on their under-belly. The Hobo builds funnel shaped webs in which to trap their prey and are found outdoors and indoors around structural areas, stacked materials and storage areas. The Hobo spider, unlike other spiders, does not climb, but they are fast runners. Threatened or provoked they are likely to attack. Hobo spiders are found throughout the Pacific Northwest.

SIGNS AND SYMPTOMS:

General signs and symptoms:
- A mark indicating a bite
- Pain in bite area
- Nausea and vomiting
- Chills or fever
- Itching or rash
- Muscle pain or cramping
- Reddish to purplish color or blister
- Increased sweating
- Difficulty breathing
- Headache
- Anxiety or restlessness

> These symptoms are also indicative of other health concerns. Diagnosis is based on history and physical signs. Spider bites and the identification of the type of spider are difficult to confirm because they usually not witnessed.

SPIDER BITE (Brown Recluse, Black Widow, and Hobo) *(continued from previous page)*

Brown Recluse
- Immediate local stinging or burning pain that may become severe after 4 hours.
- Initially, the lesion is red and swollen or blanched, and may develop a blue-gray halo around the puncture (due to hemolysis and vasospasm). The lesion may change to bluish pustules or large blistering surrounded by purpura discoloration.
- Within 12 hours, fever, chills, nausea/vomiting, scarlatiniform rash, arthralgia, diarrhea and weakness may develop. Renal failure, hemoglobinuria and shock coagulation rarely occur in children.
- Centrally, necrosis or a "sinking center" develops. The ulcer may take weeks to months to heal.

Black Widow
- Symptomatic within 20 minutes to 1 hour after bite.
- Localized to generalized severe muscle cramps, abdominal pain, weakness, and tremor may occur.
- Nausea and vomiting, dizziness, chest pain, and respiratory difficulty may follow.

Hobo
- Symptoms can be mild to severe.
- The bite may go unnoticed; however, a moderate to severe, slow healing wound will appear.
- Localized to general itching, rash, pain radiating from the site, muscle pain or cramping, and redness to purple tinge at the site may occur.
- Sweating, difficulty breathing, headache, nausea and vomiting, fever, chills, anxiety and restlessness, and elevated blood pressure may follow.

MANAGEMENT/TREATMENT:
General
- Clean the wound with mild soap and water.
- Apply ice and elevate.
- OTC analgesics for pain management.
- Seek emergency medical attention.

SPIDER BITE (Brown Recluse, Black Widow, and Hobo) *(continued from previous page)*

Brown Recluse
1. Ask about description of spider and presence of general reaction symptoms.
2. Apply ice, elevate, and seek immediate medical attention.
3. Immobilize affected area and avoid vigorous activity.
4. OTC analgesics for pain management.
5. Primary healthcare provider may begin antibiotic therapy.

Black Widow
1. Ask about description of spider and presence of general reaction symptoms.
2. Apply ice, elevate, and seek *emergency* medical attention.
3. Immobilize affected area and avoid vigorous activity.

Hobo
1. Ask about description of spider and presence of general reaction symptoms.
2. Wash area with soap and water.
3. Apply cold compress or ice (covered) to site.
4. Elevate affected area.
5. DO NOT attempt to remove venom.
6. Seek immediate medical attention.

FOLLOW UP:
- Re-assess in 48 hours; may need referral for debridement.
- Continue to monitor. Wound may need skin grafting.
- Educate regarding poisonous spider recognition:
  Brown Recluse: About one inch long, non-hairy, yellowish-tan to dark brown, and have a violin pattern on their back. They prefer dark, dry spaces (under porches, attic, closet, woodpiles. They are not aggressive but bite defensively.

  Black Widow: The Southern species are about ½-inch long, shiny, black, globular shape with distinctive red hourglass shape on the underside. The Northern species have a row of red spots down the middle of the upper surface of the abdomen and 2 cross bars on the underside. The Black Widow spider is nocturnal, prefers dark corners and crevices, and bites defensively.

SPIDER BITE (Brown Recluse, Black Widow, and Hobo) *(continued from previous page)*

FOLLOW UP: *(continued)*

<u>Hobo</u>: Hobo spiders do not have banded legs and have distinct, yellow markings on their under-belly. The Hobo builds funnel shaped webs in which to trap their prey and therefore are found outdoors and indoors around structural areas, stacked materials and storage areas. Hobo spiders do not climb, but they are fast runners. Threatened or provoked they are likely to attack. Hobo spiders are found throughout the Pacific Northwest.

Healthcare provider may recommend a tetanus booster if needed.

References

American Red Cross. (2012). Bites and stings. In *Responding to emergencies: Comprehensive first aid/CPR/AED* (p.p. 321-324). USA: Krames Staywell Strategic Partnerships Division.

Balentine, J. R. (2015). *Black widow spider bite*. E Medicine Health. Retrieved from http://www.emedicinehealth.com/black_widow_spider_bite/article_em.htm

Balentine, J. R. (2014a). *Brown recluse spider bite*. E medicine Health Retrieved from http://www.emedicinehealth.com/spider_bite_brown_recluse_spider_bite/article_em.htm

Balentine, J. R. (2014b.). *Spider bite: Brown recluse spider bite*. Retrieved from http://www.emedicinehealth.com/spider_bite_brown_recluse_spider_bite/page11_em.htm#pictures_of_brown_recluse_spiders

Centers for Disease Control. *(2015). NIOSH safety and health topic: Venomous spiders*. Retrieved from http://www.cdc.gov/niosh/topics/spiders/

Mayo Clinic. (2015). *Spider bites: First aid*. Retrieved from http://www.mayoclinic.com/health/first-aid-spider-bites/FA00048

Medline Plus, U.S. National Library of Medicine. (2013). *Brown recluse spider*. Retrieved from http://www.nlm.nih.gov/medlineplus/ency/article/002859.htm

Merck Manual, Professional Edition. *Spider bites*. (2014). Retrieved from http://www.merckmanuals.com/professional/injuries_poisoning/bites_and_stings/spider_bites.html?qt=spider%20bites&alt=sh

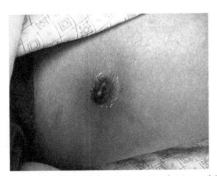

Brown Recluse Spider Bite – Merck Manual 2014

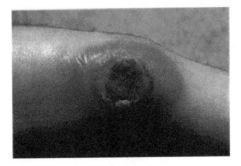

Hobo Spider Bite – Badspiderbite.com

SPRAIN AND STRAINS

DEFINITION:
A sprain is a stretched or torn ligament (fibrous tissue that connects bones to other bones). The injury can range from a stretch to a tiny tear to a complete severing of the ligament. They are often a common athletic injury of children. A strain results from pulling or overexerting a muscle or tendon (tough band of fibrous connective tissue that connects muscle to bone). Of all sprains, ankle and knee sprains occur most often.

SIGNS AND SYMPTOMS:
- History of trauma (for example, person steps down on the outside of the foot and twists the foot)
- During trauma, persons may feel a flash of heat or may describe hearing a "snap" or "pop"
- History of prior injury to same joint
- Pain/tenderness at site of injury
- Variable swelling, and/or bruising
- Limited ability to move affected part

MANAGEMENT/TREATMENT:
1. Take careful detailed history of injury, including what happened, what person felt, what person heard.
2. Follow standard precautions (infection prevention practices).
3. Assess pulse quality and capillary refill below the injured site.
4. Check range of motion and sensation (compare with corresponding area on opposite extremity).
5. Control bleeding, if necessary.
6. Avoid any movements or changes in position that cause pain.
7. Immobilize injured area.
8. Clean and bandage any open wounds.
9. Check for circulation, movement and sensation to the limb. Feel for the patient's distal pulse, skin temperature and ability to move and detect touch in the injured parts.

SPRAIN AND STRAINS *(continued from previous page)*

MANAGEMENT/TREATMENT *(continued)*

10. Institute RICE principle:

<u>R</u>est of the injured area for 48 hours	• Weight bearing may increase injury. If uncomfortable to walk, use crutches. • Review safe crutch walking technique. • Get permit to use elevator (if any). • If hall traffic is unmanageable on crutches, get permit to leave class a few minutes early. • Arrange for help to carry books.
<u>I</u>ce placed on the injured area for 20 minutes every 2 -3 hours while awake for first 24 hours	Ice cubes or frozen wet sponges can be placed in a plastic bag, wrapped in a light cloth, and applied to the painful area. Remove compression bandage while using ice.
<u>C</u>ompression with elastic bandages or if authorized, splints	• A pressure bandage may reduce swelling. Use a compression bandage, especially when the ankle is not elevated while crutch walking. • A 3" elastic ACE wrap is generally used. A more convenient material is elastic tubular bandage, a surgical dressing available from a medical or athletic supply store.
<u>E</u>levate injured part	Keep the foot higher than the hip when not mobile at least 24 hours following injury.

WHEN TO REFER TO HEALTHCARE PROVIDER:
- All injuries associated with severe pain or immediate swelling /or injured area is misshapen (may indicate fracture)
- If there are signs that circulation beyond the injured area is impaired
- Inability to bear weight
- All suspected fractures

SPRAIN AND STRAINS *(continued from previous page)*

FOLLOW UP:
- Monitor for blood flow above and below injured area; if a splint/wrap/cast has been applied, watch fingers and toes for cyanosis and coldness.
- For mild to moderate pain, a non-steroidal anti-inflammatory analgesic (ibuprofen) taken with food to limit stomach upset may be administered (if medically approved or with parent/guardian approval and per policy).
- Range of Motion (ROM) or physical therapy to retain full use of injured part.
- Advise student to not engage in physical activity until pain has subsided.

POTENTIAL COMPLICATIONS:
- Swelling may decrease blood flow to area below sprain.
- Unrecognized and inappropriately managed injury can lead to more long-term functional disability.

NOTES:
Once an ankle has been sprained, it may be susceptible to recurring sprains because of instability in the joint. The following suggestions to avoid re-injury:

- Avoid activities (exercising or sports) when tired or in pain.
- Use correctly fitted shoes and equipment.
- Warm-up and stretch before participating in exercises or sports.

References

American National Red Cross. (2011). Muscle, bone and joint injuries. Responding to Emergencies: Comprehensive First Aid/CPR/AED e-Textbook. Published online: American National Red Cross.

Mayo Clinic. (2015). *Sprains and strains*. Retrieved from http://www.mayoclinic.org/diseases-conditions/sprains-and-strains/basics/definition/con-20020958

Mayo Clinic. (2015). *Sprain: First aid*. Retrieved from http://www.mayoclinic.org/first-aid/first-aid-sprain/basics/art-20056622

Campagne, D. (2014). Overview of fractures, dislocations, and sprains. Retrieved from http://www.merckmanuals.com/professional/injuries-poisoning/fractures-dislocations-and-sprains/overview-of-fractures-dislocations-and-sprains?qt=sprains&alt=sh

Sailing, J. (2014). *Ankle injuries: Causes and treatment*. Retrieved from http://www.webmd.com/fitness-exercise/ankle-injuries-causes-and-treatments

STOMATITIS (ORAL LESION)

DEFINITION/ETIOLOGY:

Stomatitis is an inflammation of the oral mucous membrane. Lesions can occur anywhere in the mouth including the cheeks, gums, soft and hard palate, and on the tongue and lips. Oral lesions may be caused by trauma; viral, bacterial or fungal infections; poor dental hygiene; and chewing (smokeless) tobacco. Mouth sores may also occur after dental work, with braces or from accidental biting of the inside of the mouth. Certain autoimmune diseases such as Crohn's disease can affect the mucous membranes of the mouth. Mouth ulcers are also a common side effect of chemotherapy.

SIGNS AND SYMPTOMS:

Symptoms are dependent on the etiology of the oral lesion. General symptoms include:
- Oral ulcers
- Pain in the mouth

TYPE	SYMPTOMS
Aphthous Ulcer (canker sore)	• Small, oval, indurated papules with surrounding redness and a white, gray or yellow center • Often preceded by a "burning" sensation that progresses into an ulcer with surrounding redness • Usually a single lesion but may occur in a cluster of 4-5 • May experience enlarged lymph nodes
Herpes simplex virus (cold sore, fever blister)	• Vesicular lesion • Lesions are generally located on or around the outer lips • Sore crust over with scab
Oral candidiasis (thrush) – fungal (yeast) infection that occurs when there is overgrowth of Candida. Thrush may occur after a course of antibiotics or in immunocompromised individuals. Typically not seen in healthy youth.	• White patches on tongue and oral mucous membrane • Lesions may bleed when gently scraped

STOMATITIS *(continued from previous page)*

MANAGEMENT/TREATMENT:
- Do not exclude from school since the condition is not considered contagious.
- Treatment is focused on relieving symptoms.
- Rinse with salt water.
- Avoid irritating foods/liquids (spicy, salty or acidic).
- Advise careful tooth brushing to avoid the lesion(s).

FOLLOW UP:
Oral lesions may be an indication of a compromised immune system.
- Refer to healthcare provider if oral lesions are not healed in 2-3 weeks or if lesions are severe.
- Healthcare provider may consider performing a biopsy on a lesion that does not heal properly.

POTENTIAL COMPLICATIONS:
- Dehydration – encourage non-acidic fluids
- Oral cellulitis – secondary from bacterial infection
- Oral cancer

NOTES:
- If prone to mouth sores, avoid acidic and/or spicy foods.
- Practice good oral hygiene. Brush teeth (with soft bristle toothbrush) after meals/ bedtime and floss daily; change toothbrush at least 2 times per year.
- Ulcers in the mouth occur with some childhood infections including:
  - Hand, foot and mouth disease
  - Herpangina (typically caused by Coxsackie group A virus)

352

STOMATITIS *(continued from previous page)*

NOTES: *(continued)*
- Sexually Transmitted Diseases
  - Syphilis chancres may be present with primary syphilis.
  - Syphilis and Gonorrhea can also be transmitted during oral sex.
    Syphilis
    - Lesion is located at point of syphilis entry
    - Syphilis ulcer is firm, round and painless
    - Syphilis lesion may last 3-6 weeks
    Oral gonorrhea (rare) may have redness and/or ulcerative lesions on gingiva and tongue.
    - Inquire about history of engaging in oral sex
    - Refer to healthcare provider for appropriate treatment
    - Depending on school district policy – consider educating adolescent on appropriate barrier protection

References

Centers for Disease Control and Prevention (CDC). (2015). *Syphilis – CDC fact sheet*. Retrieved from http://www.cdc.gov/std/syphilis/STDFact-Syphilis.htm

John, R. & Chewey, L. (2013). Common complaints. In J. Selekman (Ed.), *School nursing: A comprehensive text* (2nd ed.) (pp. 578-640). Philadelphia, PA: F. A. Davis.

Mayo Clinic. (2015). *Canker sore*. Retrieved from http://www.mayoclinic.com/health/canker-sore/DS00354

Mayo Clinic. (2014). *Crohn's disease*. Retrieved from http://www.mayoclinic.com/health/crohns-disease/DS00104

Medline Plus, U.S. National Library of Medicine. (2014). *Canker sore*. Retrieved from http://www.nlm.nih.gov/medlineplus/ency/article/000998.htm

Medline Plus, U.S. National Library of Medicine. (2015). *Mouth ulcers*. Retrieved from http://www.nlm.nih.gov/medlineplus/ency/article/001448.htm

Merck Manual. (2014). *Stomatitis*. Retrieved from http://www.merckmanuals.com/professional/dental_disorders/symptoms_of_dental_and_oral_disorders/stomatitis.html?qt=oral%20lesions&alt=sh

WebMD. (2014). *Stomatitis*. Retrieved from http://www.webmd.com/oral-health/guide/stomatitis-causes-treatment

STRESS DISORDER, POST-TRAUMATIC

DEFINITION /ETIOLOGY:
Stress is the body's reaction to a change that requires a physical, mental, or emotional adjustment or response to a stressor. Stress includes cognitive, emotional, behavioral, and somatic symptoms due to intense fear or feelings of helplessness. Most reactions are normal responses to a serious event.

Post-traumatic disorder (PTSD):
If symptoms and behavioral problems associated with acute stress disorder continue for more than a month, and if these characteristics are associated with functional impairment or significant distress to the sufferer, the diagnosis is changed to post-traumatic stress disorder (PTSD). Symptoms of PTSD typically begin within 3 months of the traumatic incident but may not occur until years after the event.

An individual child's response to a tragedy or disaster is related to age and development, parent or guardians' responses, separation from parent or guardian(s) or peers, and disruption of routines. The severity of anxiety is usually related to proximity to the event, significant losses, and changes in lifestyle and relationships.

CAUSES:
Personal life event (death of a parent or close family member or friend; physical, emotional or sexual abuse; physical or sexual assault; fire), sudden natural disaster (e.g., tornado, hurricane, earthquake or flood) or extreme life-threatening event such as war or a terrorist event.

SIGNS AND SYMPTOMS:
Symptoms vary from person to person. General signs and symptoms associated with PTSD include:
- Intrusive memories – flashbacks (reliving the traumatic event); upsetting dreams about the disturbing event
- Avoidance and numbing – tries to avoid talking or thinking about the event, feels helpless or hopeless, avoids activities that they once enjoyed, avoids to the point of developing a phobia of person or place that reminds them of the traumatic incident
- Increased anxiety – easily startled or frightened, difficulty sleeping, irritability, anger, has trouble concentrating, focusing, guilt, shame surrounding the event

STRESS DISORDER/POST-TRAUMATIC *(continued from previous page)*

Common somatic symptoms often reported by those experiencing extreme stress include:
- Sleep disturbances
- Muscle tension
- Headache
- Gastrointestinal disturbances
- Fatigue

Preschoolers and young elementary children use "magical thinking" to explain the event. Responses may include:
- Crying or sadness
- Confusion, regression to toddler behaviors (thumb sucking, clinging, enuresis)
- Sleep disorder
- Hyperactivity or withdrawal from everyday activities
- May act out traumatic event during play

Adolescents – responses to stress may include:
- Irritable or moody
- Difficulty sleeping
- Changes in eating patterns
- Anxiety, depression
- Acting out, behavior problems
- Self-destructive behaviors
- Poor school performance, trouble concentrating

MANAGEMENT/TREATMENT:
General management, treatment for stress:
1. Get regular exercise.
2. Encourage student to share thoughts and worries.
3. Encourage student to eat a healthy, balanced diet; drink less caffeine.
4. Utilize relaxation techniques.
5. Encourage adequate sleep.
6. Help student set realistic goals.
7. Encourage student to talk to parent, guardian, school nurse, teacher, friend when they are feeling stressed.
8. Refer to healthcare provider (for possible medication and counseling) if above suggestions do not alleviate student's stress.

STRESS DISORDER/POST-TRAUMATIC *(continued from previous page)*

MANAGEMENT/TREATMENT *(continued)*

PTSD treatment includes:

1. **Medication** – antidepressants can help symptoms of depression and anxiety, help improve sleep problems, and improve concentration. Anti-anxiety medications also can improve feelings of anxiety and stress.

2. **Psychotherapy**
   - Cognitive therapy – helps person identify and change self-destructive thoughts
   - Exposure therapy – behavioral therapy technique that safely confronts the stressor that the person finds upsetting or disturbing so that they can learn to cope effectively

3. **Crisis Management**
   - The child must perceive the environment as safe.
   - Implement a crisis plan at school to deal with student tragedies or natural disasters; create mock drills so school will be familiar with plan.
   - After a crisis, restore contact with parent as soon as possible; for adolescents contact with close friends is equally important during a crisis.
   - Provide simple, honest explanations to correct distorted perceptions of what occurred.
   - Re-establish routines as soon as possible.
   - Help the child gain control of fear by choosing how to express the event in role-play, pictures and games.
   - Facilitate group activities to help children tell their stories (disasters, school tragedy).
   - Class projects related to the event or disaster may help children take control of information (cognitive coping) and recognize that their feelings are normal and shared.

FOLLOW UP:
- Monitor students for side effects from prescribed medications.
- Professional intervention is indicated when reactions interfere with usual daily activities:
  - Continuing sleep disturbance
  - Prolonged separation anxiety or clinging
  - Fears about stimuli that remind the child of the event
  - Acting out behaviors
  - Withdrawal and expressions of declining self-worth

STRESS DISORDER/POST-TRAUMATIC *(continued from previous page)*

POTENTIAL COMPLICATIONS:
- Increased vulnerability to infections
- Increased risk of accidents
- Self-destructive behaviors
- Eating disorders
- Substance or alcohol abuse
- Suicide

NOTES:
- In disasters, include children in efforts to help others more affected; helping others assists the child in regaining a sense of normalcy.

References

Cory, A., & Jovanovic, J. (2013). The student's family. In J. Selekman (Ed.), *School nursing: A comprehensive text* (2nd ed.) (pp. 383-406). Philadelphia, PA: F.A. Davis Company.

Mayo Clinic. (2014). *Post traumatic stress disorder.* Retrieved from http://www.mayoclinic.com/health/post-traumatic-stress-disorder/DS00246/DSECTION=symptoms

Medline Plus. (2014). *Post traumatic stress disorder.* Retrieved from https://www.nlm.nih.gov/medlineplus/posttraumaticstressdisorder.html

Merck Manual. (2014). *Anxiety disorders in children and adolescents.* Retrieved from http://www.merckmanuals.com/professional/pediatrics/mental_disorders_in_children_and_adolescents/anxiety_disorders_in_children_and_adolescents.html?qt=post%20traumatic%20stress%20disorder&alt=sh

National Institute of Mental Health. (2013). *Post-traumatic stress disorder (PTSD).* Retrieved from http://www.nimh.nih.gov/health/topics/post-traumatic-stress-disorder-ptsd/index.shtml

STY or STYE (Hordeolum and Chalazion)

DEFINITION/ETIOLGY:

A **hordeolum** is a sudden onset, localized, staphylococcal infection of the eyelash follicle at the margin of the eyelid, or associated sebaceous or sweat gland. A **chalazion** is an inflammatory/noninfectious nodule due to an occluded meibomian gland duct. The nodule localizes to an eyelid margin. With time, a chalazion becomes a small non-tender nodule in the eyelid center. Both conditions initially cause eyelid hyperemia and edema, and swelling. Both improve spontaneously.

SIGNS AND SYMPTOMS:

Hordeolum

- Tiny abscess (0.5-1.0 mm) on edge of eyelid
- Slight redness around abscess (may look like a pimple or boil)
- Local tenderness/pain over the affected area
- Eyelid swelling (this may make it difficult to see because eyelid can't open fully)
- Usually filled with pus
- Tearing
- Crusting around eyelids

Chalazion

- Hard, non-tender nodule
- If infected, there is painfully swollen eyelid

MANAGEMENT/TREATMENT:

Hordeolum

- Warm, moist compresses
- Improves spontaneously
- Instill ophthalmic antibiotic drops or ointment if prescribed by healthcare provider.
- DO NOT use bacitracin or other topical ointment
- DO NOT try to open (squeeze) the abscess
- Refer to healthcare provider if no improvement in 2-3 days or if redness or swelling extends beyond eyelid into face
- School exclusion not necessary

STY (STYE) *(continued from previous page)*

Chalazion
- Small chalazion disappears without intervention
- Warm, moist compresses (15-minute duration)
- Healthcare provider may order antibiotic ointment if there is secondary infection

FOLLOW UP:
- Watch for unusual spread; should heal in 3-5 days.
- If infection continues or a hordeolum (cyst) develops, refer to an ophthalmologist.
- Recheck large chalazion in 2-3 weeks for resolution.

POTENTIAL COMPLICATIONS:
- Cross-contamination - avoid rubbing eyes. This can cause development of another sty.
- Seek medical advice if vision is impaired.

NOTES:
Education:
- Encourage frequent hand washing.
- Person should keep hands away from face.
- Avoid wearing eye make-up.
- Do not share cosmetics.
- Discard all used and outdated eye make-up.
- Wash hands thoroughly before handling, cleaning or inserting/removing contact lens.

References

American Academy of Pediatrics. (2013). Sty. In S. Aronson, & T. Shope (Eds.), *Managing infectious diseases in child care and schools* (2nd ed.) (p. 159). Elk Grove Village, IL: American Academy of Pediatrics.

American Academy of Pediatrics, Committee on Infectious Diseases. (2015). Staphylococcal infections. . In D.W. Kimberlin, M. T. Brady, M.A. Jackson, & S.S. Long (Eds.), *Red Book: 2015 report of the committee on infectious diseases* (30th ed.) (pp. 715-731). Elk Grove Village, IL: American Academy of Pediatrics.

Children's Hospital of Boston. (n.d.). *Stye (hordeolum).* Retrieved from http://www.childrenshospital.org/conditions-and-treatments/conditions/stye-hordeolum

The Merck Manual. (2014). *Chalazion & hordeolum (stye).* Retrieved from http://www.merckmanuals.com/professional/eye-disorders/eyelid-and-lacrimal-disorders/chalazion-and-hordeolum-stye

Mayo Clinic. (2015). *Sty.* Retrieved from http://www.mayoclinic.com/health/sty/DS00257

SUBSTANCE ABUSE

DEFINITION/ETIOLOGY:

The use of illegal substances or the misuse of prescription or over-the-counter drugs constitutes drug abuse. Additionally, the repeated use of drugs to produce pleasure, to alleviate stress, or to alter or avoid reality (or all three) constitutes drug abuse. Drug abuse tends to be a chronic, progressive disease and can have a major impact on one's life, without intervention.

The use and abuse of drugs is associated with high-risk behaviors in adolescents, which may result in death. There are four stages of becoming dependent on a drug: experimental, seeking-out, dependency, and addiction. The transition between of stages is often a reoccurring process of regression, cessation and relapse. Common comorbid conditions associated with substance abuse are depression, anxiety disorders, bipolar and attention deficit/hyperactivity disorder.

The CDC (2012) reports deaths from opioid prescription painkillers have reached epidemic levels and is considered a major public health and public safety crisis. According to the White House (2015), the majority of drug overdoses are accidental and involve opioid prescription drugs, which are in the same class of medications as heroin. Four out of five heroin users begin by misusing opioids. The rate of overdoses involving prescription pain medication is leveling off, although it remains at an unacceptably high level. Currently, more people die from overdoses than motor vehicle accidents.

A few states passed legislation that ensures police, firefighters, first responders, school nurses and others have access to Narcan®, a drug that reverses the effects of prescription drug overdoses. Additional states are considering the enacting this legislation.

CAUSES:

Most drug abuse results from a combination of experimentation, peer pressure, and external and internal stressors. The gateway for substance abuse opens if a young person's environment causes anxiety and an illicit drug eases the pain.

Risk factors and protective factors are important in substance abuse among youth and adolescents. According to the National Institute of Drug Abuse (NIDA) (2015), risk factors can increase a person's chances for drug abuse while protective factors can reduce the risk. It is important to note that most people at risk for drug abuse never start using drugs or

SUBSTANCE ABUSE *(continued from previous page)*

CAUSES: *(continued)*

become addicted to drugs. In addition, a risk factor for one person may not be the same for another person. Risk factors and protective factors can occur at different stages of children's lives. However, risks that occur at early stages can be change by prevention interventions.

Alcohol is still the number one drug abused among young people in the United States compared to tobacco or illicit drugs (Johnston, O'Malley, Bachman, & Schulenberg, 2013). Driving while intoxicated results in the largest number of deaths in the adolescent age group. A detailed list of common drugs used is in Appendix A.

SIGNS AND SYMPTOMS:

Specific symptoms:
- Stimulants: dilated pupils, rapid pulse, talkativeness and sometimes elevated blood pressure; very high doses may cause psychotic symptoms
- Depressants: pupils normal to small, drowsiness and slurred speech (in the absence of an alcohol odor)

General signs and symptoms/behaviors of possible substance abuse include the following (National Youth Network, 2015):
- Runny or stuffy nose (constant)
- Needle tracks
- Sudden personality changes that include abrupt changes in work or school attendance, quality of work, work output, grades, discipline
- Unusual flare-ups or outbreaks of temper
- Withdrawal from responsibility
- General changes in overall attitude
- Loss of interest in what were once favorite hobbies and pursuits
- Changes in friends and reluctance to have friends visit or talk about them
- Difficulty in concentration, paying attention
- Sudden jitteriness, tremors, nervousness, and/or aggression
- Deterioration of physical appearance and grooming
- Wearing of sunglasses at inappropriate times
- Continual wearing of long-sleeved garments particularly in hot weather or reluctance to wear short-sleeved attire when appropriate

361

SUBSTANCE ABUSE *(continued from previous page)*

SIGNS AND SYMPTOMS: *(continued)*

- Association with known substance abusers
- Unusual borrowing of money from friends, co-workers or parents
- Stealing small items from employer, home or school
- Secretive behavior regarding actions and possessions; poorly concealed attempts to avoid attention and suspicion such as frequent trips to storage rooms, restroom, basement, etc.
- Change, sometimes radical, in behavior
- Slurred speech
- Memory impairment, impaired coordination
- Weight loss or gain; change in eating habits

MANAGEMENT/TREATMENT:

1. Follow the school health services program policy for suspected or known substance use among student.
2. If prescription drug overdose is suspected, give Narcan® (if available) and call 911.
3. Behavior and physical findings will dictate urgency of medical referral.
4. Notify parents (and police if an illicit substance is suspected).
5. Call 911 if condition deteriorates.

FOLLOW UP:

Once the drug of abuse is identified, a treatment plan can be developed. Polydrug use (alcohol plus marijuana, etc.) is hardest to treat. A referral to the student assistance team should be made.

SUBSTANCE ABUSE *(continued from previous page)*

POTENTIAL COMPLICATIONS:

The following table defines the five stages of substance abuse and serves as a guide for referral in non-acute cases.

Stage	Description
1	*Potential for abuse* Decreased impulse control Need for immediate gratification Availability of drugs, alcohol, inhalants Need for peer acceptance
2	*Experimentation: learning the euphoria* Use of inhalants, marijuana, and alcohol with friends Few, if any, consequences May increase to regular weekend use Little change in behavior
3	*Regular use: seeking the euphoria* Use of other drugs, e.g., stimulants, LSD, sedatives Behavioral changes and some consequences Increased frequency of use; use alone Buying or stealing drugs or money for drugs
4	*Regular use: preoccupation with the "high"* Daily use of drugs Loss of control Multiple consequences and risk-taking Estrangement from family and "straight" friends
5	*Burnout: use of drugs to feel normal* Use of multiple substances Guilt, withdrawal, remorse, depression Physical and mental deterioration Increased risk-taking, self-destructive behavior

SUBSTANCE ABUSE *(continued from previous page)*

PREVENTION:

According to the National Institute of Drug Abuse (NIDA), drug abuse is preventable. Research conducted by NIDA indicates prevention programs that involve family, schools, communities, and the media are effective in reducing drug abuse. Youth who experience a positive connection to school, family, and community are less likely to engage in risky behaviors, including alcohol and drug abuse

NOTES:

- School nurses are often asked to determine whether a student is under the influence of an illicit substance or chemical. School health services programs may need to have a policy in place for identifying students who may be under the influence of an illicit substance or chemical. The school's legal counsel or attorney should review the policy prior to approval of the policy by the school board.
- Additionally, school nurses may need specialized training and orientation for completing a student assessment for substance and chemical abuse.

References

American Academy of Pediatrics. (2011). Substance use screening, brief intervention, and referral to treatment for pediatricians. *Pediatrics 128* (5), pp. e1330 -e1340. doi: 10.1542/peds.2011-1754

Centers for Disease Prevention. (2012). Youth risk behavior surveillance-United States 2013. *Morbidity & Mortality Weekly Report,* 64 (4). Retrieved from http://www.cdc.gov/mmwr/pdf/ss/ss6304.pdf

Johnston, L. D., O'Malley, P. M., Bachman, J. G., & Schulenberg, J. E. (2013). Monitoring the Future national results on drug use: 2012. Overview, Key Findings on Adolescent Drug Use. Ann Arbor: Institute for Social Research, The University of Michigan. Retrieved from http://www.monitoringthefuture.org//pubs/monographs/mtf-overview2012.pdf

Kaul, P. (2014). Adolescent substance abuse. In W. Hay, M. Levin, R. Deterding, & M. Abzug (Eds.), *Current diagnosis and treatment pediatrics* (22nd edition) (pp. 158- 171). McGraw Hill Education, Inc. See p. 171 for more resources.

Miranda, L. (2014). Learn the 5 stages of substance abuse. Retrieved from http://www.treatmentsolutions.com/learn-5-stages-substance-abuse/

National Institute of Drug Abuse (NIDA). (2015). *NIDA for teens*. Retrieved from http://teens.drugabuse.gov

National Institute of Drug Abuse (NIDA). (2003). *Preventing drug abuse among children and adolescents – Risk factors and protective factors 2nd ed.).* Retrieved from http://www.nida.nih.gov/Prevention/risk.html

National Youth Network. (2015). *Teen substance abuse and adolescent substance abuse treatment*. Retrieved from http://www.nationalyouth.com/substanceabuse.html

Substance Abuse and Mental Health Service Administration (SAMSHA). (2015).*Talk – They hear you. Underage drinking prevention national media campaign.* Retrieved from http://www.samhsa.gov/underagedrinking/

White House, Office of the Press Secretary. (2015). *Fact sheet: Obama administration announces public and private sector efforts to address prescription drug abuse and heroin use.* Retrieved from https://www.whitehouse.gov/the-press-office/2015/10/21/fact-sheet-obama-administration-announces-public-and-private-sector

SUBSTANCE ABUSE *(continued from previous page)*

Appendix A – Drugs of Potential Abuse Among Youth and Adolescents
(Adopted from the 2012 Monitoring the Future Survey)

Monitoring the Future (MTF) is a long-term study of American adolescents, college students, and adults through age 50. The study is conducted annually by the University of Michigan's Institute for Social Research since its inception in 1975 and is supported by grants from the National Institute of Drug Abuse (NIDA). Substance abuse among American youth is rapidly changing and requires frequent assessments and reassessments. Alcohol, cigarettes (any use), and illicit drugs are the leading causes of morbidity and mortality during adolescence and adulthood. The following list summarizes drugs of potential abuse among youth and adolescents in the United States as of 2009 to 2012.

<u>Name of Drug</u>

Alcohol
Cigarettes (any use)
Smokeless Tobacco
Illicit Drugs
Cocaine
Crack Cocaine
Gamma-hydroxybutyrate (GHB)
Hallucinogens
Lysergic Acid (LSD)
MDMA (Ecstasy)

Heroin
Inhalants
Ketamine
Marijuana/Hashish
Methamphetamine
PCP
Any Prescription Drug
Rohypnol
Salvia
Steroids

(Adopted from Monitoring the Future Study: Trends in Prevalence of Various Drugs website link http://www.drugabuse.gov/related-topics/trends-statistics/monitoring-future/trends-in-prevalence-various-drugs)

SWALLOWING DISORDERS (Dysphagia)

DEFINITION/ETIOLOGY:

Swallowing disorders, also known as dysphagia, cause difficulties with feeding and swallowing. The swallowing process is very complex. Breakdown in the oral phase, pharyngeal phase or esophageal phase can cause swallowing disorders. Swallowing issues in school age children can be seen with the following diagnoses: cerebral palsy, severe developmental disabilities, meningitis, encephalopathy, gastrointestinal conditions, prematurity or low birth rate, cognitive impairment, head/neck cancer treated with radiation/chemotherapy, brain injury, spinal cord injury, muscular dystrophy, heart disease, cleft lip and/or palate, autism, head and neck abnormalities, muscle weakness in the face and neck respiratory difficulties or medications that cause lethargy or decreased appetite.

SIGNS AND SYMPTOMS:

- Coughing after eating/drinking
- Shortness of breath after eating/drinking
- Loss of pigmentation in the face after eating/drinking
- Wheezing and/or gasping during feeding
- Wet vocal quality after eating/drinking
- Feeling of food items sticking in the oral or pharyngeal phase of the swallow
- Pocketing
- Residue in oral cavity after swallowing
- Choking after eating/drinking
- Anterior loss of food/drink from the oral cavity and/or drooling
- Over-filling oral cavity with food or drink
- Student feeling of "drowning "
- Reoccurring pneumonia
- Absent swallow
- Swallow delay
- Weight loss
- Difficulty chewing or initiating swallow
- Regurgitation

SWALLOWING DISORDERS *(continued from previous page)*

MANAGEMENT/TREATMENT:
1. **If any of the above signs and symptoms are present during feeding, follow up is needed. In cases of extreme choking/respiratory symptoms, oral feeding should stop at school until student is evaluated.**
2. Collaborate with school speech language pathologist on any swallowing concerns.
3. Notify parent/guardian of symptoms and need for follow up with healthcare provider.
4. Videofluoroscopic swallow study, sometimes known as a Modified Barium Swallow Study or a Fiberoptic Endoscopic Evaluation of Swallowing (FEES) is often indicated.
5. After a complete swallow study has been completed, the student may have a change in diet level or may need to implement compensatory strategies.

Diet Levels:

Levels of Solids
1. NPO. Nothing by mouth: includes food, liquids, medication, and tooth brushing.
2. Dysphagia Level 1: Puree. Pudding-like, no chewing required.
3. Dysphagia Level 2: Mechanically Altered. Cohesive, moist, semi-solid foods, requires chewing ability.
4. Dysphagia Level 3: Soft Diet. Soft-solid foods that require more chewing ability.
5. Dysphagia Level 4: Regular Diet. All foods allowed.

Levels of Liquids
1. Thin liquids: all liquids allowed.
2. Nectar-thick liquids: slightly thickened.
3. Honey-thick liquids: Significantly thickened.
4. Pudding-thick liquids: almost solid pureed form.
5. NPO: Nothing by mouth.

SWALLOWING DISORDERS *(continued from previous page)*

Compensatory Strategies:
- Avoid straws
- Small bites
- Chin tuck
- Turn head left or right
- Slow rate while eating or drinking
- Sit upright when eating and drinking
- Crush medications
- Pills in puree
- Alternate liquids and solids
- Dry swallows after each bite of food or sip of drink
- Extra swallows with each bite of food or drink
- Present food/drink on spoon

Educational Relevance
- Safety
- Promote health to maximize attendance
- Ensure adequate nutrition/hydration during the school day
- Skill development

POTENTIAL COMPLICATIONS:
1. Silent aspiration
2. Aspiration
3. Pneumonia
4. Weight loss
5. Decreased enjoyment of eating or drinking orally

In some cases, nasogastric feedings are initiated until signs and symptoms are resolved. Placement of gastro feeding tube (G-tube or button) may be indicated if oral feeding will be limited or NPO for extended period of time.

SWALLOWING DISORDERS *(continued from previous page)*

NOTES:
The school nurse may suspect swallowing disorders with:
- Students with frequent coughing, gasping for air and wet vocal quality at mealtime
- Students with cognitive impairments, autism, cerebral palsy and other nervous system disorders
- Students that present dehydrated and malnourished
- Students with recurring pneumonia

The school nurse is the key professional to:
- Report signs and symptoms of swallowing difficulty to parents and speech language pathologist.
- Educate teachers on diet levels and insure students are consistently receiving their solid and liquid diet levels.
- Initiate individualized staff training for feeding as needed.
- Monitor medications, weight, temperature, lung sounds in at risk students.
- Implement care plan.
- Educate student on importance of following their liquid and solid diet levels.
- Participate in dysphagia management team with SLP, OT, PT, nutritionist, parent.

SAMPLE FEEDING PROTOCOLS/DYSPHAGIA PROGRAMS IN THE SCHOOL SETTING:
Feeding and Swallowing Procedures:
http://www.misd.net/SEConsult/FeedSwallow%20Manual%2009.pdf

Feeding Students in Educational Programs: http://www.douglasesd.k12.or.us/sites/douglasesd.k12.or.us/files/users/RSOI/Feeding%20Students%20in%20Educational%20Programs%20April%202015.pdf

Model School Dysphagia Program:
http://faculty.washington.edu/jul2/Readings/model.pdf

SWALLOWING DISORDERS *(continued from previous page)*

References

American Speech-Language-Hearing Association. (2015). *Feeding and swallowing disorders (dysphasia) in children.* Retrieved from http://www.asha.org/public/speech/swallowing/Feeding-and-Swallowing-Disorders-in-Children/

American Speech-Language-Hearing Association. (2015). *Pediatric dysphagia: Considerations for evaluation in the school setting.* Retrieved from http://www.asha.org/PRPSpecificTopic.aspx?folderid=8589934965&section=Assessment#Considerations_for_Evaluation_in_the_School_Setting

American Speech-Language-Hearing Association. (2015). *Swallowing disorders (dysphasia) in adults.* Retrieved from http://www.asha.org/public/speech/swallowing/Swallowing-Disorders-in-Adults/

Groher, M.E., & Cary, M.A. (2010). *Dysphagia: Clinician management in adults and children.* Maryland Heights, Missouri: Mosby Elsevier Inc.

Langmore, S. E., & Krisciunas, G. P. (2010). Dysphagia after radiotherapy for head and neck cancer: Etiology, clinical presentation, and efficacy of current treatments. *Perspectives on Swallowing and Swallowing Disorders (Dysphagia), 19*(2), 32-38. doi: 10.1044/sasd19.2.32

Mayo Clinic. (2014). *Dysphagia.* Retrieved from http://www.mayoclinic.org/diseases-conditions/dysphagia/basics/definition/con-20033444

McCullough, G., Pelletier, C., & Steele, C. (2003). National dysphagia diet: What to swallow? *The ASHA Leader, 8*(20), 16-27. doi:10.1044/leader.FTR3.08202003.16

Salzman, L. (2001). *Call for dysphagia management in the schools.* Retrieved from http://www.schoolnursenews.org/BackIssues/2001/May/OralHealth.pdf

TATTOO/BODY PIERCING

DEFINITION/ETIOLOGY:

Tattoos and body piercing are forms of body art that have been practiced for years by various cultures. The English word tattoo derived from the Polynesian word *tatau* that means, "to mark". Tattooing became a trendy fashion statement in the U.S. in the 1990s. Tattoos and body piercing can express individuality, rebellion or group membership. It may signify spiritual meaning or a life milestone, such as a new love. While most states prohibit tattooing of minors, school nurses see students with tattoos or piercings, often done by peers and outside of commercial establishments.

As a result of 2009 U.S. Senate Bill 5391, the definitions of "tattoo" and "body art" have changed. Tattoo is "to pierce or puncture the human skin with a needle or other instrument for the purpose of implanting an indelible mark, or pigment, into the skin". Body art is "the practice of invasive cosmetic adornment."

SIGNS AND SYMPTOMS:

Possible complications from tattooing that require treatment:

- Inflammation of the pierced or tattooed area
- Allergic reaction includes swelling, redness, and itching
- Severe allergic reaction can lead to anaphylactic shock
- Scars

MANAGEMENT/TREATMENT:

1. Treatment for local infection may include warm compresses, and antibacterial ointment for local infection, to a course of oral antibiotics.
2. Tattoos are considered permanent; removal can be both painful and expensive. The methods of tattoo removal include the following:
   - Surgical removal – cutting the tattoo away
   - Dermabrasion – sanding the skin (epidermis and dermis)
   - Salabrasion – using a salt solution to soak the tattooed skin
   - Scarification – removing the tattoo with an acid solution and creating a scar in its place
   - Laser therapy as regulated by the Food and Drug Administration (FDA) may also be used as a method of tattoo removal

TATTOO/BODY PIERCING *(continued from previous page)*

FOLLOW UP:

- Youth are a population at risk and influenced by media, peers, and "heroes". Most tattoos are done on a whim, so youth may not consider the long-term health risks of receiving a tattoo or the permanent marking of the skin. School personnel such as health educators and school nurses can educate students in making informed decisions about tattoos.
- Infection control may depend on certification of artists and shop inspections. If a student intends to get a tattoo or piercing, the Alliance of Professional Tattooists suggests safety measures and asking about or looking for autoclaving instruments, one-time needle and pigment use, and how the workspace is cleaned.

COMPLICATIONS:

Tattoos and body piercings may be popular but pose definite health risks.

- When proper sterilization and safety procedures are not exquisitely followed, tattooing can transmit blood-borne pathogens including Hepatitis B and C, and HIV.
- Body piercing can also present the risk of scarring (formation of granulomas or keloids.
- Skin infections.
- Allergic reactions: Tattoo dyes — especially red, green, yellow and blue dyes — can cause allergic skin reactions, such as an itchy rash at the tattoo site. This can occur even years after receiving the tattoo.

REFERENCES:

Alliance of Professional Tattooist. (n.d.). *Guidelines for getting a tattoo.* Retrieved from http://www.safe-tattoos.com/pamphlets/basic.html

Bowden, V.R., & Greenberg, C. S. (2014). Adolescence. In V. R. Bowden, & C.S. Greenberg (eds.), *Children and their families: The continuum of care* (3rd edition) *(p. 231-232).* Philadelphia, PA: Lippincott Williams and Wilkins.

Centers for Disease Control and Prevention. (2013). *Body art – Follow regulations.* Retrieved from http://www.cdc.gov/niosh/topics/body_art/stateRegs.html

Mayo Clinic. (2015). *Tattoos: Understanding risks and precautions.* Retrieved from http://www.mayoclinic.com/health/tattoos-and-piercings/MC00020

Senate Bill 5391. (2009). *Regulating tattooing and body piercing.* Retrieved from http://www.washingtonvotes.org/2009-SB-5391

Tielisch - Goddard, A. (2008). Adolescent body art: Piercings and tattoos in the school nurse's office. *NASN School Nurse,* 23(3), 16-17. doi: 10.1177/104747570802300309

TIC DISORDERS AND TOURETTE SYNDROME

DEFINITIONS/ETIOLOGY:

A *tic* is a sudden, rapid, recurrent, non-rhythmic, stereotyped motor movement or vocalization. Any part of the body can be involved—face, neck, hands, legs. The person can hold a tic back for a little while but the condition is involuntary. Many children have mild tics that disappear over time without intervention.

- *Tourette Syndrome* is an inherited, neurological disorder characterized by repeated, involuntary body movements and vocal sounds. It may be accompanied by obsessions, attention problems, learning disabilities and impulsivity. The onset is before age 18, usually between 4 and 8 years with an average onset of 6 years of age. The cause of Tourette Syndrome is unknown, but research suggests that it is very complex.

TICS

Tics are classified as **transient or chronic** (Tourette Syndrome) and are most common during adolescence.

TRANSIENT

- The essential feature of Transient Tic Disorder is the presence of single or multiple motor tics and/or vocal tics using limited muscle groups. The tics occur many times a day, nearly every day for at least 4 weeks, but for no longer than 12 consecutive months.

TOURETTE

The full name of the disorder is Gilles de la Tourette Syndrome (GTS). The essential features of Tourette Syndrome are:

- Multiple motor tics and one or more vocal tics involving several muscle groups appear simultaneously or at different periods.
- Tics occur many times a day (usually in bouts), nearly every day or intermittently for a period of more than one year, and during this period, there is never a tic-free period of more than 3 consecutive months.
- The disorder is not due to direct physiological effects of a substance (e.g., a stimulant) or a general medical condition (e.g., post-viral encephalitis).
- It causes marked distress or significant impairment in social, occupational, or other important areas of functioning.

TIC DISORDERS AND TOURETTE SYNDROME *(continued from previous page)*

The type, number, frequency, complexity and severity of tics change over time. Motor tics typically involve the head and frequently, other parts of the body (torso, upper and lower limbs). Vocal tics include words or sounds, such as clicks, grunts, yelps, barks, sniffs, snorts and coughs. Complex sounds such as obscenities occur in only 10% of cases.

SIGNS AND SYMPTOMS:

Tics vary greatly between and within individuals. Some clinical features include:

- Simple motor tics with brief, sudden, and meaningless muscle movements, e.g. eye blinking, nose twitching, or shoulder shrugging (usually the first to appear).
- May only appear when tired, stressed or anxious and have 30-100 tics per minute.
- Complex motor tics are more purposeful and involve several muscle groups, e.g. touching other people or objects, retracing steps when walking, and various complex hand gestures.
- Vocal tics may be simple or complex and range from meaningless sounds (clearing throat, sniffling, or barking) to sudden utterance of words, phrases, and complete sentences (echolalia or coprolalia).
- Tic intensity can vary from barely visible and audible tics to extremely forceful and loud expressions.
- Tics may severely interfere with everyday activities including social relationships and school performance.

MANAGEMENT/TREATMENT:

1. Identification and careful diagnosis of the disruptive effects of tics.
2. Minimize stress and teach relaxation techniques.
3. Rewards and punishments are not indicated or helpful.
4. Educate staff and student to understand the disorder. GTS does not diminish intellect.
5. Refer to support groups.
6. Medications are used when tics significantly interfere with functioning and for co-morbid conditions (e.g., ADHD, obsessive-compulsive disorder, anxiety).
7. Medication side effects include tremors, depression, weight gain, decreased cognitive abilities and heart problems.
8. Severe tics lasting for more than a year may need intervention from a mental healthcare provider.

TIC DISORDERS AND TOURETTE SYNDROME *(continued from previous page)*

SCHOOL NURSE FOLLOW UP:
- Communicate with parents/guardians regarding health needs and special accommodations during school (may need a Section 504 plan).
- Participate as a member of the multidisciplinary team to promote health and academic success.
- Schedule the student for a break in the nurse office during the school day where he/she can allow tics to happen. This gives the student a break from trying to control the tics all day in school and this break allows the student to then return to class with fewer or less obvious tics.
- Provide information and educate school staff.
- Follow up on individualized healthcare plans, emergency plans, and health goals are necessary for continuity of care in school and at home.
- Provide support and try to build self- esteem in student.
- Provide an emotionally and physically safe environment.
- Monitor symptoms in various situations and report to licensed healthcare provider.

NOTES:
Co-morbidities include Attention Deficit/Hyperactivity Disorder and Obsessive-Compulsive Disorder.
Migraines, learning disabilities, sleep difficulties, anxiety and mood swings may also accompany this disorder.

RESOURCES

Tourette Syndrome Association's website is www.tsa-usa.org.

National Tourette Syndrome Association, Tourette Syndrome in the Classroom School & Community at http://www.tsa-usa.org/news/ED_DVD_TSA_Free_Offer.html

TIC DISORDERS AND TOURETTE SYNDROME *(continued from previous page)*

References

Giordano, K. (n.d.). Tourette syndrome education: *Getting help at school.* Retrieved from http://www.tsa-usa.org/ Education/getting_help_at_school.htm

Kedia, S., Knupp, K., Schreiner, T., Yang, M.L., Levisohn, P.M., & Moe, P.G. L.D. (2014). Neurologic & muscular disorders. In W. Hay, M. Levin, R. Deterding, & M. Abzug (Eds.), *Current diagnosis and treatment pediatrics* (22nd edition) (pp. 830-832). McGraw Hill Education, Inc.

Mayo Clinic. (2012). *Tourette syndrome.* Retrieved from http://www.mayoclinic.com/health/tourette-syndrome/DS00541

Selekman, J., Diefenbeck, C., Guthrie, S. (2013).Mental health concerns. In J. Selekman (Ed.), *School nursing: A comprehensive text* (2nd ed.) (pp.952-954). Philadelphia, PA: F.A. Davis.

National Institute of Neurological Disorders and Stroke. (2014). *Tourette syndrome fact sheet.* Retrieved from http://www.ninds.nih.gov/disorders/tourette/detail_tourette.htm#220493231

TICK-BORNE DISEASES (including Rocky Mountain Spotted Fever) AND TICK REMOVAL

DEFINITION/ETIOLOGY:

A tick is a small, blood-sucking, parasitic arachnid that lives in moist or humid environments, particularly in or near wooded or grassy areas. Ticks live on the blood of large animals such as deer, but can also attach to humans. Once a tick attaches to a host, it will move to a warm, moist location such as the armpit, groin, or hair. Ticks vary in size, can range from very large to very small, and are almost impossible to see.

Ticks attach as one moves by bushes, plants, or grass in tall wooded areas or fields. Tick bites can cause a variety of health conditions ranging from harmless to serious. While most ticks are harmless and do not carry disease, some ticks can carry bacteria which can lead to diseases such as Colorado tick fever, Rocky Mountain spotted fever, and Tularemia.

*For information on Lyme disease, refer to guideline on LYME DISEASE

Disease	Rocky Mountain Spotted Fever*
Cause	Rickettsia rickettsii
Transmission	Various species (dog, wood ticks)
Exposure risk	Bite 4-6 hours; crushing with fingers
Incubation	2-14 days
Early signs	Sudden onset of fever, lasting 2-3 weeks, severe headache, nausea, muscle pain
Other signs	May have a maculopapular rash on limbs 2-5 days after fever, by day 3 rash may spread to trunk/face; may have petechiae day 6 or later.
Complications	Multisystem involvement, shock, 15% fatality if untreated

*May be reportable to the health department

TICK-BORNE DISEASES (including Rocky Mountain Spotted Fever)
AND TICK REMOVAL *(continued from previous page)*

SIGNS AND SYMPTOMS:

Initially, the tick bite is usually painless and remains that way after the tick stops the blood meal and falls off the skin. Later, the following signs and symptoms may develop at the site of the tick bite:

- Itching
- Burning
- Redness
- Localized pain in some individuals

Some individuals develop sensitivity or an allergic reaction to tick bites and may experience:

- Rash
- Shortness of breath
- Swelling
- Numbness
- Paralysis

Other symptoms may be rare or infrequent immediately after or during a tick bite and require **immediate medical attention**. These symptoms include:

- Fever
- Shortness of breath
- Weakness
- Vomiting
- Swelling
- Weakness or Paralysis
- Headache
- Confusion
- Palpitations

TICK-BORNE DISEASES (including Rocky Mountain Spotted Fever)
AND TICK REMOVAL *(continued from previous page)*

MANAGEMENT/TREATMENT:
1. Try to establish source and duration of tick adherence. Be familiar with the types of ticks in the area that carry disease.
2. Cleanse the site and then remove the tick with a small, fine-tipped forceps or tweezers grasp the tick as close to the skin as possible, pulling upward with a firm, steady pressure to keep the tick intact.
3. Re-cleanse the site.
4. Place tick in small vial or plastic bag and mark with student's name, address, date, site of attachment. Have the tick identified by lab, health department, or veterinarian. If unable to retain the tick for identification, flush the tick in toilet; do not burn or dispose of in waste can.
5. Inform parent/guardian of signs that need a healthcare provider's attention following a tick bite.
6. Monitor student for signs of illness for up to one month.

FOLLOW-UP:
Educate about tick avoidance (clothing, DEET repellents, and pet protection), frequent checks, and careful removal.

NOTES:
- Children should be taught to seek the help of an adult for tick removal.
- If the tick must be removed using fingers, use a barrier such as a tissue or leaf to avoid contact with possible infected fluids.
- Do not pick, crush, or burn the tick as it may release infected tissues or fluids.
- Do not attempt to smother the tick with substances such as petroleum jelly or nail polish. Smothering is not an effective technique for tick removal as the tick has enough oxygen to complete the feeding (adopted from Lyme Disease Foundation, Inc.).

Check state and local health department websites for details pertinent to the occurrence and types of ticks in your school's location.

TICK-BORNE DISEASES (including Rocky Mountain Spotted Fever)
AND TICK REMOVAL *(continued from previous page)*

References

American Academy of Pediatrics. (2013). Lyme disease (and other tick-borne diseases). Scabies. In S. Aronson, & T. Shope (Eds.), *Managing infectious diseases in child care and schools* (2nd ed.) (p. 115-116). Elk Grove Village, IL: American Academy of Pediatrics.

American Academy of Pediatrics, Committee on Infectious Diseases. (2015). Lyme disease. In D.W. Kimberlin, M. T. Brady, M.A. Jackson, & S.S. Long (Eds.), *Red Book: 2015 report of the committee on infectious diseases* (30th ed.) (pp. 516-525). Elk Grove Village, IL: American Academy of Pediatrics.

American Academy of Pediatrics, Committee on Infectious Diseases. (2015). Rocky mountain spotted fever. In D.W. Kimberlin, M. T. Brady, M.A. Jackson, & S.S. Long (Eds.), *Red Book: 2015 report of the committee on infectious diseases* (30th ed.) (pp. 682-684). Elk Grove Village, IL: American Academy of Pediatrics.

Centers for Disease Control and Prevention (CDC). (2015a). *Stop ticks.* Retrieved from *http://www.cdc.gov/features/stopticks/*

Centers for Disease Control and Prevention (CDC). (2015b). *Ticks.* Retrieved from *http://www.cdc.gov/ticks/index.html*

Centers for Disease Control and Prevention (CDC). (2015c). *Lyme disease.* Retrieved from http://www.cdc.gov/lyme/

Centers for Disease Control and Prevention (CDC). (2013). *Rocky mountain spotted fever (RMSF).* Retrieved from http://www.cdc.gov/rmsf/

Davis, Charles. (2014). *Ticks.* Retrieved from http://www.medicinenet.com/ticks/article.htm

Lymedisease .org. (n.d.). *Tick removal.* Retrieved from https://www.lymedisease.org/lyme-basics/ticks/tick-removal/

Medline Plus, U.S. National Library of Medicine. (2015). *Tick removal.* Retrieved from http://www.nlm.nih.gov/medlineplus/ency/article/007211.htm

University of Maryland Medical Center. (2013). *Tick bite – overview.* Retrieved from *http://www.umm.edu/ency/article/002856.htm*.

TUBERCULOSIS (PRIMARY OR CHILDHOOD)

DEFINITIONS/ETIOLOGY:

Tuberculosis (TB) is caused by *Mycobacterium tuberculosis*, an acid-fast bacillus (AFB). It is the leading cause of death throughout the world. Mycobacterium are usually slow growing and have waxy cell wall that are resistant to digestion. Many mycobacterium are intracellular parasites. Additional information related to TB definitions and etiology includes the following:

- **Childhood or Primary TB** is *M. tuberculosis* infection in older infants and children, contracted from prolonged household case contact. It is usually an asymptomatic infection. The diagnosis is confirmed only by a positive tuberculin skin test (TST).
- **Tuberculin Skin Test** also known at the Mantoux test or purified protein derivative (PDD) is the standard for identifying infected persons. The Mantoux test is read 48-72 hours after being placed.
- **Positive tuberculin skin test**: The classifications of reactions (measuring *induration*, not redness) are:
  - Induration ≥ 5mm: Positive if patient is at high risk, such as household contact with TB disease, clinical evidence of TB, abnormal chest radiograph, or HIV+.
  - Induration ≥ 10 mm: Positive if patient is at moderate risk, e.g., children younger than 4 years of age, or born in high-prevalence regions, or those who travel to these regions, children with other medical conditions (e.g. Hodgkin's disease, Lymphoma, Diabetes, or chronic renal failure).
  - Induration ≥ 15mm: Positive if patient is 4 years of age or older without any risk factor.
- **Latent tuberculosis infection (LTBI)** is defined as TB infection in a person who has a positive TST result but no physical finding of TB disease; chest radiograph findings are normal or reveal evidence of healing infection.
- **Tuberculosis disease** is defined as disease in a person with TB infection having symptoms, signs, or radiographic manifestations.

CAUSES:

All cases of TB are passed from person to person through airborne transmission of droplets. Inhalation of droplets can occur from an adult or adolescent with contagious, cavity, pulmonary tuberculosis. When a person with TB infection coughs, sneezes, or talks, tiny droplets of saliva or mucus are expelled in the air and can be transmitted through inhalation by another person.

TUBERCULOSIS (PRIMARY OR CHILDHOOD) *(continued from previous page)*

CAUSES *(continued)*
- The incubation period from infection to development of a positive TST is 2-10 weeks. The risk of developing of TB disease is highest during the 6 months after infection and remains high for 2 years.
- Once the infectious particles are inhaled and reach the alveoli, small sac-like structures develop in the air spaces in the lungs and the macrophage cell engulfs the TB bacteria.
- The TB bacteria are then transmitted to the lymphatic system and bloodstream and the spread to other organs occurs.
- The TB bacteria begin to multiply in organs with high oxygen pressures, e.g. the upper lobes of the lungs, kidneys, bone marrow, and meninges.
- TB disease occurs when the bacteria cause clinically detectable disease.
- Persons who have inhaled the TB bacterium but show no signs of clinically detectable disease are referred to as infected. Persons infected with TB have no symptoms of disease because the immune system has walled off the organism in an inflammatory focus known as a granuloma.
- The skin test for TB will often be positive in people infected with TB, but the disease cannot be transmitted to others while in the latent phase of TB infection.

EVIDENCE-BASED RECOMMENDATIONS FOR SCREENING FOR CHILDREN AND ADOLESCENTS
- Screen for risk factors of TB and LTBI.
- Test with a TST only if more than one of the following risk factors is present:
  - Contact with adult with active TB disease
  - Foreign birth
  - Travel to a country with high prevalence of infection
  - Household member with latent tuberculosis infection (LTBI)

SIGNS AND SYMPTOMS:
- Common symptoms of TB may include fever, cough, chest x-ray abnormalities, loss of appetite, weight loss, night sweats, nonproductive cough, failure to thrive, and difficulty gaining weight.
- Most children and adolescents with tuberculosis infection have no symptoms (asymptomatic).
- Children and adolescents with continued exposure or weakened immunity can develop symptoms such as fatigue, malaise, low-grade fever, and symptoms resulting from lymph node enlargement, especially in the center of the chest (hilar node).

TUBERCULOSIS (PRIMARY OR CHILDHOOD) *(continued from previous page)*

SIGNS AND SYMPTOMS: *(continued)*
- In 6-8 weeks, the body's defenses wall off the infection with scar tissue. There are no further consequences other than positive TST. This is the typical course of childhood or primary TB.
- About 5% of children with a delayed diagnosis or no treatment can develop a serious form of TB.

MANAGEMENT/TREATMENT:
Medical treatment of TB includes the following recommendations:

- Treatment is recommended for all children and adolescents diagnosed with LTBI, because young children are at higher risk for progression to TB disease.
- Multiple antimicrobial drugs are available for treatment of TB.
- First line drugs are isoniazide (INH), rifampin (RIF), pyrazinamide (PZA), and ethambutol (EMB).
- Children are usually treated with isoniazid (INH), daily by mouth for 9 months.
- For children less than 4 years of age with a close contact, INH should be initiated, even if the TST result is first negative. TST should be retested 12 weeks after the last contact. If the result is negative, INH may be discontinued.
- Second line drugs include both the aminlglycosides (streptomycin, kanamkin, amikacin, and capreomycin) and fluroquinolones (levofloxacin, moxifloxacin).

Management for schools of TB includes the following recommendations:

- Suspected or known tuberculosis must be reported to the Public Health Department immediately, because early reporting may help minimize the spread of TB.
- **With rare exception, primary TB is non-contagious; student may remain in school, even though a person at home has active TB**. Comply with healthcare provider orders, health department guidance and school policy.
- Children with LTBI can participate in all activities whether they are receiving treatment or not.
- Educate faculty and staff to understand relative risk.
- Cooperate with the Public Health Department and the school physician (if available) to assist students with skin testing and/or x-rays of students and staff when these tests are recommended.

TUBERCULOSIS (PRIMARY OR CHILDHOOD) *(continued from previous page)*

FOLLOW UP:
- Promote and monitor adherence to treatment of LTBI in all students.
- Provide education about the importance of adhering to completing treatment and the potential side effects of INH. These side effects include hepatitis, gastrointestinal disturbances, and peripheral neuropathy.
- If a student demonstrates any symptom of liver toxicity, stop treatment immediately and refer the student to the healthcare provider for assessment.

NOTES:
- Exposure to an infected adult is the most common risk factor in children.
- TB is preventable through effective management and treatment. Treatment of TB in a single person prevents latent infection from becoming active disease. Treatment is also effective in controlling the spread of disease among large populations.
- The TB vaccine, bacilli Calmette-Guerin (BCG), may often be used in foreign countries to prevent the spread of disease among children. However, the vaccine does not protect against pulmonary tuberculosis and often results in a false positive TST.

References

American Academy of Pediatrics. (2015). Tuberculosis. In L. K. Pickering, C. J. Baker, D. W. Kimberlin, & S. S. Long (Eds.), *Red Book: 2015 report of the committee on infectious diseases, (30th ed.)* (pp. 805-831). American Academy of Pediatrics: Elk Grove Village, IL.

American Academy of Pediatrics. (2013). *Tuberculosis (tb)*. In S. Aronson, & T. Shope (Eds.), *Managing infectious diseases in child care and schools (2nd ed.)* (p. 163-164). Elk Grove Village, IL: American Academy of Pediatrics.

Batra, V. (2015*). Pediatric tuberculosis*. Retrieved from http://emedicine.medscape.com/article/969401-overview

Centers for Disease Control and Prevention (CDC). (2015). *Tuberculosis*. Retrieved from http://www.cdc.gov/tb/?404;http://www.cdc.gov:80/tb/publications/factsheets/testing/skintest.htm

Frederico, M.J., Baker, C.D., Balasubramaniam, V., Deboer, E.M., Deterding, R.R. ...& Zelmanick, E.T. (2014). Respiratory tract & mediastinum. In W. Hay, M. Levin, R. Deterding, & M. Abzug (Eds.), *Current diagnosis and treatment pediatrics* (22nd edition) (pp. 567-568). McGraw Hill Education, Inc.

Herchline, T.E. (n.d.). *Tuberculosis*. Retrieved from http://emedicine.medscape.com/article/230802-overview

Merck Manual. (2014). *Tuberculosis*. Retrieved from http://www.merckmanuals.com/professional/infectious_diseases/mycobacteria/tuberculosis_tb.html

Ogle, J.W., & Anderson, M.S. (2014). Infections: Bacterial & spirochetal. In W. Hay, M. Levin, R. Deterding, & M. Abzug (Eds.), *Current diagnosis and treatment pediatrics* (22nd edition) (pp. 1335-1338). McGraw Hill Education, Inc.

UPPER RESPIRATORY INFECTION or "COMMON COLD"

DEFINITION/ETIOLOGY:
Common cold – viral infection of the upper respiratory tract (affects the nose, throat, ears and eyes). More than 200 viruses can cause a cold. The rhinovirus is the most common pathogen that causes upper respiratory infections. The incubation period is generally 24-72 hours. Symptoms typically last 7 – 10 days although a mild cough may continue into the second week. The virus is spread by airborne droplets, hand to hand contact or by sharing contaminated objects.

SIGNS AND SYMPTOMS:
- Runny nose – nasal drainage initially clear; after few days mucous becomes whitish or yellowish in color; as the cold progresses the mucous may change to a greenish color (this is normal)
- Sneezing
- Watery eyes
- Sore (or scratchy/itchy) throat
- Cough
- Mild headache
- Mild joint pain
- Earache (may result from the URI virus or from a secondary bacterial infection)
- May have a low grade fever although temperature is usually normal

MANAGEMENT/TREATMENT:
There is no cure for an upper respiratory infection. Treatment is supportive.
1. Limit exercise if cough is troublesome. Coordinate with PE teacher.
2. Exclude from school if student has severe cough, and is disruptive to learning.
3. Educate about hygienic use and disposal of tissues and thorough hand washing.
4. Educate to not pick at nose and to blow nose gently.
5. Encourage fluids.
6. Diet as tolerated.
7. Do not use aspirin under age 18. Aspirin can play a role in causing Reye's Syndrome.
8. If giving acetaminophen or ibuprofen, follow medication orders.
9. Nasal antihistamines/decongestants may provide nasal relief. Parent/guardian(s) should follow healthcare provider/pharmacist's guidelines.
10. Watch for adverse side effects even with over-the-counter medicines taken at home; antihistamines can cause drowsiness; decongestants can cause excitability.
11. Refer to healthcare provider if temperature is > 100.4°
12. If lasts more than 10-14 days, another diagnosis may be explored by the healthcare provider.

UPPER RESPIRATORY INFECTION or "Common Cold" *(continued from previous page)*

FOLLOW UP:
- Refer to healthcare provider for persistent cough or complications: earache, fever, vomiting, headache, loss of appetite, sore throat, dehydration, etc.

POTENTIAL COMPLICATIONS:
Complications are rare. Potential complications include:
- Sinus infection
- Ear infection
- Bronchitis
- Wheezing – colds may exacerbate asthma

NOTES:
Educate parent/guardians and staff regarding the importance of:
- Good handwashing.
- Covering nose and mouth with a tissue when coughing or sneezing, and proper disposal of tissues; wash hands or use alcohol-based hand sanitizer after blowing nose or touching nasal secretions.
- To prevent the spread of germs, teach children to cough or sneeze into their shoulder or elbow if a tissue is not available.
- Keep fingers away from eyes and nose to prevent the spread of the virus.
- Educate parent/guardian that antibiotics will not cure the common cold; a cold is caused by a virus; an antibiotic may be needed for secondary bacterial infections (ear infection, etc.).
- Exposure to cold temperature (outdoor recess, etc.) does not make a person more susceptibility to an upper respiratory infection.

References

American Academy of Pediatrics. (2013). Upper respiratory infection (common cold). In S. Aronson, & T. Shope (Eds.), *Managing infectious diseases in child care and schools (2ⁿᵈ ed.)* (pp. 165-166). Elk Grove Village, IL: American Academy of Pediatrics.

Centers for Disease Control and Prevention. (2015). *Common cold and runny nose*. Retrieved from http://www.cdc.gov/getsmart/antibiotic-use/URI/colds.html

John, R., & Chewey, L. (2013). *Common complaints*. In J. Selekman (Ed.), *School nursing: A comprehensive text* (2ⁿᵈ ed.) (pp.578-640). Philadelphia, PA: F. A. Davis.

Mayo Clinic. (2013). *Common cold*. Retrieved from http://www.mayoclinic.com/health/common-cold/DS00056

Merck Manual. (2014). *Common cold*. Retrieved from http://www.merckmanuals.com/professional/infectious_diseases/respiratory_viruses/common_cold.html?qt=UpperRespiratory Infection&alt=sh

URTICARIA (Hives)

DEFINITION/ETIOLOGY:
Urticaria, also known as hives, is a skin condition identified by pruritic red wheals that are transient with well-defined borders and central pallor. Angioedema occurs in about 50% of the cases that affects the face, lips, mouth, upper airway and extremities, although it can also affect other body locations. Acute urticaria can last six weeks or less and chronic urticaria lasts six weeks or longer. The lesions may occur singularly or in groups on any part of the skin. Urticaria can affect up to 25% of the population during their lifetime.

CAUSES:
Urticaria is triggered by an inflammation in the skin due to mast and basophil cells releasing histamine and other chemicals into the blood stream. The resulting erythema, fluid extravasation and swelling of the superficial dermis cause the urticarial wheal. Triggers for urticaria can be difficult to pinpoint and the underlying cause may be difficult to identify. Below are some known causes of urticaria:

- Food allergens (egg, milk, soy, peanut and wheat in infants; fish, seafood and nuts in older children)
- Food pseudoallergens (food or food additives that contain histamine or cause the release of histamine)
- Viral, bacterial and fungal infections
- Parasitic infection
- Drug hypersensitivities (antibiotics and nonsteroidal anti-inflammatory drugs are the most frequent triggers)
- Latex
- Anxiety
- Connective tissue diseases
- Physical triggers such as, heat, cold, vibration, water, pressure and exercise that raises the core body temperature
- Inhalants (e.g., pollens, dust)
- Contact substances (e.g., dust, plants)

URTICARIA (Hives) *(continued from previous page)*

SIGNS AND SYMPTOMS:

The defining characteristic of urticaria is that the wheals are migratory and transient, lasting less than 24 hours and resolving with no residual skin lesion. Children with urticaria tend to rub the skin with their palm rather than scratching the skin as seen with contact dermatitis. Below are characteristics of the wheals in urticaria:

- Circular, oval or irregular varying in size from 1/2 cm to 2-3 cm
- Clear in center with surrounding redness
- Tenderness
- Pruritic
- Can intensify with heat
- Characteristically short-lived, but reappear often in other parts of body
- May be accompanied by swelling of lips, eyes, fingers, genitalia
- Never contagious
- **LARYNGEAL EDEMA (hoarseness and difficulty breathing) IS THE MOST SERIOUS COMPLICATION and requires immediate establishment of an airway and a call to 911.**

MANAGEMENT/TREATMENT:

1. Cool moist compresses to help control itching.
2. Avoid implicated foods or other suspect triggers.
3. Antihistamines.
4. Notify parents/guardians about the occurrence of hives. Communicate any known or contributing causes of the urticaria.
5. Carefully monitor a child with hives for signs and symptoms of a progressive and serious allergic reaction (potentially anaphylaxis).

FOLLOW UP:

1. Ensure policies are in place for supporting students with allergies and allergic responses.
2. Provide appropriate training to school staff.
3. Individualized emergency plan for students with known allergies.
4. Avoid triggers at school.

URTICARIA (Hives) *(continued from previous page)*

References

American Academy of Dermatology. (2013). *Hives*. Retrieved from http://www.aad.org/dermatology-a-to-z/diseases-and-treatments/e---h/hives

American College of Osteopathic Dermatology. (2013). *Urticaria (hives)*. Retrieved from http://www.aocd.org/skin/dermatologic_diseases/urticaria.html

Columbia University College of Physicians and Surgeons, Department of Pediatrics. (n.d.). *Hives*. Retrieved from http://www.cumc.columbia.edu/pediatrics/patient-care/allergy-immunology/research/hives

Mayo Clinic. (2014). *Chronic hives*. Retrieved from http://www.mayoclinic.com/health/chronic-hives/DS00980

Schaefer, P. (2011). Urticaria: Evaluation and treatment. *American Family Physician 83*(2), 1078-1084. Retrieved from http://www.aafp.org/afp/2011/0501/p1078.html

Tsakok, T., Du Toit, G. Flohr, C. (2014). Pediatric urticaria. *Immunology and Allergy Clinics of North America 34*, 117-139. Retrieved from http://dx.doi.org/10.10.16/j.iac.2013.09.008http://acaai.org/allergies/types/skin-allergies/hives-urticaria

Schosesler, S. & White, M.V. (2013) Recognition and treatment of anaphylaxis in the school setting: The essential role of the school nurse. *The Journal of School Nursing 29*(6), 407-415.doi: 10.1177/1059840513506014.

VARICELLA (Chickenpox)

DEFINITION/ETIOLOGY:
Chickenpox (varicella) is an acute, highly contagious, generalized viral disease that is caused by the zoster virus (VZV). Transmission occurs through contact with respiratory droplets/secretions and direct contact. It is vaccine preventable. Most cases appear in children under age 10.

SIGNS AND SYMPTOMS:
- Usually a history of exposure
- Sudden onset of slight fever, mild constitutional symptoms and a characteristic skin eruption beginning on scalp, face or trunk
- Itchy, fluid filled blister like rash
- New bumps continue to appear for several days thus you can have all stages simultaneously (macular rash, vesicle, scab)
- Contagious 1-2 days before the rash appears while experiencing symptoms of fever, malaise, decrease appetite and headache
- No longer contagious when all blisters have formed scabs
- See also chart on *Rashes*

MANAGEMENT/TREATMENT:
1. Treatment is supportive with management of itching with antihistamines, calamine lotion or oatmeal baths; acetaminophen for fever; and antistaphylococcal penicillin or cephalosporins for bacterial superinfections.
2. Exclusion from school until all lesions are scabbed over and dry (5-7 days; longer for immunocompromised persons to assure all blisters are crusted). Incubation period averages 14-16 days for new exposures, but may range 10-21 days.
3. Immunosuppressed individuals are particularly at risk and may develop life threatening disease (students with leukemia or HIV). Alert parents of students with immunity problems that their child may have been exposed to chickenpox at school.
4. Also, alert school staff members who may be immunocompromised or pregnant of the outbreak of chickenpox.
5. Advise parent or guardian to:
   - DO NOT give aspirin or products containing salicylates due to the link with Reye's Syndrome.
   - Oatmeal baths in lukewarm water may be comforting to the itching rash.
   - Trim fingernails to reduce secondary infections from scratching.

VARICELLA (Chickenpox) *(continued from previous page)*

POTENTIAL COMPLICATIONS:
- Complications are uncommon, but may include dehydration from vomiting or diarrhea.
- Secondary bacterial infections may occur from scratching the blister.
- Complications that are more serious include chicken pox lesions in the throat, eyes and mucous membranes, pneumonia and encephalitis.

NOTES:
- Varicella tends to be more severe in adolescents and adults.
- Remind all parents that a vaccine (or proof of disease) is required for school entry.
- Adults may get "shingles" if they have had chicken pox.
- 95% of adults have had chickenpox (even if they do not remember it).
- After exposure to a person with shingles, someone can get chickenpox if they have not been vaccinated or have never had chickenpox.
- Persons vaccinated can still get chickenpox. However, the symptoms are usually milder. They usually recover more quickly and have less than 30 pox. These cases are often harder to diagnosis. Someone with even a mild case can still spread the chickenpox virus.

References

American Academy of Pediatrics, Committee on Infectious Diseases. (2015). Varicella-zoster virus infections. In D.W. Kimberlin, M. T. Brady, M.A. Jackson, & S.S. Long (Eds.), *Red Book: 2015 report of the committee on infectious diseases* (30th ed.) (pp.846-850). Elk Grove Village, IL: American Academy of Pediatrics.

Centers for Disease Control and Prevention (CDC). (2011). *About chickenpox*. Retrieved from http://www.cdc.gov/chickenpox/about/index.html

Centers for Disease Control and Prevention (CDC). (2014a). *Chickenpox fact sheet*. Retrieved from http://www.cdc.gov/vaccines/vpd-vac/varicella/fs-parents.html

Centers for Disease Control and Prevention (CDC). (2014b). *Chickenpox and pregnancy*. Retrieved from http://www.cdc.gov/pregnancy/infections-chickenpox.html

Immunization Action Coalition. (2015). *Varicella state mandates on immunizations and vaccine-preventable diseases*. Retrieved from http://www.immunize.org/laws/varicella.asp

Levin, M.J., & Weinberg, A. (2014). Infections: Viral and rickettsial. In W. Hay, M. Levin, R. Deterding, & M. Abzug (Eds.), *Current diagnosis and treatment pediatrics* (22nd edition) (pp. 1246-1249). McGraw Hill Education, Inc.

Mayo Clinic. (2013). *Chickenpox*. Retrieved from http://www.mayoclinic.org/diseases-conditions/chickenpox/basics/definition/con-20019025

Mayo Clinic. (2014). *Shingles*. Retrieved from http://www.mayoclinic.org/diseases-conditions/shingles/basics/causes/con-20019574

Medline Plus, US National Library of Medicine. (2013). *Chickenpox*. Retrieved from http://www.nlm.nih.gov/medlineplus/ency/article/001592.htm

Medline Plus, US National Library of Medicine. (2014). *Reye Syndrome*. Retrieved from http://www.nlm.nih.gov/medlineplus/ency/article/001565.htm

National Reye's Syndrome Foundation. (n.d,). *Reye's and chickenpox*. Retrieved from http://www.reyessyndrome.org/chickenpox.html

Selekman, J., & Coates, J. (2013). Disease prevention. In J. Selekman (Ed.), *School nursing: A comprehensive text* (2nd ed.) (pp. 505-506). Philadelphia: F.A. Davis.

WARTS (Verrucae Vulgaris)

DEFINITIONS/ETIOLOGY:

Warts are non-cancerous epidermal skin growths caused by the *Human Papillomavirus* (HPV). There are many different types of warts. Types include common, flat, plantar and genital. Warts affect all age groups, but are more common in children. Most warts are asymptomatic.

SIGNS AND SYMPTOMS:

Type	Location	Symptoms
Common warts	Often appear on hands and/or fingers	• Small, grainy flesh-colored, white, tan or pink lesions • Lesions may be rough to touch
Flat	Appear on face or legs	• Flat topped, slightly raised lesions, smoother than other warts • Tend to grow in clusters or several in the area
Plantar	Found on soles and balls of feet	• Small, fleshy colored lesion • Callus on the balls of feet or soles of feet (wart has grown inward) • May have black "seeds" • May have mild pain
Genital	• Sexually transmitted disease; lesions grow on penis (tip or shaft), exterior female genitals, vulva, walls of vagina, anus, and cervix; genital warts can appear in the mouth after oral sex with an infected person. • Transmitted during sexual intercourse or skin to skin contact • Can be transmitted by asymptomatic infected persons	• More common in women • Itching, burning or discomfort around lesions • Small and flat (may be so small that they are not visible)

WARTS *(continued from previous page)*

MANAGEMENT/TREATMENT:
Most warts resolve spontaneously. If treatment is indicated:
- Over-the-counter (OTC) medication (salicylic acid)
  - OTC medication is typically effective if the individual is motivated to adhere to treatment
  - Can take several weeks for the medication to be effective
  - Can erroneously mistake cancerous lesion for wart
- Cryotherapy (freezing) – may take several treatments
- Excision – virus may remain in tissue even though the lesion has been removed
- Laser surgery

See healthcare provider if wart is located on face or genitals.
Seek medical advice if not sure it is a wart or is bothersome, painful or other symptoms are present.

Do not treat genital warts with OTC wart removers

FOLLOW UP:
- To avoid the spread of warts, educate child/youth to avoid picking at own wart (autoinoculation); avoid touching someone's wart.
- If district allows, educate teens on avoiding risky sexual behaviors.
- Refer diabetic students with plantar warts to a healthcare provider for treatment – poor healing could lead to nerve damage.

POTENTIAL COMPLICATIONS:
- Autoinoculation
- May spread to other people
- Cervical cancer is linked to genital warts

NOTES:
- Monitor wart lesions – skin cancer may look like a wart.
- Educate students and staff to wear flip-flops in public showers, locker rooms and on pool decks.
- Prevention – Gardasil® vaccine is available to protect from certain strains of HPV that cause genital warts.

WARTS *(continued from previous page)*

References

American Academy of Dermatology. (2015). *Warts. Tips for management.* Retrieved from https://www.aad.org/dermatology-a-to-z/diseases-and-treatments/u---w/warts/tips/warts-tips-for-managing

Mayo Clinic. (2015). *Common warts.* Retrieved from http://www.mayoclinic.org/diseases-conditions/common-warts/basics/definition/con-20021715

Mayo Clinic. (2015). *Genital warts.* Retrieved from http://www.mayoclinic.org/diseases-conditions/genital-warts/basics/definition/con-20019380

Mayo Clinic. (2015). *Plantar warts.* Retrieved from http://www.mayoclinic.org/diseases-conditions/plantar-warts/basics/definition/con-20025706

Medlineplus/ U.S. National Library of Medicine. (2015). *Warts.* Retrieved from http://www.nlm.nih.gov/medlineplus/warts.html

Merck Manual. (2014). *Warts.* Retrieved from http://www.merckmanuals.com/professional/dermatologic_disorders/viral_skin_diseases/warts.html

Selekman, J. & Kahn, P. (2013). High-risk behaviors. In J. Selekman (Ed.), *School nursing: A comprehensive text* (2nd ed.) (pp. 1118-1154). Philadelphia, PA: F. A. Davis.

SECTION II

CLINICAL PROCEDURES

BLOOD GLUCOSE MONITORING

DEFINITION:
Blood glucose monitoring measures the amount of glucose (sugar) in a drop of blood utilizing a blood glucose meter.

PURPOSE:
For students with diabetes it is important to measure the blood glucose during the school day as an indicator of whether the student is maintaining a good balance of food, insulin and exercise. These readings will help guide insulin dosages and food intake. Severe low and high blood glucose levels can be a medical emergency and may require prompt treatment. A student's individualized healthcare plan (IHP), based on the healthcare provider's orders, will provide standard times for testing, generally before meals and snacks. In addition, testing should be done whenever the student may feel that they are low or high, and as needed prior to recess, times of high activity or before leaving school for the day is taking the school bus. The healthcare provider will also provide goals or target ranges for appropriate blood glucose levels for the student.

EQUIPMENT:
- ✓ Blood glucose meter
- ✓ A lancet, automatic lancet or lancet pen
- ✓ Alcohol swab or pad
- ✓ Testing strips
- ✓ Cotton swabs or 2x2 gauze pads
- ✓ Sharps container

PROCEDURE:
1. Perform hand hygiene and apply clean gloves.
2. Student should perform hand hygiene.
3. Select finger or alternate site to be used for testing and clean with an alcohol swab/pad for 5-10 seconds. *Meters, capable of testing a small volume of blood, can use an alternate site (forearm, thigh, or palm). It must be understood that the readings obtained from the small volume of blood may not be as accurate as readings from blood samples from the If fingertips.*
4. Fingertip/alternate sites should be rotated.
5. Allow finger/alternate site to dry completely. Do not fan or blow on the site to hasten the drying process.

BLOOD GLUCOSE MONITORING *(continued from previous page)*

PROCEDURE *(continued)*

6. Hold the lancet device firmly against the side of the student's finger. Avoid pad of the finger which has a denser nerve supply. If using an alternate site, follow manufacturer's directions. Do not milk or massage finger site to increase the blood flow to the area before puncture. Milking the finger may hemolyze the specimen and introduce excess tissue fluid.
7. Push the release mechanism on the device. Remove device.
8. <u>Gently</u> squeeze the finger or alternate site, as needed, to obtain a first drop of blood
9. Use gauze pad to wipe away the first drop of blood.
10. <u>Gently</u> squeeze the finger or alternate site, as needed, to obtain the required volume of blood for testing.
11. Test the second drop of blood. Touch and hold the testing strip to the drop of blood. The test strip will wick the blood sample into the strip. The meter will signal when an adequate blood volume sample has been collected. Do not scrape blood onto the test strip as this may result in an inaccurate test measurement. Refer to the specific meter manufacturer's instructions to assure an adequate blood volume is collected for testing.
12. Record the reading in the student's personal blood glucose log and the student's health record.
13. Dispose of the lancet using proper guidelines for disposal.

NURSING CONSIDERATIONS:
1. This procedure may be performed by the school nurse or may be delegated to unlicensed personnel who have been properly trained and are supervised.
2. All students with diabetes should have an individualized healthcare plan (IHP) to address their needs. This plan may be part of a Section 504 plan.
3. Blood glucose self- monitoring should be encouraged for students who have the capability to do this, allowing them to spend less time out of class. The IHP should include a plan for communication between the student and the school nurse that enables a response to blood glucose levels out e the normal range for that student.
4. Blood glucose testing may be done in the health office, in a classroom, or other area of the school.
5. Schools must adhere to universal precautions to reduce the transmission of blood borne pathogens.

BLOOD GLUCOSE MONITORING *(continued from previous page)*

NURSING CONSIDERATIONS: *(continued)*

6. Fingerstick devices, meters, and test strips should not be shared. This is an infection control issue.
7. Meters that can test blood samples from alternate site must be able to test small volume blood samples.

References

American Diabetes Association. (2015) *Checking Your blood Glucose.* Retrieved from http://www.diabetes.org/living-with-diabetes/treatment-and-care/blood-glucose-control/checking-your-blood-glucose.html

Centers for Disease Control and Prevention. (2012). *Infection prevention during blood glucose monitoring and insulin administration.* Retrieved from http://www.cdc.gov/injectionsafety/blood-glucose-monitoring.html

Connecticut State Department of Education. (2014). *Clinical guidelines for Connecticut school nurses: Blood glucose monitoring.* Retrieved from http://www.sde.ct.gov/sde/cwp/view.asp?a=2663&q=334270

Connecticut State Department of Education. (n.d.) *Guidelines for blood glucose self-monitoring in Connecticut schools.* Retrieved from http://www.sde.ct.gov/sde/lib/sde/pdf/publications/glucose/glucose_guidelines.pdf

Einis, S., Kinne, J., Raymond, M., Reardon, K., Srivatsa, A., & Warman, K. Y. (2014). Diabetes. In S. M. Porter, P. A. Branowicki, & J. S. Palfrey (Eds.), *Supporting students with special health care needs: Guidelines and procedures for schools* (3rd ed.) (pp. 387-451). Baltimore, MD: Brookes Publishing Co.

Mayo Clinic. (2014). *Blood sugar testing: Why, when and how.* Retrieved from http://www.mayoclinic.org/diseases-conditions/diabetes/in-depth/blood-sugar/art-20046628?pg=1

Mayo Clinic. (2014). *Diseases and conditions diabetes.* Retrieved from http://www.mayoclinic.org/diseases-conditions/diabetes/in-depth/blood-sugars/art-20046628?pg=2

Perry, A., Potter, P., & Ostendorf, W. (2014). Specimen collection. In *Clinical nursing skills and techniques,* (8th ed). (pg. 1085-1090). St. Louis, MO: Elsevier/Mosby

Record, E., & Ballard, L. (2013). The child with endocrine dysfunction. In M. Hockenberry (Ed,), *Wong's essentials of pediatric nursing,* (9th ed.) (pp. 995 and 1003-1004). St. Louis, MO: Elsevier/Mosby

U.S. Department of Health and Human Services. (2012). *Helping the student with diabetes succeed A guide for school personnel.* Retrieved from http://ndep.nih.gov/media/NDEP61_SchoolGuide_4c_508.pdf

U.S. Food and Drug Administration. (2015). *Blood glucose monitoring devices.* Retrieved from http://www.fda.gov/medicaldevices/productsandmedicalprocedures/InVitroDiagnostics/GlucoseTestingDevices/default.htm

CATHETERIZATION (URINARY): Insertion or reinsertion of urinary catheter

DEFINITION:
Urinary Catheter: A tube used to empty or drain the bladder. Catheters are sized in units called French, where one French equals 1/3 of 1 mm. Catheters vary from 12 (small) FR to 48 (large) FR (3-16mm) in size.

Intermittent (Short-Term) Catheters: An intermittent catheter would be used when the catheter only needs to be used intermittently. These catheters are removed after the flow of urine has stopped.

Indwelling Urethral Catheters: An indwelling urinary catheter is used when the catheter is left in the bladder. An indwelling catheter collects urine by attaching to a drainage bag. A newer type of catheter has a valve that can be opened to allow urine to flow out.

Urethra: The urethra is the tube that carries urine out of the body from the bladder.

PURPOSE:
To ensure emptying of the bladder for students who are unable to void independently and/ or completely.

EQUIPMENT:
- ✓ Gloves
- ✓ Clean or sterile straight catheters
- ✓ Collection bag and tubing
- ✓ Receptacle for collection
- ✓ Water based lubricant (do not use a petroleum lubricant such as Vaseline)
- ✓ Disposable pad (i.e. Chux®) or disposable towel
- ✓ Soap and water or disposable wipes
- ✓ Sterile water (for indwelling catheters)
- ✓ 10 cc syringe (for indwelling catheters)

CATHETERIZATION (URINARY) *(continued from previous page)*

PROCEDURE:

Male Clean Intermittent Catheterization

Position: Male students may be catheterized standing, sitting on a toilet, lying down or in a wheelchair.

- Wash hands.
- Open the catheter utilizing clean technique.
- Hold sides of penis with non-dominant hand at a straight angle from the body.
- Clean the urethra and the tip of penis with wipes or mild soap and water.
- Retract the foreskin if uncircumcised.
- Generously coat the distal end of the catheter with a water soluble lubricant
- Have the student take a deep breath and slowly insert the catheter into the urethra until there is a good flow of urine. Depending on the size of the student, you may advance the catheter ½ to 1 inch more.
- If resistance is met prior to the flow of urine, have the student take another deep breath and gently advance further. Some resistance of the catheter is normal. If necessary, have the student bear down or adjust student's position. You may need to reposition on the penis.
- If the student is experiencing pain or the catheter is not advancing notify the parents/healthcare provider. When the urine flow has ended, remove the catheter slowly, rotating the catheter, pausing if the urine flow begins. When the bladder is empty pinch off the catheter and withdraw it from the urethra. Measure urine if indicated and observe urine for color, mucus or odor.
- Document results and time. If the catheter can be used again, wash, rinse, dry and store in an appropriate container.
- Wash hands.

CATHETERIZATION (URINARY) *(continued from previous page)*

Female Intermittent Clean Catheterization

Position: Female students may be catheterized sitting on a toilet, lying down or in a wheelchair. When catheterizing on the toilet, have the student sit on the back of the toilet seat with legs straddled.

- Wash hands.
- Put on gloves.
- Open the catheter utilizing clean technique.
- Position the student to expose the urethral opening.
- Clean the vulva from front to back.
- Generously coat the distal end of the catheter with a water-soluble lubricant.
- Use your non-dominant hand to separate the labia minora to visualize the urinary meatus.
- Have the student take a deep breath, insert the catheter until there is a good flow of urine, and advance the catheter slightly.
- If necessary, have the student bear down or adjust position.
- If you are unable to get a flow of urine, check for catheter placement. The catheter may be in the vagina. If it is remove, discard and use a clean catheter. When the urine flow has ended remove the catheter slowly, rotating the catheter, pausing if flow begins. When the bladder is empty pinch off the catheter and withdraw it from the urethra.
- Measure if indicated and observe urine for color, mucus or odor.
- If the catheter can be used again, wash, rinse, dry and store in an appropriate container.
- Document results and time.
- Wash hands.

CATHETERIZATION (URINARY) *(continued from previous page)*

Indwelling Catheters
Generally, indwelling catheters only require emptying of the collection bag as it accumulates and measuring the output if indicated. In the event it becomes dislodged, the nurse may be responsible for reinsertion.

Reinsertion of indwelling catheters male catheterization
- Hold sides of penis with non-dominant hand at a straight angle from the body.
- Clean the urethra and the tip of penis with the wipes or mild soap and water.
- Retract the foreskin if uncircumcised.
- Generously coat the distal end of the catheter with a water-soluble lubricant.
- Have the student take a deep breath and slowly insert the catheter into the urethra until urine begins to flow.
- Depending on the size of the student, you may advance the catheter ½ to 1 inch more.
- Inflate the balloon with the ordered amount of sterile water.
- If resistance is met prior to the flow of urine, have the student take another deep breath and gently advance further. Some resistance of the catheter is normal.
- If the student is experiencing pain or the catheter is not advancing notify the parents/healthcare provider.
- Gently pull catheter until inflation balloon is snug against bladder neck.
- Attach the catheter to the drainage system.
- Wash hands.

Reinsertion of indwelling catheters female catheterization
- Wash hands.
- Put on gloves.
- Position the student to expose the urethral opening.
- Clean the vulva from front to back.
- Generously coat the distal end of the catheter with lubricant.
- Use one hand to separate the labia minora to visualize the urinary meatus.
- Have the student take a deep breath and insert the catheter until urine begins to flow and advance the catheter slightly.
- Inflate the balloon with the appropriate amount of sterile water.
- Gently pull catheter until inflation balloon is snug against bladder neck.
- Attach the catheter to the leg bag or other drainage system.
- Wash hands.

CATHETERIZATION (URINARY) *(continued from previous page)*

NURSING CONSIDERATIONS:

1. A RN or LPN generally only does this task. Nurses should check with their state laws and State Board of Examiners for Nursing regarding whether catheterization can be delegated to an unlicensed staff member.
2. This should be done for all students in a private location with little possibility of interruption.
3. If frank bleeding or edema is present, the healthcare provider should be notified.
4. If insertion is difficult or the decision is made that insertion is not to be done, the student should be diapered to prevent soiling.
5. Be aware of the student's medications that affect changes in his/her urine.
6. Note the baseline status of the student's urine color, amount and pattern of continence.
7. Depending on the student's ability, promote independence and teach him/her how to perform the procedure.
8. The facilities may need to be wheelchair accessible or have special equipment such as a raised toilet or hand rails.
9. Catheters come in different sizes; the same sized catheter should be inserted each time.

References

Connecticut State Department of Education. (2014). *Clinical guidelines for Connecticut school nurses: Catheterizations.* Retrieved from http://www.sde.ct.gov/sde/cwp/view.asp?a=2663&q=334188

Department of Emergency Medicine, University of Ottawa. (2003). *Urinary catheter insertion.* Retrieved from http://www.med.uottawa.ca/procedures/ucath/

Grant, R.H., & Dunleavey, M.J. (2014). Clean intermittent catheterization. In S. M. Porter, P. A. Branowicki, & J. S. Palfrey (Eds.), *Supporting students with special health care needs: Guidelines and procedures for schools* (3rd ed., pp. 279-291). Baltimore, MD: Brookes Publishing Co.

Selekman, J., Bochenek, J., & Lukens, M. (2013). Children with chronic conditions. In J. Selekman (Ed.), *School nursing: A comprehensive text* (2nd ed., pp. 1042-1044). Philadelphia, PA: F.A. Davis Company.

ENTERAL TUBE FEEDINGS

DEFINITION/ETIOLOGY:
Enteral Nutrition: Nutrition administered in the gastrointestinal tract.

Bolus Feedings: The administration of liquid into a feeding tube using gravity.

Tube Feeding Pump: A mechanical pump that administers a designated amount of liquid over a prescribed amount of time. A tube feeding bag and tubing is also utilized.

Nasogastric Tubes (NGT): Tubes inserted through the nose and into the stomach. They can be inserted and removed for each feeding or can stay in place for a predetermined amount of time. Some tubes can be weighted for additional security for staying in place.

Gastrostomy Tube (GT): The most common type of tube in children and utilized in the school setting. A surgically implanted tube is placed through the stomach wall with one end accessible on the abdomen. The "mic-key" is a common type utilized. It may also be referred to as a "button". The tube remains in place at all times and is capped between feedings to prevent leakage of stomach contents. It stays flush with the abdomen and tubing is connected for feeding or medication administration.

Gastro-jejunostomy Tube (G-JT): Inserted surgically through the stomach wall, it passes through the pylorus and ends in the jejunal segment of the small intestine. They may be double lumened with one lumen that ends in the stomach and the other lumen that land in the jejunum. These are placed in students who cannot tolerate food or liquid in their stomachs. The lumen in the stomach is often utilized for medication administration.

Jejunostomy Tube (JT): Inserted surgically through the abdominal wall and into the jejunal section of the small intestine.

PURPOSE:
To deliver a liquid formula/medication directly to the duodenum, jejunum or stomach. Generally, the purpose of such a feeding method is to provide nutrition to a student who is unable to eat orally or to supplement oral feedings to provide nutrients and calories.

ENTERAL TUBE FEEDINGS *(continued from previous page)*

EQUIPMENT:
- ✓ Prescribed formula (room temperature)
- ✓ Tube feeding bag and tubing (as indicated by order)
- ✓ Syringe (generally 30 or 60 cc)
- ✓ Feeding pump (as indicated by order)

PROCEDURE:

> **If the student begins to cough, choke or have a color change, stop the feeding and re-check tube placement.**

Nasogastric Tube
- Wash hands.
- Prepare feeding. Ensure the NG tube is in the stomach. Check that the position of a black mark on the tube is the same length from the nose for each use. You may also inject 5cc of air into the NGT while listening with a stethoscope over the stomach for the sound of air entering the stomach. Check with the healthcare provider's orders to ascertain if this is necessary.
- Position student (to prevent aspiration):
  1. On right side with head elevated minimum of 30°, OR
  2. Lying on back 45° OR
  3. In a sitting position.
     - ○ The student should remain in an elevated or upright position for 30 minutes after the feeding (avoid lying flat).
- Check for residuals, if ordered. Slowly withdraw the gastric juice, formula or medication from the stomach with a syringe, assess, return the fluid and document.
- Attach syringe and administer the feeding via gravity or feeding pump as ordered. If performing a bolus feeding, hold the syringe 4-6 inches above abdomen or per orders. Raising or lowering the height of the syringe will help control the rate of intake.
- When feeding is complete, detach the syringe and flush with a water utilizing a syringe.
- Disconnect and cap the tube.
- Wash syringe and other reusable equipment with soapy water and store in a clean area.
- Document.

ENTERAL TUBE FEEDINGS *(continued from previous page)*

Gastrostomy Tube Feeding
- Wash hands.
- Prepare feeding.
- Ensure tube placement is appropriate. Mic-key tubes should be level with the skin and not leaking. They should be able to rotate 360°.
- Position to student (to prevent aspiration) on:
  - Right side with head elevated minimum of 30°, lying on back 45° or in a sitting position.
  - Student should remain in this position for 30 minutes after feeding.
- Check for residuals, if ordered. Slowly withdraw the gastric juice, formula or medication from the stomach with a syringe, assess, return the fluid and document.
- Fill the extension tubing with water or formula, clamp and attach to the mic-key button by connecting and locking it into place. If using a pump, prime the pump before connecting tubing to GT to the attaching to the mic-key.
- Insert the syringe into the open end of the extension set.
- Pour the food into the syringe until it is half-full. Unclamp the extension set to begin feeding. Hold the tip to the syringe no higher than the child's shoulders. If the food is not flowing, squeeze the tube in downward strokes to bring the food down.
- When feeding is complete, flush with water. Pinch the tubing and detach the syringe. Cap and disconnect tubing.
- Wash syringe and other reusable equipment with soapy water and store in a clean area.
- Document.

Medication Administration
- Prepare the medication as prescribed.
- The medicine should be liquid, or finely crushed and dissolved in water, so that the tube does not get blocked.
- Medication is more effective if given before feeding. Medication should never be mixed in the formula. Always flush before and after giving medication to make sure all medication goes in the stomach and is not left in the feeding tube.
- Clamp or pinch off the tube prior to opening to air to avoid reflux of gastric secretions.
- Attach syringe and administer medications unclamping the tube.

ENTERAL TUBE FEEDINGS *(continued from previous page)*

NURSING CONSIDERATIONS:

1. An RN or LPN generally initiates tube feedings. School nurses should check with their individual state delegation laws regarding whether G-tube feedings can be delegated to an unlicensed staff member. If so, competency based training should be done with the appropriate level of supervision.

2. Tube feedings in school require a healthcare provider's order or treatment authorization which would include the type of formula, infusion type, rate and frequency, as well as flushing instructions.

3. Consider securing the GT/NG tube for young or special needs students. Secure by placing a piece of tape around the tube and pinning to clothing or putting the tube under the student's clothing.

4. Administer a bolus feeding over 15-30 minutes unless otherwise specified. A slow drip feeding is delivered continuously over a set number of hours.

5. Assess the insertion site for skin integrity with each use, as rashes tend to occur with leaking around the stoma site. A barrier ointment or use of a dry dressing may be utilized.

6. Aspiration of feeding into the lungs is a risk with enteral feedings. Ensuring and securing proper placement of the tubing is essential.

7. If there is any nausea, vomiting or cramping the feeding rate may need to be slowed or the formula may be too cold.

8. A healthcare provider's order may include venting the GT (open the cap to air). This procedure allows the release of air and makes the student comfortable.

9. Open formula may be stored in the refrigerator for 24 hours and then discard.

10. If a mic-key tube dislodges, nurses should be trained in insertion of a new tube. Keep an additional mic-key at school. Insertion involves filling an internal balloon with 5cc of water for securing the tube to the side of the stoma.

11. Before attempting to dislodge a blockage try rolling the tube between fingers in a milking motion towards the site of insertion. If unsuccessful in removing the blockage, warm water seems to work best. Fill a syringe with warm water and try to slightly move the plunger slightly back and forth. If the blockage remains, contact the parent.

ENTERAL TUBE FEEDINGS *(continued from previous page)*

NURSING CONSIDERATIONS: *(continued)*

12. If the student is does not receive any food by mouth consider oral stimulation during the feeding.

13. Students with tube feedings can be fed anywhere and as long as the setting is appropriate to the student's desire for privacy or the desire to be with their peers. Either the cafeteria or if the student prefers the health room can be utilized. If frequent feedings are needed the student may be fed in the classroom.

14. Students with tube feedings should have an Individualized Healthcare Plan (IHP) tailored to the individual student's needs.

15. Depending on the age and capabilities of the student, have him or her assist with the feeding by holding the syringe or pouring fluid into it.

References

Cleveland Clinic. Center for Human Nutrition and Digestive Disease Institute. (n.d.). *Tube feeding instructions for home.* Retrieved from http://my.clevelandclinic.org/ccf/media/files/Digestive_Disease/center-human-nutrition/home-enteral-nutrition-booklet.pdf

Connecticut State Department of Education. (2014). *Clinical guidelines for Connecticut school nurses: Enteral tube feedings.* Retrieved from http://www.sde.ct.gov/sde/cwp/view.asp?a=2663&q=334284

Donoghue, E. (2010). *Managing chronic health needs in childcare and schools a quick reference guide.* Elk Grove Village, Ill.: American Academy of Pediatrics.

Hootman, J. (2004). Procedures. *Quality nursing interventions in the school setting: Procedures, models, and guidelines* (Rev. ed.). Scarborough, ME: National Association of School Nurses.

Perkins, J.M., & Paul, F. (2014). Tube feeding. In S. M. Porter, P. A. Branowicki, & J. S. Palfrey (Eds.), *Supporting students with special health care needs: Guidelines and procedures for schools* (3rd ed.) (pp. 211-249). Baltimore, MD: Brookes Publishing Co.

Simons, S., & Remington, R. (2013). The percutaneous endoscopic gastrostomy tube: A nurse's guide to PEG tubes. *MEDSURG Nursing, 22*(2), 77-83.

U.S. National Library of Medicine. (2014). *Gastrostomy feeding tube – bolus.* Retrieved from http://www.nlm.nih.gov/medlineplus/ency/patientinstructions/000165.htm

Williams, N. T. (2008). Medication administration through enteral feeding tubes. *American Journal of Health-System Pharmacist, 65,* pp.2347-2357. Retrieved from http://www.ajhp.org/content/65/24/2347.short

Wisconsin Department of Public Instruction. (2015). *School nursing and health services training: Nursing procedures (WISHeS).* Retrieved from http://www.wishesproject.org/?page_id=50

TRACHEOSTOMY CARE (Tracheostomy Suctioning and Tracheostomy Change)

DEFINITION:

A tracheostomy is a surgical opening into the trachea. It is often referred to as a "trach". The opening is called a stoma, and a tracheostomy tube is inserted into the stoma. The trach tubes are primarily made of specialized plastic, and come in a variety of brands and sizes. Tracheostomies may be temporary or long term. Common indications for tracheostomies include:

- bronchopulmonary dysplasia (BPD, which can be a sequalae of severe prematurity),
- central hypoventilation syndrome,
- chronic pulmonary diseases,
- congenital anomalies,
- degenerative neuromuscular diseases (such as Muscular Dystrophy); and
- spinal cord injuries.

Many children with tracheostomies also require support from a ventilator, either all of the time or for parts of the day.

PURPOSE:

The primary goal of tracheostomy care is airway maintenance. It will allow long-term access to a ventilator and provides access to clear the trachea of secretions. Tracheostomy tube change is not a routine procedure in the health office but may be needed if the tube is blocked with secretions and is impeding respiration.

EQUIPMENT:

Tracheostomy Change

- ✓ Extra trach tube, with obturator placed inside
- ✓ Additional extra trach tube, one size smaller than normal, with obturator placed inside
- ✓ Clean trach ties
- ✓ Scissors
- ✓ Water-soluble jelly or lubricant
- ✓ Suction equipment with correct size catheters
- ✓ Ambu bag and mask.
- ✓ Oxygen (if part of school health plan)
- ✓ Gloves
- ✓ Trach dressing
- ✓ Delee mucus trap
- ✓ Bulb syringe

TRACHEOSTOMY CARE (Tracheostomy Suctioning and Tracheostomy Change)
(continued from previous page)

Tracheostomy Suctioning
- ✓ Tracheostomy Suctioning machine
- ✓ Suction catheter of prescribed size
- ✓ Disposable clean gloves
- ✓ Ambu bag and mask
- ✓ Tracheostomy adapter and mask
- ✓ Saline ampules or sterile water

The school nurse should develop an Individualized Healthcare Plan (IHP) outlining the procedure, along with emergency interventions.

PROCEDURE:
I. **RESPIRATORY ASSESSMENT. Tracheostomy may need to be suctioned if you observe the following after checking placement of trach tube:**
   - Increased respiratory rate
   - Trouble breathing
   - Noisy respirations
   - Visible mucus
   - Restlessness
   - "Wet" sounding breathing
   - Color change, particularly blue or pale around the mucous membranes and nail beds
   - Increased heart rate
   - Skin feels moist or "clammy" to the touch

II. **SUCTIONING:**
   - Clean technique is recommended for home/school.
   - Shallow suctioning: this method is used when mucus is visible at the opening of the trach. This may occur after the child coughs. A Yankauer catheter or even a bulb syringe may be used to remove the mucus.
   - Premeasured depth suctioning: Measure the length of the trach tube and add ¼ inch. Make a note of this on the child's Individualized Healthcare Plan. When suctioning, only advance the catheter as far as the premeasured length. It is beneficial to use pre-marked suction catheters.
   - Deep suctioning: The catheter is advanced beyond the tip of the tracheal tube until resistance is felt. This procedure usually is not needed in the school setting and requires specific orders from the licensed healthcare provider. If deep suctioning necessary, it should be performed by a licensed nurse.

TRACHEOSTOMY CARE (Tracheostomy Suctioning and Tracheostomy Change)
(continued from previous page)

SUCTIONING *(continued)*

PROCEDURE

1. Wash hands.
2. Glove.
3. Set up equipment.
4. Position student as is recommended. Most students are suctioned while seated
5. Explain the procedure to the student using developmentally appropriate language
6. Encourage the student to cough to loosen secretions
7. If ordered, insert several drops of saline into the tracheostomy and use the ambu bag to disperse
8. Turn on suction machine, check by tip of catheter into cup of sterile water/saline.
9. Advance the catheter to pre-measured length into trach tube.
10. Cover the air vent with your thumb to apply suction, gently twirl the catheter as you withdraw the catheter from the trach tube. This should take 5 seconds or less.
11. Allow student to rest for approximately 30 seconds between suctioning
12. After each suction pass, rinse the tubing in the cup of sterile water/saline.
13. Notify parent/guardian if:
    - increased need for suctioning,
    - a color change in the mucus such as green or yellow; or
    - bleeding from the trach.
14. Replace artificial nose after suctioning.

Note: If oral suctioning is also required, the oral cavity may be suctioned with the trach catheter, but a catheter used in the oral cavity cannot be used to suction the trach.

TRACHEOSTOMY CARE (Tracheostomy Suctioning and Tracheostomy Change)
(continued from previous page)

III. **TRACHESTOMY TUBE CHANGE:**
- Indications for trach change or replacement should be written into the individualized healthcare plan.
- Maintain a "go bag" containing emergency supplies for trach change. This bag should travel with the child and must be checked daily upon arrival to school. It is recommended that a checklist be developed for documentation.

PROCEDURE

1. Wash hands.

2. Assemble equipment.

3. Glove.

4. Explain the procedure to the student utilizing appropriate developmental language

5. Position the child. Small children may be positioned on their backs with a blanket under their shoulders.

6. Open tracheostomy tube package and insert obturator.

7. Attach holders to tube (some students may have velcro or fabric ties).

8. Lubricate the end of the tracheostomy tube with water-soluble lubricant or sterile saline.

9. Suction nose and mouth if needed.

10. Give two to four breaths with the ambu bag as needed.

11. Have a second person hold the tracheostomy in place while removing the ties.

12. With the new tube in hand have the second person remove the tube.

13. Insert the new tube at a right angle rotating it downward.

14. Immediately remove obturator.

15. Observe the student for signs of distress.

16. Secure with tracheostomy holder.

17. Assess breath sounds and chest movement.

TRACHEOSTOMY CARE (Tracheostomy Suctioning and Tracheostomy Change)
(continued from previous page)

Nursing Considerations

1. Assessment of the stoma site:
   a. Assessment of the site may be done as you carry out routine trach care.
   b. Incorporate the type of care recommended by the provider (i.e. cleaning with soap and water or half strength hydrogen peroxide) into the individualized healthcare plan.
   c. The area around the stoma should be kept clean and dry. Many children use a trach dressing and the dressing should be changed when it becomes moist.
   d. Notify parent/guardian if there is an increased need for dressing changed secondary to increased drainage, redness at the stoma site, "crusting" at the site or any type of skin breakdown or signs/symptoms of infection.

2. Emergency Go Bag should always be with the student (during recess, field trips, school bus).

3. The tracheostomy holders should be loose enough to slip one finger between the tube holders and the neck.

4. A small amount of bleeding may occur around the stoma, if persistent or unusual notify parents.

References

Brubaker, C. & Selekman, J. (2013). Skills needed by children who are technology dependent. In J. Selekman (Ed.), *School nursing: A comprehensive text* (2nd ed.) (pp. 1028-1032, 1047-1053). Philadelphia, PA: F.A. Davis.

Connecticut State Department of Education. (2014). *Clinical guidelines for Connecticut school nurses: Tracheostomy care and suctioning.* Retrieved from http://www.sde.ct.gov/sde/cwp/view.asp?a=2663&q=334188

Perlman, L. & Rosen, D. (2014). Respiratory care. In S. M. Porter, P. A. Branowicki, & J. S. Palfrey (Eds.), *Supporting students with special health care needs: Guidelines and procedures for schools* (3rd ed.) (pp. 313-387). Baltimore, MD: Brookes Publishing Co.

Selekman, J., Bochenek, J., & Lukens, M. (2013). Children with chronic conditions. In J. Selekman (Ed.), *School nursing: A comprehensive text* (2nd ed.) (pp. 700-783). Philadelphia, PA: F.A. Davis.

SECTION III

SCHOOL NURSE MANAGEMENT

DISASTER PREPAREDNESS

OVERVIEW/DEFINITION:
Disaster preparedness is the ongoing and continuous cycle of planning, preparing, training and evaluating in order to effectively respond to any disaster or emergency within the school or community. Disasters in the school setting can be the result of natural disasters, such as a hurricane, blizzard, flood or tornado, or human-generated disasters, such as accidents, school shootings, hazardous explosions, or fire. Disasters and emergencies can involve individual students, staff and visitors or large numbers of persons within the school community. By definition, a disaster is any event that causes human suffering and requires resources beyond the normal amount and outside assistance to recover (Lundy & James, 2016; Stanhope & Lancaster, 2015).

ANTICIPATED CONCERNS/PROBLEMS:
- Physical Injuries – immediate and long-term
- Psychological Conditions – immediate and long-term
- Socioeconomic shifts – loss of resources, employment, homes, food and water sources

MANAGEMENT/POTENTIAL INTERVENTIONS:
Planning: the purpose of planning is to prevent and mitigate problems resulting from any disaster. The creation of a school or district-wide disaster plan, based on input from all stakeholders (i.e., school officials, agencies involved in emergency responses as well as community members), is essential to effective preparation and response. The school nurse has a critical role in planning and responding to disasters and as such is an essential member of the planning and response team.

The key elements of a disaster plan are:
- Establish lines of authority during the event.
- Establish communication methods both internally and externally.
- Determine where or how resources and equipment needed will be obtained based on student/staff needs and existing building resources.
- Identify access to human resources that may be needed during or after a disaster.
- Identify of roles and responsibilities of team members (by title and not person to avoid changing the plan when persons leave or change positions within the organization).

DISASTER PREPAREDNESS *(continued from previous page)*

Planning *(continued)*

- Establish transportation patterns to evacuate or control access and gridlock at the site.
- Determine documentation procedures and how records will be managed (health and resources).
- Designate evacuation routes (within the building and away from the site).
- Plan for evacuation of students with special needs (in wheelchairs, visually or hearing impaired, developmental or emotional disabilities, etc.).
- Establish search and rescue plans with local emergency responders.
- Plan for provision of acute care including collection site, triage plans, and roles of healthcare providers and laypersons.
- Consider shelter management in the event that the staff and students remain on site for more than a few hours (e.g., food, water, medications, etc.).
- Determine any special considerations needed for any children or staff with special healthcare needs or chronic conditions.
- Establish debriefing plans during the recovery phase.
- Evaluate the plan routinely through disaster drills and review of response in any actual events.

Note: Disaster plans should be based on routine procedures whenever possible to avoid confusion (e.g., evacuation of the building may be designed in a way that is similar to evacuations during fires so the route is familiar to staff and students).

Preparedness requires conducting regular disaster drills based on the school disaster plan, evaluating the outcomes of the drill or an actual event, reviewing and revising the plan using information gathered during the drill or an actual event, training of school personnel for specific responsibilities (e.g., triage training for the school nurse or media training for the designated spokesperson), and a review of the current evidence on effective disaster management.

Response requires an immediate and organized approach to the disaster based on the established disaster plan. The school nurse may be involved in the acute management of victims including assessment of the situation, triage, establishing the collection area for victims if they can be moved, administering first aid and nursing care, directing others

DISASTER PREPAREDNESS *(continued from previous page)*

Response *(continued)*

to assist in the management of care, determining resources and equipment needed, establishing and providing psychological care and counseling to indirect victims, such as witnesses to the event, family members, and community members. During the event, the school nurse may also need to respond to or delegate any routine healthcare needs of the students.

Recovery is the process of returning to optimal functioning after an event. It is suggested that even for the most well-prepared person, the results of a disaster can be devastating and have long-term effects. How individuals and communities affected by the disaster recover are impacted by many factors: duration of the event, degree of injury, witnessing graphic scenes, disruption of social and economic structures within the community, and the characteristics of the group (s) impacted. The school nurse along with mental health professionals will need to address the psychological needs of the community and intervene to assist the transition back to pre-disaster functioning. The school nurse may also be involved in managing any new acute or chronic physical health needs as a result of the disaster.

FOLLOW-UP:
As noted in the preparedness phase of disaster response, reviewing and revising the disaster plan is an important follow-up to any actual disaster. Debriefing is key to helping the first responders and disaster team members recover from the event too. Recognizing event and occupational stressors is a necessary step for nurses to identify what care and assistance they may need to recover.

NOTES: Disaster preparedness is not a one-time activity; being prepared requires ongoing assessment and collaboration regarding student and faculty needs, resources, staffing, equipment and clear lines of communication with the community- wide response team.

Children affected by disasters do not have the same coping skills as adults and may need additional support and intervention. Common concerns in children following a disaster are new fears, phobias, sleep disturbances, fear of being alone, increased dependency, hypersensitivity to noise and weather, and developmental regressions.

DISASTER PREPAREDNESS *(continued from previous page)*

Resources:

Caring for Children in Disasters: http://www.cdc.gov/childrenindisasters/schools.html

References

Centers for Disease Control and Prevention. (2015). *Emergency preparedness*. Retrieved from http://emergency.cdc.gov/index.asp

Lundy, K. & Janes, S. (2016). *Community health nursing: Caring for the public's health* (3rd ed.). Burlington, MA: Jones and Bartlett.

National Association of School Nurses. (2014). *Emergency preparedness and response in the school setting – the role of the school nurse* (Position Statement). Retrieved at http://www.nasn.org/PolicyAdvocacy/PositionPapersandReports/NASNPositionStatementsFullView/tabid/462/ArticleId/117/Emergency-Preparedness-and-Response-in-the-School-Setting-The-Role-of-the-School-Nurse-Revised-June.

Stanhope, M., & Lancester, J. (2014). *Foundations of nursing in the community* (4th ed.). St. Louis: Elsevier/Mosby.

U.S. Department of Homeland Security. (2015). *Planning and preparing for disasters*. Retrieved from http://www.dhs.gov/topic/plan-and-prepare-disasters

DO NOT ATTEMPT RESUSCITATION (DNAR)

OVERVIEW/DEFINITION:

Due to medical advances along with federal laws such as IDEIA, an increased number of children with life-threatening, complex and chronic medical conditions attend school. Chronic conditions include terminal and irreversible illnesses, congenital diseases and anomalies, malignancies and injuries. There are developmental, psychosocial, and emotional benefits for the child to continue to attend school. School attendance maintains a sense of community and normalcy for the student and family.

Parents/guardians, in collaboration with schools and healthcare providers, make difficult end of life decisions about steps to be taken in the event that respiratory/cardiac arrest occurs at school. Schools may receive *Do Not Attempt Resuscitation* (DNAR) orders from the healthcare provider and parents/guardians requesting that life support procedures be withheld in the event respirations and heartbeat have ceased and that the student be allowed to die without emergency intervention. This also may be referred to as *Do Not Resuscitate* (DNR) or *Allow Natural Death* (AND) orders. It is important to note that a DNAR order is not an order to stand by and not intervene, but rather to provide supportive and comfort measures that are integrated into the plan of care. Spiritual and emotional needs also should be addressed in the plan.

ANTICIPATED CONCERNS/PROBLEMS:

- Schools face difficult decisions in the presence of DNAR directives that are framed by medical, emotional, legal, and ethical issues for the educational setting. These directives reflect the need of school districts to have local, school-based policies and guidelines.
- Acceptance of the DNAR order vary according to state.
- Staff's attitudes and cultural beliefs concerning dying.

421

DO NOT ATTEMPT RESUSCITATION (DNAR) *(continued from previous page)*

MANAGEMENT/ INTERVENTIONS:
- Identification of federal, state, and local laws related to DNAR directives in the educational setting and the care of medically fragile children at school. (General Counsel at the state Department of Education is a good resource to define federal, state, and local laws and the ability of schools to comply with "do not attempt resuscitation" directives in the school district).
- Local policy development and the development of guidelines that support policy should include both members of the school community (i.e. attorney for the school board of education, school administrator, the school nurse, other members of the school services team), and members of the medical community (e.g., Emergency Medical Services [EMS], and funeral director).
- Obtain release of information and DNAR order.
- Organize team meeting including school staff, parents/guardians, and palliative care team. Other community members that may be considered: clergy, local EMS, funeral home director, healthcare provider.
- Conduct student assessment and assessment of staffing needs.
- Develop an Individualized Healthcare Plan. Components to consider:
  - Disease-directed treatment
  - Symptom control
  - Copy of the DNAR order
  - Specific explanation of what actions may be taken by staff members
  - Specific comfort measures such as holding the child, providing oxygen, keeping student warm (AAP, 2010)
  - Address spiritual needs
  - Clear instructions on classroom management should child's health status change, i.e. a code that elicits quick staff response, privacy considerations for student
  - Education of identified school staff to include defining staff roles and accommodations for bus transportation
- Develop a plan to provide and support staff and student's peers.

FOLLOW-UP:
- Re-evaluate the plan annually, at minimum.
- Implement the plan to provide support to school staff and student's peers.

DO NOT ATTEMPT RESUSCITATION (DNAR) *(continued from previous page)*

NOTES:

- An article, *Do Not Attempt Resuscitation (DNAR) Orders in School Setting* (NASN School Nurse, March 2013) provides a comprehensive checklist for planning for a DNAR order for a child at school. See reference list for complete information.

References

Adelman, J. (2010). The school based do-not-resuscitate order. *DePaul Journal of Health Care Law, Winter,* 197- 214.

American Academy of Pediatrics. (2010). Policy statement: Honoring do-not-attempt resuscitation requests in schools. *Pediatrics, 125,* 1073-1077. doi: 10.1542/peds.2010-0452

National Association of School Nurses. (2014). Do not attempt resuscitation (DNAR) (Position Statement). Retrieved from http://www.nasn.org/PolicyAdvocacy/PositionPapersandReports/NASNPositionStatementsFullView/tabid/462/ArticleId/640/Do-Not-Attempt-Resuscitation-DNAR-The-Role-of-the-School-Nurse-Adopted-January-2014

Selekman, J., Bochenek, J., & Lukens, M. (2013). Do not resuscitate orders. In J. Selekman (Ed.), *School nursing: A comprehensive text (2nd ed.)* (pp. 713-714). Philadelphia, PA: F.A. Davis.

Weise, K. L. (2010). Do-not-attempt-resuscitation orders in public schools. *American Medical Association Journal of Ethics, 12*(7), 569-572. Retrieved from http://virtualmentor.ama-assn.org/2010/07/pfor1-1007.html

Zacharski, S., Minchella, L., Gomez, S., Grogan, S., Porter, S., & Robarge, D. (2013). Do not attempt resuscitation (DNAR) orders in school settings: Special needs nurses review current research and issues. *NASN School Nurse, 28*(2), 71-75. doi: 10.177/1942602X12472540

EMERGING INFECTIOUS DISEASES IN SCHOOLS

OVERVIEW/DEFINITION:

Emerging infectious diseases refer to infectious diseases new to the horizon for the medical community, school nurses, and the general population. Schools provide a unique opportunity for the spread of disease and the potential for an outbreak. School nurses are a vital link in the healthcare system and are essential for mitigating the risk of an outbreak through screening, monitoring, communication and educational efforts.

An outbreak is defined as an epidemic (the occurrence of cases of illness clearly in excess of normal expectancy over a specific time period in a community, geographic region, building or institution) (Brockmeyer, Gracek, Krasnitski, & Soto, 2014; Warner & Salemeh, 2014).

Recent examples of emerging infectious diseases include Enterovirus D68, Ebola Virus Disease (EVD), H1N1 and each year's seasonal flu virus. The same containment and prevention principles can guide school nurses through emerging infections.

ANTICIPATED CONCERNS/PROBLEMS:

The close proximity of large numbers of students and staff in both school and on school buses as well as developmental behaviors of young children allow for easy transmission of many infectious diseases. In addition, children are one of our most vulnerable population due to their limited immune systems.

MANAGEMENT/ INTERVENTIONS:

Preparation

- Establish partnerships and collaborations with key stakeholders including state and local health departments. Have contact information readily available.
- Understand the Family Educational Rights and Privacy Act (FERPA) and how, what and in what circumstances information can be shared.
- Maintain adequate supplies for infection control, e.g. personal protective supplies (soap, masks, gowns, gloves).
- Have baseline illness and absenteeism data from several months, at different times of the year to provide a framework for comparison of future spikes in illness.
- Keep a list in each building of "at risk" populations (e.g. immune depressed, medically complex). These individuals or families should be informed of any potential outbreak or incidence and be encouraged to consult with their healthcare provider.

424

EMERGING INFECTIOUS DISEASES IN SCHOOLS *(continued from previous page)*

Preparation *(continued)*

- Have templates of letters or informational blasts prepared that provide consistent, accurate and clear messages in the event that information regarding outbreaks, school closures or other important information will need to be shared with your school community.
- Educate staff, students and parents about signs and symptoms of influenza and other existing conditions of concern.
- Educate staff, students and parents about best hygiene practices for prevention.

Surveillance

- Know baseline illness and absenteeism rates of a school population during seasonal periods to give perspective on increasing trends to identify an outbreak.
- Identify clusters of ill children, for example, ill children from one classroom or school bus.
- Identify threshold absenteeism rates that alert a potential outbreak.
- Share information regarding changes in absenteeism with the local health department.
- Inquire about travel history of students and families.

Preventive Education for Staff, Students and Families

- Dissemination of education regarding proper disease prevention, including proper techniques of handwashing, should be reinforced and heightened during times of an outbreak or increase in illness.
- Have materials available in multiple languages available for students for whom English is a second language.
- Encourage students and staff to stay home when sick.
- Students with chronic health concerns such as asthma should work with their healthcare providers to ensure optimal health during an outbreak.

EMERGING INFECTIOUS DISEASES IN SCHOOLS *(continued from previous page)*

Communication
- Coordinate communications with families and the school community with the local health department.
- Have clear accurate information to minimize misinformation and anxiety.
- Keep school websites updated with current information.
- Consider the use of a public information officer for press releases, media alerts and other public service announcements.
- Refer to FERPA guidelines for specific information regarding outbreaks. It is generally sufficient to report that a child in a particular school or class has been diagnosed rather than identifying the child.

FOLLOW-UP:
School nurses must continually familiarize themselves with the most current information regarding emerging diseases and be prepared to take action when it presents. Early planning is essential in the event of an outbreak and the same strategies and principles discussed above will help address whatever emerging disease is on the horizon.

References

Brockmeyer, J. Gacek, P. Krasnitski, J., & Soto, K. (October, 2014). *Outbreaks and incidents: The role of the school nurse*. Oral presentation: CT School Nurse Conference. Presentation conducted at conference hosted by CT State Department of Education.

Levasseur, S. (2014). *Enterovirus D68 and ebola virus disease- surviving the unknown*. Nashville, TN: School Health Alert.

National Association of School Nurses. (2014). *Enterovirus, EV68: What you need to know*. Retrieved from http://schoolnursenet.nasn.org/nasn/nasnradio

U.S. Department of Education (USDE). (2009). *Family Educational and Privacy Act (FERPA) and H1N1*. Retrieved from http://www2.ed.gov/policy/gen/guid/fpco/pdf/ferpa-h1n1.pdf

Warner, K., & Salemeh, B. (2014). Epidemiology in community health care. In J. Allender, C. Rector, & K. Warner (Eds.), *Community and public health nursing (8th ed.)* (pp. 216-245). Philadelphia, PA: WoltersKluwer/Lippincott Williams & Wilkins.

ENVIRONMENTAL HEALTH

OVERVIEW/DEFINITION:

Environmental health is a division of public health that addresses how physical, chemical and biological factors affect a person's health. Examples of environmental exposures that a child might encounter in the school setting include: poor indoor air quality, chemical exposure (secondary to pest management, cleaning products, etc.), injuries/death due to building code violations, playground injuries, air pollutants (such as exhaust fumes), heating and cooling ventilation, etc.

ANTICIPATED CONCERNS/PROBLEMS:

Environment-related diseases affect a child's current and future health and potentially the child's academic success.

> Children are more vulnerable to environmental exposures and usually suffer more harm from exposure to these toxic substances than adults due to physiological, metabolic and behavioral differences.

Environmental toxin exposure has been linked to the following:
- Asthma (allergens/pesticides/pollutants/poor indoor air quality/ventilation, etc.)
- Lead poisoning—cognitive deficits, aggressive behaviors, learning disabilities, hearing problems, headaches, ADHD symptoms
- Birth defects secondary to mother's exposure to environmental toxicants (mercury, PCBs, pesticides)
- Childhood cancer (pesticides)

Signs and symptoms that children/youth may present with after exposure to environmental toxins (e.g. molds, pesticides, exhaust, cleaning solutions):
- Shortness of breath
- Cough
- Chest tightness
- Wheezing
- Headache
- Rash

ENVIRONMENTAL HEALTH *(continued from previous page)*

MANAGEMENT/POTENTIAL INTERVENTIONS:
Create a healthier environment:

1. Implement and enforce "no idling" of bus and car engines while waiting to pick up children.
2. Maintain school grounds (cut grass) after school hours.
3. Clean school buildings with "green cleaners".
4. Inspect air and water quality routinely.
   a. Change furnace filters every 3 months.
   b. Test water sources for lead.
5. Maintain adequate lighting and ventilation in classrooms/buildings.
6. Minimize the use of fragrances (perfumes/air fresheners).
7. Reduce indoor allergens.
   a. Minimally, vacuum classroom carpets weekly with vacuum cleaner equipped with high-efficiency particulate air (HEPA) filter.
   b. Steam clean carpets every 8 weeks.
8. Avoid classroom pets.
9. Inspect and maintain playground structures to promote safety and minimize injuries.
10. Consider using organic lawn products.
11. Pest prevention – improve school sanitary conditions to avoid insect infestation.
12. Minimize the use of chemical pesticides.
    a. Pesticide application – as a last resort use least toxic pesticide.
    b. Many states require school districts to notify parents/guardians prior to pesticide application.
    c. Post signs notifying parents/guardians of upcoming pesticide application.
    d. Students/staff should not be allowed into the building within 2 hours of pest extermination; follow product health warnings.

ENVIRONMENTAL HEALTH *(continued from previous page)*

FOLLOW-UP:
Role of the school nurse:
- Be alert to maintenance (building and playground) concerns that could be contributing to environmental health issues; notify appropriate staff regarding potential issues.
- Track and identify building trends in health problems that may be linked to environmental toxins.
- Participate in school committees that advocate for reducing exposures to environmental contaminants.
- Advocate for moderation in the use of fragrances; may need to intervene if odors become too strong.

POTENTIAL COMPLICATIONS:
- Lead poisoning resulting in cognitive impairment
- Asthma/allergies: respiratory distress/death
- Cancer/death

Notes:
Children living in poverty are especially vulnerable to environmental toxic exposures. Pollutants, such as lead (paint chips, lead dust, etc.), molds, pollution (commerce, diesel exhaust, etc.) are more prevalent in lower socioeconomic communities. They may lack the resources and finances needed to reduce their child's exposure to the toxins. The school nurse may need to act as a liaison between the school, community, and healthcare provider to meet the health needs of the most vulnerable.

RESOURCES
EPA Programs Supporting Schools - http://www2.epa.gov/iaq-schools/epa-programs-supporting-schools

Institute of Medicine. (2011). *Climate change, the indoor environment, and health* http://www.iom.edu/Reports/2011/Climate-Change-the-Indoor-Environment-and-Health.aspx

ENVIRONMENTAL HEALTH *(continued from previous page)*

References

Children's Environmental Health Network. (2012). *Educational brief on children's environmental health.* Retrieved from http://www.cehn.org/files/EducationalBriefonChildrensEnvironmentalHealth1112.pdf

Environmental Protection Agency. (2015). *Frequently asked questions about improved academic performance.* Retrieved from http://www2.epa.gov/iaq-schools/frequently-asked-questions-about-improved-academic-performance

Environmental Protection Agency. (2014). *Idle free schools.* Retrieved from http://www2.epa.gov/region8/idle-free-schools

Environmental Protection Agency. (2012a). *Student health and academic performance.* Retrieved from http://www2.epa.gov/sites/production/files/2014-08/documents/student_performance_findings.pdf

Environmental Protection Agency (EPA). (2012b). *Voluntary guidelines for states: Development and implementation of a school environmental health program.* Retrieved from www.epa.gov/sc3/ehguidelines/downloads/OCHP_Healthy%20SchoolsFactsheet.pdf

Environmental Protection Agency (EPA). (2012c). *School citing guidelines.* Retrieved from www.epa.gov/schools/siting/downloads/School_Siting_Guidelines.pdf

National Association of School Nurses [NASN]. (2014). *Environmental health concerns in the school setting: The role of the school nurse* (Position Statement). Retrieved from http://www.nasn.org/PolicyAdvocacy/PositionPapersandReports/NASNPositionStatementsFullView/tabid/462/ArticleId/642/Environmental-Health-in-the-School-Setting-The-Role-of-the-School-Nurse-Adopted-January-2014

Proctor, S. (2013). Standards of practice. In J. Selekman (Ed.), *School nursing: A comprehensive text* (2nd ed.) (pp. 48-78). Philadelphia, PA: F. A. Davis.

SCHOOL REFUSAL

OVERVIEW/DEFINITION:

School nurses encounter numerous children and adolescents that have trouble attending school or difficulty remaining in school for the entire day. This can be for a myriad of reasons and the school nurse can be an integral part of the school team in addressing these issues.

- Prevalence is greater than many childhood behavioral disorders
- Most common in 10-13 year olds
- Not linked to gender, race or socioeconomic status

Definitions

School Refusal Behavior: Child initiated refusal to attend school and/or difficulties remaining in school the entire day. An umbrella term that may refer to different kinds of attendance problems

School Phobia (outdated term): Fear-based, intense anxiety about being in school

School Refusal: Emotionally based absenteeism (anxiety or depression)

Separation Anxiety: Excessive worry and difficulty separating from parent on the part of a child and possibly a parent

Truancy: Illegal absence from school or unexcused absence without parental knowledge

Habitual Truancy: Applied to students who are referred for court in violation of state attendance law

Absenteeism: Legitimate or illegitimate absence from school or class

School Withdrawal: Parents withdrawal of a child from a school either legally or illegally

SCHOOL REFUSAL *(continued from previous page)*

ANTICIPATED CONCERNS/PROBLEMS:

Students with chronic school refusal are at a high risk for drop out. If poor attendance is allowed to persist, the impact undermines academic achievement and social emotional skills. Students who are chronically absent have lower reading and math skills as well as weaker social emotional skills than their peers (Chang, Gomperts & Boissiere, 2014). Students with anxiety-based refusal have high rates of physical complaints including stomachaches, headaches and complaints of being tired. School nurses can be instrumental is helping to determine whether these are a result of a true medical condition or attempts at school avoidance.

<u>Warning Signs</u>

- Frequent unexcused or excused absences
- Frequent tardiness
- Absence on significant days
- Frequent requests to call home
- Worrying about a parent while at school
- Parent who frequently calls to "check on" child during school
- Frequent requests to go to the nurse's office
- Crying in school

MANAGEMENT/INTERVENTIONS:

- Use data to monitor who is at risk for poor attendance and intervene early.
- Notify school administrators of students with excessive visits to the health office or high absenteeism rates.
- Connect struggling students with positive and engaging supports.
- Work with educational colleagues to regularly discuss students with attendance issues.
- Provide parent and student education about appropriate health reasons for staying home from school.
- Support and assist parents as needed, to get students into the school building.
- Consider home visits from a team of educators when students are refusing to come to school.
- Assist families of students with anxiety and depression to seek counseling to learn cognitive behavioral strategies to manage their feelings.

SCHOOL REFUSAL *(continued from previous page)*

NOTES:

Early identification and intervention is key. Once students get too far behind in school and feel they have missed too much school it becomes more difficult to get them back in school. Often the longer they are out of school the more difficult it is to return. Homebound tutoring should be discouraged. Sometimes partial days or slow reintroduction back into school may be utilized as a tool for re-entry.

Assisting parents in setting up consistent morning routines and ignoring pleas to stay home and inappropriate behaviors may be helpful.

References

Bernstein, B.E., & Balentine, J.R. (2015). *School refusal.* Retrieved from http://www.emedicinehealth.com/school_refusal/article_em.htm

Bernstein, B.E. (2014). *Separation anxiety and school refusal.* Retrieved from http://emedicine.medscape.com/article/916737-overview

Burstein, A., Talmi, A., Stafford, B., & Kelsay, K. (2014). Child & adolescent psychiatric disorders & psychosocial aspects of pediatrics. In W. Hay, M. Levin, R. Deterding, & M. Abzug (Eds.), *Current diagnosis and treatment pediatrics* (22nd edition) (pp. 202-204). McGraw Hill Education, Inc.

Chang, H., Gomperts, J. & Boissiere, L. (2014). Chronic absenteeism can devastate k-12 learning. *Education Week, October 7, 2014, 34*(7), 22-23. Retrieved from http://www.edweek.org/ew/articles/2014/10/08/07chang.h34.html

Wimmer, M. B. (2013). *Evidenced-based practices for school refusal and truancy* (2nd ed.). Bethesda, MD: National Association of School Psychologists.

SCHOOL-SPONSORED TRIPS

OVERVIEW/DEFINITION: School-sponsored trips, sometimes called field trips, are trips designed to support and enhance a student's education outside of the school-day or school-site. Students may be off the school grounds for a few hours, overnight, days and may be out-of-state or the country. It is important to clearly distinguish between school-sponsored trips and other extra-curricular activities. School-sponsored trips are approved by the local board of education and are part of the students' education and school curricula.

ANTICIPATED CONCERNS/PROBLEMS:
- Student safety while away from the school campus.
- Management of chronic conditions, including medication administration and health procedures.
- Emergency responses when off-site.
- Recognition of practice issues and nursing responsibilities whether a nurse is attending or not.
- Delegation to unlicensed assistive personnel (UAP) when no licensed staff accompany the trip or plans for accommodating health needs when delegation to UAPs is not allowed.

MANAGEMENT/POTENTIAL INTERVENTIONS:
Planning Considerations

1. Notification Process: School nurses should be notified during the initial approval process of the proposed trip and before the final administrative approval is obtained. This notification process allows the school nurse to determine:
   - student health needs;
   - feasibility of providing needed care;
   - staffing needs;
   - accessibility of proposed experience for all students (i.e., accommodating students with special healthcare needs);
   - unique needs based on location;
   - training needs; and
   - nursing licensure procedures in the destination state.

2. Nursing Assessment: School nurses are uniquely positioned to conduct an assessment of a variety of areas in order to promote a safe and rewarding experience for students and staff. The assessment areas to consider include:

434

SCHOOL-SPONSORED TRIPS *(continued from previous page)*

<u>Nursing Assessment (continued)</u>

- Healthcare needs of students –identified health concerns, medications, procedures, conditions requiring monitoring as well as self-care abilities of students.
- Staffing needs – does a nurse need to attend the trip, can it be an RN or LPN, can students manage their own care or can nursing care be delegated to UAPs (i.e., teacher or other school personnel)?
- Provisions for meals/food – will food be offered, any special dietary needs, what accommodations are needed?
- Nursing licensure considerations – if nurse attending what are the destination state licensure requirements (is it one of the Nurse License Compact (NLC) state and is the nurse licensed under the NLC; if not, does the nurse need a temporary license or does that licensing board offer a *visiting nurse* status)? If the nurse is not attending, can nursing responsibilities (e.g., medication administration or blood glucose monitoring) be delegated, to whom, and what are the training and supervision requirements?

3. <u>Training and Supervision</u>: If the school nurse or other nursing personnel are not attending the school-sponsored trip, then training of the UAPs by the nurses is an essential component as well as the nurse determining if the UAP is competent and safe to provide the nursing interventions. The training should include all aspects of the UAPs responsibilities including return demonstrations. For example, if the UAP will be administering medication, the training should include the six rights of medication administration, what to do if the student experiences side effects or the medication is not effective, who to notify in the event of emergency, and how to document the situation.

   Supervision of the UAPs also needs to be established prior to the trip. Considerations include:
   - Communication with the school nurse or school physician; who to contact when they are not available; who to contact in an emergency; and
   - Observations of skills performed by UAP prior to trip.

SCHOOL-SPONSORED TRIPS *(continued from previous page)*

Emergency Procedures:
Emergency plans established prior to the school-sponsored trip allows for effective management of an emergent situation and increased potential for a positive resolution. Emergency plans should include lines of authority among the staff present; communication between the staff present and the school administration at the school building or district level; communication with school medical personnel as needed; communication with families; plans for emergency transportation of student (s) as needed, such as 911 or use of a local emergency department; emergency equipment/supplies for the staff on the trip; and any training needed, such as first aid or CPR training prior to the trip.

FOLLOW-UP:

Upon return from a school-sponsored trip, a brief discussion between the school nurse, staff participating on the trip and school administration is useful to evaluate what worked well as well as suggestions for improvement on subsequent trips. If an unanticipated event or emergency occurred while away, a more in-depth discussion may be needed.

NOTES:
- Ability to practice nursing in any given state is determined by the Nurse Licensure Compact (25 states participate and allow for multi-state licensure) or the nursing licensure board in your home state and the state of trip destination. Nurses need to determine prior to administering nursing care during the school-sponsored trip if their license is valid in the destination state.
- Nurses not attending the trip and delegating to UAP to provide care in the destination state need to be aware of what responsibilities may be delegated in that particular state and care must be provided according to those requirements.
- All students have the right under federal laws (Section 504 of the Rehabilitative Act of 1973 and the Individuals with Disabilities Education Improvement Act [2004]) to participate in school-sponsored trips, if the student needs cannot be accommodated, and then the district must cancel or alter the trip.

SCHOOL-SPONSORED TRIPS *(continued from previous page)*

References

Connecticut State Department of Education. (2014). *Field trips: Guidance for school nurses.* Retrieved from http://www.sde.ct.gov/sde/lib/sde/pdf/publications/field_trips/fieldtrips.pdf

Erwin, K., Clark, S., & Mercer, S. (2014). Providing health services for children with special healthcare needs on out-of-state field trips. *NASN School Nurse, 29*(2), 84-88.

National Association of School Nurses. (2014). *School-sponsored before, after and extended school year programs: The role of the school nurse.* (Position statement). Silver Springs, MD: author.

National Council of State Boards of Nursing (2015). *Nurse licensure compact.* Retrieved from: https://www.ncsbn.org/nurse-licensure-compact.htm

Kentucky Department of Education (2015). *Field trips and medication administration.* Retrieved from: http://education.ky.gov/districts/SHS/Pages/Field-Trips-and-Medication-Administration.aspx

SECTION IV

MANAGEMENT OF
VULNERABLE POPULATIONS

CHILD MALTREATMENT

OVERVIEW/DEFINITION:

Child maltreatment is any act or series of acts of commission or omission by a parent or other caregiver (e.g., clergy, coach, and teacher) that results in harm, potential for harm, or threat of harm to a child. Child abuse is an act of commission. Commission is a deliberate or intentional act in which there is harm, potential harm or the threat of harm but harm to the child is unintentional. Child neglect is an act of omission. Omission, an act of negligence is failure to protect or meet the child's basic physical, emotional, medical, safety or educational needs. Both are components of family violence defined as physical, emotional or sexual abuse and includes physical or emotional neglect.

> **Law designates School Nurses as mandatory reporters of suspected child abuse/neglect.**

ANTICIPATED CONCERNS/PROBLEMS:

Risk Factors for Child Abuse/Neglect

Child	• Children under the age of 1 year (50% of fatalities) • Children under the age of 3 years (75% of fatalities) • Males (60% are abused) • Caucasians (45% are abused) • Special needs children (sometimes place extra burdens on parents)
Adult	• Most common abuser is the parent/guardian • Women under 40 years of age are the highest abusers • Abused as a child • Young parents, low education, numerous children, poverty, and/or a single parent • Lack of parenting skills, understanding children's needs and child development • Additional transient adult caregivers in the home, substance abuse, individual or family history of mental health and/or physical health issues • Belief that discipline considered child maltreatment is appropriate • Limited social network, lack of family support and/or self esteem • An unwanted pregnancy or the child does meet their expectations
Family	Dysfunctional families that may include violence between spouses
Community	• Transient neighborhoods, with violence • High poverty • Unemployment rates

CHILD MALTREATMENT *(continued from previous page)*

Signs/Symptoms of Abuse:
All forms of abuse
- Behavior and personality changes
- Changes in relationship with peers, family members and school personnel
- Changes in school attendance and performance
- Apprehensive of certain situations and people

Physical Abuse
- Bruises, cuts, burns, fractures healing at different stages
- Marks from a belt, rope or chain located on the face, arms, back, legs and buttocks
- An increase in chronic health condition symptoms may be related from withholding medication
- Wincing indicating pain with movement
- Parts of a handprint on the body
- Behaviors inconsistent with developmental age

Emotional Abuse
- Low self-esteem, low self-image, cries, feelings of shame or guilt
- Trust issues, avoids eye contact, withdrawn
- Social, emotional or academic delay
- Inappropriate behavior (aggressive, destructive, cruel, engages in improper sexual activities)
- Attempts suicide
- Lack of attachment to the parent
- Older children may experiment with substance abuse

Sexual Abuse
- Genital area may or may exhibit signs of trauma (redness, bruises, bleeding, swelling)
- Sexually transmitted infection, urinary tract infection, difficulty sitting or walking
- Somatic complaints (headache, stomachaches, etc.), bedwetting, night terrors
- Feelings of, hostility, guilt, anger, shame, eating disorders

CHILD MALTREATMENT *(continued from previous page)*

MANAGEMENT/POTENTIAL INTERVENTIONS:
- Physical exam and comprehensive history
- Removal of child from the abusive situation if necessary
- Mental health therapy from a trained professional
- Art therapy
- Group or family treatment
- Treatment pursuant to type of abuse may include a physical exams, x-rays, MRI, CT, urine cultures

FOLLOW UP:
- Establish trusting relationship with parent.
- Prevent further injury.
- Emphasize the importance of counseling and follow up care.
- Support the victims of child maltreatment.
- Homecare teaching (family treatment and parenting classes).
- Educate staff regarding signs and symptoms of child maltreatment.
- Identify students with indicators of maltreatment.
- Provide safety education to children.
- Provide community resources to victims and families.
- Collaborate with community to raise awareness to reduce incidence.
- Expected school nurse outcomes include a developing nurturing environment for the child, normal growth and development, positive sense of self-esteem, stress relief for parents and absence of episodes of abuse.

NOTES:
- Each state provides its own definitions of child abuse and neglect based on minimum standards set by federal law.
- Follow state and school district mandatory guidelines for reporting child abuse/neglect.
- When obtaining information about the injury document the child's and parent's response verbatim.
- Abuse or neglect may negatively affect a child's health and mental status throughout life.

CHILD MALTREATMENT *(continued from previous page)*

RESOURCES

Child Welfare Information Gateway, Developing and Sustaining Prevention Programs at https://www.childwelfare.gov/preventing/developing/index.cfm

References

Ball, J., Binder, R., & Cowen, K. (Eds.). (2012). Assessment and management of social and environmental influences. *Principles of Pediatric Nursing: Caring for Children (5th ed.)* (pp. 461-462). Upper Saddle River, NJ: Pearson Education, Inc.

Centers for Disease Control. (2015). *Child maltreatment-definition.* Retrieved from http://www.cdc.gov/violenceprevention/childmaltreatment/definitions.html

Children's Bureau. (2015). *Child maltreatment-data tables.* Retrieved from http://www.acf.hhs.gov/programs/cb/resource/child-maltreatment-2010-data-tables

Selekman, J., Pelt, P., Garnier, S., & Baker, D. (2013). Youth violence. In J. Selekman (2nd Ed.), *School nursing: A comprehensive text* (pp. 1103-1110). Philadelphia: F.A. Davis.

DEVELOPMENTAL DISABILITIES

OVERVIEW/DEFINITION:

Developmental disabilities (DD) are a diverse group of physical, cognitive, psychological, sensory and speech impairments that are identified prenatally up 18 years of age and are likely to continue throughout life. They result in considerable limitations in three or more of the following areas: comprehension and language skills (receptive and expressive language), learning, self direction, self care, mobility and the ability to function independently without coordinated services (capacity for independent living and economic self sufficiency). Developmental Disabilities may have a severe adverse effect on educational outcomes.

Type	Description/Characteristics
Autism Spectrum Disorders	• Significantly affects verbal and nonverbal communication and social interaction.
ADHD	• There are 3 main symptoms, the inability to focus, hyperactivity and impulsivity. Maybe managed with medication and /or a behavior plan.
Cerebral Palsy	• The inability to control muscle responses and/or a weakness of the muscle. AFO's (braces) and splints help support the feet and legs for walking and for use of hands.
Intellectual Development Disabilities (IDD)	• Considered a condition, but actually a symptom of numerous different conditions. • Average IDD is sub average intelligence (I.Q.>55-70 range) with deficits in adaptive behavior and manifested during a developmental period. • Common IDD's are Fragile X syndrome, Fetal Alcohol syndrome, Down syndrome, Angelman syndrome, Prader Willie syndrome and toxoplasmosis. • IDD's can be diagnosed during pregnancy through blood tests (amniocentesis or chorionic villus). • After birth, intelligence quotient (I.Q.) test determine diagnosis in addition to observing behavior and assessing adaptive skills. • Children with intellectual disabilities may become functional adults; they are able to learn, but do so slowly, and with difficulty.
Learning Disabilities	• Specific types of learning problems, dyscalcula (math), dysgrahia (writing) and dyslexia (reading).
Hearing	• Unable to process communication through hearing with or without implication, may be permanent or fluctuate.

DEVELOPMENTAL DISABILITIES *(continued from previous page)*

Type	Description/Characteristics
Vision Impairment	• Depends on what part of the eye is affected, the eye condition; and how much correction is possible through glasses, contacts, surgery or medicine. • Senses of smell, touch, taste, and hearing are heightened.
Vision and Hearing Impaired	• Causes severe developmental, communication and educational needs which may require a specific program to accommodate blind and deaf students.

Developmental disabilities may be caused by:
- Traumatic Brain Injury (TBI) and other child maltreatment manifestations (shaken baby syndrome or head trauma)
- Prenatal or after birth nutrition or growth problems
- Prenatal or after birth infections
- Chromosome abnormalities
- Poor maternal diet, lack of prenatal care, substance abuse or OTC drugs
- Prematurity
- Environmental toxins (lead poisoning, infections)

ANTICIPATED CONCERNS/PROBLEMS:
- Vary depending on condition
- Delay in developmental milestones (walking, talking, etc.)
- Speaking difficulty or talking later, can't remember things
- Unable to follow or understand rules of social behavior
- Difficulty solving problems or understanding outcomes of action
- IDD's that show up sooner may indicate a more severe disability

MANAGEMENT/POTENTIAL INTERVENTIONS:
- No cure is available
- Treatment specific to disability
- Accessing educational related services resources; physical therapy, occupational therapy, therapeutic speech therapy or nursing services
- Early intervention for children birth -3 years of age
- Development of an Individualized Family Service Plan (IFSP)
- Special education services 3-21 of age (a couple of states extend services)
- Development of an Individualized Educational Plan (IEP)
- Transitional planning for school to community

DEVELOPMENTAL DISABILITIES *(continued from previous page)*

MANAGEMENT/POTENTIAL INTERVENTIONS: *(continued)*
- Communication devices and computer technology
- Special equipment depending on condition (standers, bikes, braces, wheelchairs, adaptive seating, eating utensils, sensory stimulation etc.)

FOLLOW UP:
- Investigate instructional and classroom accommodations
- Provide interventions based on need of the student and evaluate the impact of the outcomes
- Hearing and vision screening (minimize sensory deficits)
- Dental care (prevent periodontal disease)
- Immunizations (deficiencies in immune system)
- Use multi sensory approach
- Promote good nutrition
- Alert parents of signs of illness (ear and upper respiratory infections)
- Assist with transition planning from school to the community (IEP planning for transitioning must begin before the age of 16)

NOTES:
- The average I.Q. is 100, IDD can range from mild 55-70 , moderate 40-54, severe 25-39, and profound less than 25

Laws:
- The Individuals with Disabilities Education Improvement Act (IDEIA) directs how educational services available through the state, school district and public agencies are provided to infants, toddlers, children and youth with disabilities http://idea.ed.gov/

- Section 504 of the Rehabilitation Law is prohibits educational discrimination on the basis of disability providing students with disabilities services who do not qualify for IDEIA http://www.hhs.gov/ocr/civilrights/resources/factsheets/504.pdf

- The American Disabilities Act (ADA) provides equality for people with disabilities (education, employment, transportation, access to buildings, etc.) http://www.ada.gov/

DEVELOPMENTAL DISABILITIES *(continued from previous page)*

RESOURCES:

Administration of Community Living, Administration of Intellectual Developmental Disabilities at http://www.acl.gov/Programs/AIDD/Index.aspx

Early Childhood Technical Assistance at http://www.ectacenter.org/contact/ptccoord.asp

Early Intervention at http://www.parentcenterhub.org/repository/ei-overview/

National Dissemination Center for Children with Disabilities at http://nichcy.org/

Partnering with Your Child's School: A Guide for Parents at http://www.hscfoundation.org/aboutus/publications/partnering_with_schools_english_guide.pdf

References

American Psychiatric Association (APA). (2013). *Diagnostic and statistical manual of mental disorders (DSM-V)* (5th ed.) Washington, DC. Author.

Autism Science Foundation. (2014). *How common is autism?* Retrieved from *http://www.autismsciencefoundation.org*

Ball, J., Binder, R., & Cowen, K. (Eds.). (2012).Alterations in mental health and cognition. *Principles of Pediatric Nursing: Caring for Children (5th Ed.)* (pp. 931-939). Upper Saddle River, NJ: Pearson Education, Inc.

Blom, M., Crawford, L., & Whitehead, S. (2013).intellectual disabilities. In J. Selekman (Ed.), *School nursing: A comprehensive text* (2nd ed.) (p.p. 899-923). Philadelphia: F.A. Davis.

Centers for Disease Control. (2013). *Developmental disabilities.* Retrieved from http://www.cdc.gov/ncbddd/developmentaldisabilities/index.html

MedlinePlus. (2013). *Developmental disabilities.* Retrieved from http://www.nlm.nih.gov/medlineplus/developmentaldisabilities.html

National Dissemination Center for Children with Disabilities. (2015.). *Disabilities.* Retrieved from http://nichcy.org/disability

O'Brian, P., G., Kennedy, & W., Z. (2013). Clients with intellectual and developmental disabilities. In D.R. Falvo, & K.A. Ballard (Eds.), *Psychiatric mental health nursing*, (pp. 605-603). New York, NY: Jones and Bartlett Learning.

Selekman, J., Bobhenek, J. & Lukens, M. (2013).Children with chronic conditions. In J. Selekman (Ed.), *School nursing: A comprehensive text* (2nd ed.) (p. 702). Philadelphia: F.A. Davis.

The U.S. Equal Employment Opportunity Commission. (n.d.). *Questions & answers about persons with intellectual disabilities in the workplace and the Americans with Disabilities Act (ADA).* Retrieved from: http://www.eeoc.gov/laws/types/intellectual_disabilities.cfm

U.S. Department of Education. (2014). *36th annual report to Congress on the implementation of the Individuals with Disabilities Education Act*, 2007.Washington, DC: Author. Retrieved from http://www2.ed.gov/about/reports/annual/osep/index.html

U.S. Department of Education (2010). Thirty –five years of progress in educating children with disabilities through IDEA. Retrieved from http://www2.ed.gov/about/offices/list/osers/idea35/history/index_pg10.html

HOMELESSNESS

OVERVIEW/ DEFINITION:

The law[1] defines homeless children and youth as those who lack a fixed, regular, and adequate nighttime residence. According to the National Center on Family Homelessness (2011), homeless families comprise roughly 1/3 of the total homeless population. Approximately 1.6 million children will experience homelessness over the course of a year. In any given day, researchers estimate that more than 200,000 children have no place to live.

The McKinney Homeless Assistance Act (1987) was created in response to findings that half of the homeless children were not regularly attending school. The McKinney Act ensures homeless children receive free transportation to and from school. The Act further requires schools to register homeless children even if they lack normally required documents, such as immunization records or proof of residence.

Homeless children live in shelters, cars, homes of parents' friends or relatives or strangers, shared single-family quarters, motels on a weekly pay basis, tents and under bridges. Attendance suffers with length-of-stay rules in shelters, short stays in relatives' homes, and parent's relocation to seek work. They may have no storage for possessions such as donated clothing, no place to study or do homework, and irregular sleep and eating times.

CAUSES OF HOMELESSNESS (FOR FAMILIES):
- Lack of affordable housing
- Poverty
- Unemployment

ANTICIPATED CONCERNS/PROBLEMS:
- Chronic health conditions (asthma, chronic otitis media, anemia, etc.)
- Behavioral problems
- Developmental delay
- Early initiation of substance abuse
- Social isolation
- Mental health problems (anxiety, depression, and withdrawal)
- Tuberculosis

---

[1] McKinney-Vento Homeless Education Assistance Improvements Act of 2001 (U.S.C. 42).

HOMELESSNESS *(continued from previous page)*

MANAGEMENT/POTENTIAL INTERVENTIONS:

States and communities are expected to remove barriers to enrollment, attendance, and success of these children, including preschool age children. Potential barriers include:

1. **Barriers to enrollment** - Lack of birth certificate, guardianship papers, previous school record transfer, lack of residence address for school assignment, and immunization records.

2. **Barriers to attendance** - Transportation, family mobility, poor health (e.g., untreated asthma), inadequate food, no clean clothing, no school supplies.

3. **Barriers to success** - Difficulty getting evaluation for special education or gifted programs, transportation and materials for extra-curricular events, counseling services and/or after-school care.

INTERVENTIONS: SCHOOL NURSE ROLE

1. **Enrollment**
   a. Follow laws with respect to admitting homeless children and secure up-to-date immunizations and records as quickly as possible.
   b. Refer to local healthcare provider or health department if immunization status is incomplete.

2. **Attendance (School Nurse Concerns)**
   a. Assess for undiagnosed or untreated problems; e.g., poor growth, chronic infections, reactive airway disease, wounds, gastrointestinal problems, speech problems, physical and mental health conditions.
   b. Coordinate with public health and community clinics for complete treatment including immediate access to immunizations.

3. **TB test follow up:**
   a. Secure tuberculosis testing promptly (in accord with state or local requirements) as homeless children and youth are at greater risk of exposure.
   b. Assure that positive TB skin tests are adequately evaluated, and if medication is needed, assist the parent to assure medication completion.

HOMELESSNESS *(continued from previous page)*

INTERVENTIONS: SCHOOL NURSE ROLE *(continued)*

4. **Provide support**
   a. These children often experience violence in their lives. They may experience more anxiety; monitor need for social work services. Refer if services are needed.
   b. Coordinate with shelters and social services for clothing (possibly facilitating showering and changing at school), school meals, school supplies and after-school homework centers, adjusted assignments or tutoring to assure completion of schoolwork.
   c. A backpack or packet with class pictures, preserved samples of quality work, and stamped post cards to stay in touch with classmates helps to meet mental health needs of children who change schools.

References

Abdoo, D., Brady, M, Diamond, J., & Dunn, A. (2013). Role relationships. In C. Burns, M. Brady, A. Dunn, NB Starr, C. Blosser, eds. *Pediatric primary care* (5th ed.) (pp. 319-321). St. Louis, MO: Saunders Elsevier.

McKinney-Vento Homeless Education Assistance Improvements Act of 2001 (U.S.C. 42). Retrieved from http://www.ed.gov/policy/elsec/leg/esea02/pg116.html

National Center on Family Homelessness. (2011). *The characteristics and needs of families experiencing homelessness.* Retrieved from http://www.familyhomelessness.org/media/306.pdf

National Coalition for the Homeless. (2012). *Homeless families with children.* Retrieved from http://www.nationalhomeless.org/factsheets/families.html

Substance Abuse and Mental Health Services Administration. (2015). Homelessness resource center. Retrieved from http://homeless.samhsa.gov/

LESBIAN, GAY, BISEXUAL, AND TRANSGENDER (LGBT) YOUTH

OVERVIEW/DEFINITION:

Sexual orientation refers to an enduring pattern of emotional, romantic, and sexual attractions to men, women, or both sexes. Additionally, sexual orientation may refer to a person's sense of identity based on attractions, related behaviors, and membership in a community of others who share similar attractions (APA, 2013). Sexual orientation is often discussed in relation to the following three categories:

1. Homosexual – having emotional, romantic, or sexual attractions to members of the same sex, i.e. "Gay" refers to men who have emotional and physical attraction to men; and "Lesbian" refers to women who have emotional and physical attraction to women.
2. Heterosexual – having emotional or physical attraction to members of the opposite sex.
3. Bisexual – men or women having emotional or physical attraction to both sexes.

Transgender students have a gender identity that is different from their sex at birth and whose gender expression is different from the way males or females are expected to act or behave.

Homosexuality is not a psychiatric disorder. Approximately 9 million Americans identify as lesbian, gay, bisexual or transgender (Gates, 2011). Homosexuality, bisexuality, and questioning one's own sexual orientation are no longer considered health conditions/ disorders that need or respond to treatment or remediation (NASN, 2012).

The fact that gay, lesbian, bisexual and transgender youth are more likely to attempt suicide or leave school to avoid ill treatment by adults or peers calls for educational leadership to teach that discrimination, hatred and intolerance are unacceptable. When harassment is based on a student's sex or sexual orientation, failure to address it properly and promptly violates the law.

All adults in schools share the responsibility to help all youth develop into well-adjusted adults and to create a safe school and community environment that respects individual difference. Health education about tolerance and acceptance of diversity in the school and about sexual activity and sexually transmitted diseases.

LESBIAN, GAY, BISEXUAL, AND TRANSGENDER (LGBT) YOUTH *(continued from previous page)*

POTENTIAL CONCERNS/PROBLEMS:
- Lesbians may be at risk for depression and suicide (Mayo Clinic, 2014a).
- Men who have sex with men (MSM) are at increased risk of sexually transmitted disease, depression, and poor body image (Mayo Clinic, 2014b).
- Other potential complications:
  - Human Immunodeficiency Virus/Acquired Immunodeficiency Syndrome (HIV/AIDS)
  - Human Papilloma Virus (HPV)
  - Stigma
  - Suicide
  - Sexually transmitted diseases (STDs)
  - Substance abuse (club drugs)
  - Body image and disordered eating
  - Homelessness
  - Domestic violence and victimization

MANAGEMENT/POTENTIAL INTERVENTIONS:
1. Use gender neutral, non-judgmental language. Avoid the term "sexual preference" as this suggests choice (which current research does not support); sexual orientation is preferred.
2. Ensure confidentiality.
3. Educate students to the risk of unsafe behaviors, e.g., risky sexual activity, alcohol abuse, driving while intoxicated, etc., while accepting the person who views him or herself as gay, lesbian or bisexual.
4. Suggest keeping a private journal to write about stresses and challenges, personal strengths, and possible solutions or ambitions. Journaling helps separate minor from major issues.
5. Be non-judgmental when asking questions about sexual activity or orientation in order to be effective in encouraging the student to share concerns and behaviors.
6. Offer to help or refer those who need help telling parents or who are having trouble in school or with peers.
7. Provide training to all staff in LGBT issues.
8. Encourage Gay, Straight Alliance school based support groups.

LESBIAN, GAY, BISEXUAL, AND TRANSGENDER (LGBT) YOUTH *(continued from previous page)*

MANAGEMENT/POTENTIAL INTERVENTIONS: *(continued)*

9. Develop a network of community resources for youth and their parents for social and emotional support.
10. All students, including transgender, gay and lesbian students have a right to privacy; this includes keeping a student's transgender/sexual orientation private.
11. School personnel should use the name/pronoun appropriate to the student's gender identity regardless of the student's assigned birth sex.
12. Students should have access to the restroom/locker room that corresponds to their gender identity. Students may also be provided a private, non-stigmatizing alternative such as the use of the health room bathroom.

FOLLOW UP:

- Observe for depression and suicidal ideation.
- Observe for and support a safe environment.
- Provide support to ensure health education principles are implemented.

NOTES:

Guidelines for Health Education include:

- Do not refer to homosexuality as a medical term by limiting the mention of lesbian and gay issues in health education and HIV prevention curricula.
- Avoid "sexualizing" or defining homosexuality only by sexual activity; heterosexuals do not define themselves by their sex lives.
- In HIV and AIDS prevention education, all students need to recognize risk-taking behaviors; worldwide, heterosexual transmission is significant.
- Reduce "them" versus "us" thinking and behavior. In-service and professional development can help educators reflect on their own biases, deal with their feelings, and recognize actions that covertly reinforce stereotypical ideas about LGBT youth.
- Encourage vaccination which can offer protection from hepatitis A and hepatitis B, serious liver infections that can spread through sexual contact. The HPV vaccine is available to women and men up to age 26.

LESBIAN, GAY, BISEXUAL, AND TRANSGENDER (LGBT) YOUTH *(continued from previous page)*

Characteristics of successful school programs include:

- Keep disclosure in confidence.
- Use inclusive language, e.g., "parent" (not mother, father), "seeing anyone" or "date" (not boy or girlfriend), that conveys acceptance.
- Include LGBT issues in discussing multicultural issues.
- Establish and enforce policies that protect students from harassment, violence and discriminatory jokes or slurs by adults or students.
- Support students whose families include people in the LGBT community.

Resources
American Psychological Association (APA)
http://www.apa.org/

Lesbian, Gay, Bisexual, and Transgender Concerns Office (LGBTCO)
750 First Street N.E.
Washington, DC 20002
http://www.apa.org/pi/lgbt/index.aspx Centers for Disease Control (CDC)

LGBT Youth Resources
http://www.cdc.gov/lgbthealth/youth-resources.htm

National Gay and Lesbian Task Force
1325 Massachusetts Ave NW, Suite 600
Washington, DC 20005
Phone: (202) 393-5177
TTY: (202) 393-2284
Fax: (202 393-2241
http://www.ngltf.org/

LESBIAN, GAY, BISEXUAL, AND TRANSGENDER (LGBT) YOUTH *(continued from previous page)*

References

American Psychological Association. (2015). *Sexual orientation and homosexuality*. Retrieved from http://www.apa.org/helpcenter/sexual-orientation.aspx

Connecticut Safe School Coalition (2012). *Guidelines for Connecticut schools to comply with gender identity and expression non-discrimination laws*. Retrieved from http://www.ct.gov/chro/lib/chro/Guidelines_for_Schools_on_Gender_Identity_and_Expression_final_4-24-12.pdf

Centers for Disease Control and Prevention. (2014). *Lesbian, gay, bisexual, and transgender health: About LGBT health*. Retrieved from http://www.cdc.gov/lgbthealth/about.htm

Gabel, J. (2015, November 4). Transgender students in K-12 Navigating accommodations and avoiding litigation [Webinar]. *In Education Admin Web Advisor.*

Gates, G. L. (2011). *How many people are lesbian, gay, bisexual and transgender?* Williams Institute of the UCLA School of Law. Retrieved from http://williamsinstitute.law.ucla.edu/wp-content/uploads/Gates-How-Many-People-LGBT-Apr-2011.pdf

Institute of Medicine (US) & the Committee on Lesbian, Gay, Bisexual, and Transgender Health Issues and Research Gaps and Opportunities. (2011). *The health of lesbian, gay, bisexual, and transgender people: Building a foundation for better understanding*. Washington, DC: The National Academy Press. Retrieved from http://www.ncbi.nlm.nih.gov/books/NBK64806

Mayo Clinic. (2014a). *Health issues for lesbians*. Retrieved from. http://www.mayoclinic.org/healthy-lifestyle/womens-health/in-depth/health-issues-for-lesbians

Mayo Clinic. (2014b). *Health issues for gay men: Tips to stay healthy*. Retrieved from http://mayoclinic.com/health/health-issues-for-gay-men/MY00738

National Association of School Nurses [NASN] (2011). *Sexual orientation and gender identity/expression* **(sexual minority students)**: *School nurse practice* (Position Paper). Retrieved from http://www.nasn.org/PolicyAdvocacy/PositionPapersandReports/NASNPositionStatementsFullView/tabid/462/ArticleId/47/Sexual-Orientation-and-Gender-Identity-Expression-Sexual-Minority-Students-School-Nurse-Practice-Rev

Riley-Lawless, K. (2013). Demographics of children and adolescents. In J. Selekman (Ed.), *School nursing: A comprehensive text* (2nd ed.) (pp. 331-332). Philadelphia, PA: F.A. Davis.

SUICIDE IDEATION/THREATS

OVERVIEW/DEFINITION:

Suicidal ideation is reoccurring thoughts of committing suicide. Suicide and suicidal ideas are very difficult to predict; however, it does occur in children as young as 8-years-old (Stuart, 2013). For youth between the ages of 10 and 24, suicide is the third leading cause of death. It results in approximately 4600 lives lost each year. The top three methods used in suicides of young people include firearm (45%), suffocation (40%), and poisoning (8%) (Center for Disease Control Youth Suicide and Prevention, 2015). Almost three million children between the ages of 12 to 17-years old have thought about suicide and of these children, one third have made an actual attempt (Stuart, 2013). Risk factors for childhood suicide include depression, sexual abuse, prior suicide ideas or plans, being bullied, substance abuse, impulsive or aggressive behavior, and access to firearms (Varcarolis, 2013). Culture and family factors influence the possibility that youth consider suicide as an option for handling distress, depression or hopeless feelings. There are many contributing factors linked to suicidal ideation. Aggravating factors may include:

- History of mental disorder, including depression
- Chronic medical condition such as seizure disorder or diabetes
- Fewer social and personal supports than peers
- Youth who attempt suicide report more negative life events (disappointments and losses)
- May have experienced a significant loss: relationship breakup, death of someone close, physical disability, or loss of status/perceived humiliation (losing a competitive event or admission to a group/school)
- Family history of psychiatric disorder or suicide

ANTICIPATED CONCERNS/PROBLEMS:

WARNING SIGNS OF SUICIDE
- Changed eating and sleeping habits
- Withdrawal from friends, family and everyday routine
- Personality changes
- Acting out, rebellion, running away
- Violent behavior/explosive rage
- Substance/alcohol use
- Difficulty focusing/concentrating

SUICIDE IDEATION/THREATS *(continued from previous page)*

<u>WARNING SIGNS OF SUICIDE</u> *(continued)*
- Hinting that "nothing matters" and "I won't be a problem much longer"
- Preoccupation with death/dying
- Throwing or giving personal items away
- Sense of hopelessness or dramatically upbeat following a period of depression
- Talking about suicide ("I wish I was never born" and "I wish I was dead")
- Existence of specific suicide plan

MANAGEMENT/POTENTIAL INTERVENTIONS:
1. **Emergency situations**
   - **Refer immediately for crisis intervention.**
   - Suicidal attempts necessitate an immediate psychological evaluation.
   - Assure a safe environment (this may mean psychiatric hospitalization).
   - Medical treatment for underlying mental health conditions (depression, bipolar disease, schizophrenia).

2. **Nonemergency situations**
   - Psychotherapy (counseling)
   - Medications – antidepressants, antipsychotic medications, anti-anxiety medications
   - Treatment for underlying mental health conditions

3. **General guidelines**
   When the child / adolescent expresses feelings of sadness, hopelessness, and despair or grief, it is important to assess for possible risk of physical harm to themselves. Begin the assessment with more general questions; if you hear affirmative answers, continue with more specific probing questions such as the following:
   - Have you ever felt so blue you thought of killing yourself?
   - Do you feel like hurting yourself now?
   - Do you have a plan to hurt yourself?
   - If yes, how would you do it? If present, act immediately; provide constant supervision, set a contract, and call for local crisis assistance, notify parent/guardian(s)
   - What would happen if you were dead?
   - How would other people react if you were dead?
   - Recognize and approach the student directly; *talking about suicide does not increase the risk.*

SUICIDE IDEATION/THREATS *(continued from previous page)*

General guidelines *(continued)*
- Encourage verbalizing feelings (rather than internalizing); provide support.
- Suspend judgments, arguments and moral views of suicide; and listen for immediate risk.
- Be aware of others likely to identify with a student who is known to have attempted suicide and who may imitate the action; assure that a trained school person checks their well-being.

FOLLOW UP:
- Participate in interdisciplinary team to assure that student has a plan for support and successful return to school.
- Review crisis plan to address the needs of any student who indicates intent to commit suicide.
- Provide general health education for all students about mental health, including depression and related risk and protective factors for suicide.

Possible Complications
- Consumed by suicidal thoughts – may not be able to function in daily activities
- Unsuccessful suicide attempt may leave person with permanent and/or debilitating injuries such as organ failure or brain damage
- Death

NOTES:
- About a third of those who attempt suicide have additional problems such as mood disorders, delinquent behavior, concern about sexual orientation, or substance abuse.
- Many people who commit suicide have had at least one previous attempt, and half had prior contact with a mental health professional.
- Educate staff/parents on the warning signs of suicide.

SUICIDE IDEATION/THREATS *(continued from previous page)*

References

American Psychiatric Association (APA). (2013). *Diagnostic and statistical manual of mental disorders (DSM-V)* (5th ed.) Washington, DC. Author.

Center for Disease Control and Prevention (CDC). (2013a). *Suicide prevention.* Retrieved from http://www.cdc.gov/ViolencePrevention/suicide/index.html

Center for Disease Control and Prevention (CDC). (2013b). Mental health surveillance among children — United States, 2005–2011. *Morbidity and Mortality Weekly Report (MMWR, 62*(2), 1-35. Retrieved from http://www.cdc.gov/mmwr/preview/mmwrhtml/su6202a1.htm

Mayo Clinic. (2015). *Suicide and suicidal thoughts.* Retrieved from http://www.mayoclinic.org/diseases-conditions/suicide/basics/definition/con-20033954

Merck Manual. (2013). *Suicidal behavior.* Retrieved from http://www.merckmanuals.com/professional/psychiatric_disorders/suicidal_behavior/suicidal_behavior.html?qt=suicide&alt=sh

Selekman, J., Diefenbeck, C. & Guthrie, S. (2013). *Mental health concerns.* In J. Selekman (Ed.), *School nursing: A comprehensive text* (2nd ed.) (pp. 927-969). Philadelphia, PA: F A Davis Company.

Stuart, G. W. (2013). Special populations in psychiatry: Child psychiatric nursing. In G. W. Stuart (Ed.), *Principles and practices of psychiatric nursing, p.*678. St. Loius, MO: Elsevier, Mosby.

Varcarolis, E. (2013). *Essentials of psychiatric mental health nursing: A communication approach to evidence based care,* (2nd ed). St Louis, MO Elsevier.

TEEN PREGNANCY/PREGNANCY PREVENTION

OVERVIEW/DEFINITION:

In 2013, 273,105 babies were born to women aged 15–19 years, for a live birth rate of 26.5 per 1,000 women in this age group. This is a record low for U.S. teens in this age group, and a drop of 10% from 2012. Birth rates fell 13% for women aged 15–17 years, and 8% for women aged 18–19 years. While reasons for the declines are not clear, teens seem to be less sexually active, and more of those who are sexually active seem to be using birth control than in previous years (CDC, 2015). Non-Hispanic black youth, Hispanic/Latino youth, American Indian/Alaska Native youth, and socioeconomically disadvantaged youth of any race or ethnicity have the highest rates of teen pregnancy and childbirth. Black and Hispanic teens together comprised 57% of U.S. teen births in 2013 (CDC, 2015).

The National Association of School Nurses (NASN) believes that the school nurse is in a prime position to support the health and wellbeing of pregnant and parenting students and contribute to their lifelong success by linking them to resources and advocating for policies and practices that promote high school graduation. It is the position of NASN that school nurses have a vital role in the development and implementation of evidenced-based policies, nursing care procedures, educational programs and materials for students and their parents relating to pregnancy prevention, teen parenting and school completion. School nurses track pregnancy trends, review the school's human growth and development curriculum, assist in the selection of high-quality educational materials and programs based on the age, culture, and level of risk of the target population, and evaluate the short-term and long-term outcomes of the school's programs (NASN, 2011, p.1).

Pregnant and parenting students in public schools are protected against discrimination by law and are eligible for a free and appropriate education in the least restrictive environment.

It is important that the school nurse follow state and federal laws regarding adolescent reproductive health issues, confidentiality rights and consent. Additionally the school nurse must be knowledgeable about child protection laws in regard to minors' suspected sexual abuse and pregnancy (some states have mandates that require reporting to Child Protective Services should a girl of a specific age or younger be suspected of being pregnant).

TEEN PREGNANCY/PREGNANCY PREVENTION *(continued from previous page)*

SIGNS AND SYMPTOMS of PREGNANCY
If the youth has had sexual intercourse and experiences the following symptoms:
- Missed period
- Short, scant period
- Sore, tender or swollen breasts
- Nausea and/or vomiting
- Fatigue
- Frequent urge to urinate
- Mood swings

SOCIAL AND ENVIRONMENTAL RISKS FOR TEEN PREGNANCY
- Poverty
- Not living with biological parent
- Growing up in a single family home
- Poor self esteem
- School failure
- No future plans
- Minority race/ethnicity
- Childhood victimization
- Depression/ Stress

MANAGEMENT/POTENTIAL INTERVENTIONS:
1. Be non-judgmental when asking questions about sexual activity or exploitation in order to be effective in encouraging the student to share concerns and behaviors.
2. Encourage student to seek pregnancy testing and counseling services.
3. Develop supportive relationships with the pregnant student and their parent/ guardian.
4. Provide the student with local and community resources.
5. Understand the legal statutes that protect minor consent and confidentiality.
6. Encourage students to involve parents/guardians or another responsible adult in pregnancy.
7. If confirmed pregnancy encourage student to seek prenatal care/counseling and testing for sexually transmitted infections.
8. Work with multidisciplinary school team to provide necessary accommodations to support the pregnant student in the school setting.

TEEN PREGNANCY/PREGNANCY PREVENTION *(continued from previous page)*

9. Plan for re-entry into school after pregnancy with the multi-disciplinary school team.
10. Monitor for mental health problems such as depression, substance abuse and posttraumatic stress disorder in pregnant and parenting teens.
11. Provide educational programs to pregnant teens including fathers to promote positive parenting or refer to community agencies.

POTENTIAL COMPLICATIONS:
1. Pregnant teens and their babies are at higher risk of health problems. Possible complications for pregnant teens, especially those younger than age 15, include:
   - Premature labor
   - Anemia
   - High blood pressure
   - Possible complications for a baby born to a teen mother include:
     o Premature birth
     o Low birth weight
2. Childbearing during early adolescence has been associated with decreased likelihood of completing school, advancing education, and being employed and increased dependence on public assistance. In addition, many adolescent mothers have a second pregnancy. Recent studies suggest that background factors such as economic status, lifetime adversities and family support or conflict/violence are more influential on maternal and child outcomes than maternal age alone (The National Campaign to Prevent Teen and Unplanned Pregnancy, 2015).

PREGNANCY PREVENTION
1. The school nurse plays a role in teen pregnancy prevention along with school health educators and school counselors. Effective reproductive health education has been shown to delay sexual activity and increase the use of condoms and other contraception for sexually active adolescents (NASN, 2012). School nurses are challenged to examine their communication skills and views of youth behavior to determine how they can best contribute to teen pregnancy prevention efforts. This may include advocating for research-based comprehensive sex education and participating in sex education policy development. School nurses need to ensure that district policy adheres to state legal statutes and that the needs of students with disabilities are met. Additionally, supporting student's achievement, attendance and involvement can help in pregnancy prevention.

TEEN PREGNANCY/PREGNANCY PREVENTION *(continued from previous page)*

NOTES: Some teens may be prescribed contraceptives by a healthcare provider.

Contraceptive Method	Description	Comments
Sexual abstinence	Practice of refraining from some or all aspects of sexual activity	
Withdrawal	The penis is taken out of the vagina before ejaculation.	Twenty-two (22) women out of 100 using this method will get pregnant within 1 year, and this can be much higher for teens.
Condoms (male and female)	Latex, polyurethane, and silicone rubber (some with spermicidal agents) placed over the erect penis or in the vagina.	Typical use failure rate: 18-21%.
Oral Contraceptives	Hormonal Methods. Sometimes referred to as the "pill. The pill contains the hormones estrogen and progestin. It is taken daily to keep the ovaries from releasing an egg. The pill also causes changes in the lining of the uterus and the cervical mucus to keep the sperm from joining the egg.	Typical use failure rate: 9%.
Progestin Injection (Depo-Provera ®-medroxyprogesterone)	A progestin-only injectable given every three months; like the pill, it suppresses ovulation. Injection protects against endometrial cancer and iron-deficiency anemia.	Typical use failure rate: 6%.
Contraceptive Implant (Implanon® or Nexplanon®	A subdermal implant of six sustained-release silastic capsules containing levonorgestrel; provides protection for five years.	Failure rates similar to Depo-Provera® **at** <1%.
Spermicides - (nonoxynol-9)	Spermicides increase the contraceptive efficacy of condoms significantly.	Twenty-eight out of 100 women who use spermicide alone for birth control will get pregnant within the first year, a high failure rate. Also provides some protection against HIV.

TEEN PREGNANCY/PREGNANCY PREVENTION *(continued from previous page)*

Contraceptive Method	Description	Comments
Emergency contraception (E.C.) (also known as oral postcoital contraception) - Plan B One-Step® and Next Choice® are the most common brands of emergency contraception.	An oral pill that contains levonorgestrel, a female hormone that prevents ovulation (the release of an egg from an ovary). Levonorgestrel also causes changes in the cervical mucus and uterine lining, making it harder for sperm to reach the uterus and harder for a fertilized egg to attach to the uterus. It is used to prevent pregnancy after unprotected sex or failure of other forms of birth control. Because implantation defines an established pregnancy and because EC is used before, implantation occurs, it should be considered contraception and not an abortifacient.	Package labeling indicates that both of these products should be taken within 72 hours of unprotected intercourse; however, data supports that use up to 120 hours after intercourse may prevent pregnancy. No physical exam or pregnancy testing is required prior to the use of these products. Plan B One-Step® is available for purchase at pharmacies without a prescription by those who are age 17 and over; a prescription is needed for those under than 17.
Contraceptive vaginal ring (Nuvaring®)	A soft plastic vaginal ring worn for 3 weeks and taken out for 1 week to allow menses.	Typical use failure rate: 9%.
Transdermal contraceptive patch (ortho evra)	A patch worn for 3 weeks and removed for one week to allow for menses.	Typical use failure rate: 9%.
Other methods	IUD, diaphragm and cervical cups, sponge.	

TEEN PREGNANCY/PREGNANCY PREVENTION *(continued from previous page)*

References

American Academy of Pediatrics /Healthychildren.org. (2014*), Adolescent health*. (2014). Retrieved from https://www.healthychildren.org/English/ages-stages/teen/dating-sex/Pages/Birth-Control-for-Sexually-Active-Teens.aspx

Centers for Disease Control and Prevention. (2015). *Teen pregnancy the importance of prevention.* Retrieved from http://www.cdc.gov/teenpregnancy/about/index.htm

Center for Disease Control. (2012, April 6). HIV, other STD, and pregnancy prevention education in public secondary schools – 45 states, 2008 – 2010. *Morbidity and Mortality Weekly Report 61*(13), 222-228. Retrieved from http://www.cdc.gov/mmwr/preview/mmwrhtml/mm6113a2.htm?s_cid=mm6113a2_x

Fisher, M. M., & Alderman, E., Kreipe, R., & Rosenfeld, W. (Eds.). (2011). Growth and development. *Textbook of adolescent health care* (pp. 253-473, 506-513). Elk Grove Village, IL: American Academy of Pediatrics.

Hodgkinson, S. Beers, L., Southammakosane, C., & Lewin, A. (2014). Addressing the mental health needs of pregnant and parenting adolescents. *Pediatrics, 133*(1), 114-122. *doi: 10.1542/peds.2013-0927*

Kaiser Family Foundation. (*2014). Sexual health of adolescents and young adults in the United States.* Retrieved from http://www.kff.org/womenshealth/3040.cfm

Martin, J.A., Hamilton .B.E., Osterman, M.J.K., Curtin, S.C., & Mathews, T. J. (2015). Births: Final data for 2013. *National Vital Statistics Report 2015, 64*(1). Retrieved from http://www.cdc.gov/nchs/data/nvsr/nvsr64/nvsr64_01.pdf

Mayo Health Clinic. (2015). *Teen pregnancy.* Retrieved from http://www.mayoclinic.com/health/teen-pregnancy/MY00820

National Association of School Nurses. *(2011). Pregnant and parenting students, the role of the school nurse* (Position Statement). Silver Spring, MD: Author.

National Association of School Nurses. (2012). *School health education about human sexuality* (Position Statement). Silver Spring, MD: Author.

Nierengarten, M.B. (2015). Contraception guidelines for adolescents. *Contemporary Pediatrics, 32(6)*, 24 -26. *doi: 10.1542/peds.2014-2299*

Office on Women's Health. (2012, July 16). *Birth control methods fact sheet.* Retrieved from http://www.womenshealth.gov/publications/our-publications/fact-sheet/birth-control-methods.html#b

The National Campaign to Prevent Teen and Unplanned Pregnancy. (2015). Retrieved from https://thenationalcampaign.org/

Schaffer, M.A. & Mbibi, N. (2014). Public health nurse mentorship of pregnant and parenting adolescents. *Public Health Nursing, 31*(5*), 428-437.* doi: 10.1111/phn.12109

CPSIA information can be obtained
at www.ICGtesting.com
Printed in the USA
BVHW050433210120
569579BV00001B/1